Accelerating Progress in Obesity Prevention
SOLVING THE WEIGHT OF THE NATION

Committee on Accelerating Progress in Obesity Prevention
Food and Nutrition Board

Dan Glickman, Lynn Parker, Leslie J. Sim,
Heather Del Valle Cook, and Emily Ann Miller, *Editors*

INSTITUTE OF MEDICINE
OF THE NATIONAL ACADEMIES

THE NATIONAL ACADEMIES PRESS
Washington, D.C.
www.nap.edu

THE NATIONAL ACADEMIES PRESS   500 Fifth Street, NW   Washington, DC 20001

NOTICE: The project that is the subject of this report was approved by the Governing Board of the National Research Council, whose members are drawn from the councils of the National Academy of Sciences, the National Academy of Engineering, and the Institute of Medicine. The members of the committee responsible for the report were chosen for their special competences and with regard for appropriate balance.

This study was supported by Grant No. 61747 between the National Academy of Sciences and the Robert Wood Johnson Foundation and a grant between the National Academy of Sciences and the Michael & Susan Dell Foundation. Any opinions, findings, conclusions, or recommendations expressed in this publication are those of the author(s) and do not necessarily reflect the view of the organizations or agencies that provided support for this project.

Library of Congress Cataloging-in-Publication Data

Institute of Medicine (U.S.). Committee on Accelerating Progress in Obesity Prevention.
  Accelerating progress in obesity prevention: Solving the weight of the nation / Committee on Accelerating Progress in Obesity Prevention, Food and Nutrition Board, Institute of Medicine of the National Academies ; Dan Glickman . . . [et al.], editors.
    p. ; cm.
  Includes bibliographical references.
  ISBN 978-0-309-22154-2 (pbk.) — ISBN 978-0-309-22155-9 (e-ISBN)
  I. Glickman, Dan. II. Title.
  [DNLM: 1. Obesity—prevention & control—United States. 2. Environment Design—United States. 3. Needs Assessment—United States. 4. Program Development—United States. WD 210]

  362.1963′98—dc23
                                                        2012007112

Additional copies of this report are available from the National Academies Press, 500 Fifth Street, NW, Keck 360, Washington, DC 20001; (800) 624-6242 or (202) 334-3313; http://www.nap.edu.

For more information about the Institute of Medicine, visit the IOM home page at: **www.iom.edu.**

WEIGHT OF THE NATION is a trademark owned by the U.S. Department of Health and Human Services (DHHS/CDC). Use of this trademark is not an endorsement by DHHS/CDC of a particular company or organization.

Cover photo credits: yellow squash (first column, first row) by DC Central Condition; people running up stairs (fourth column, second row) by Osman Meran; man pushing a stroller on the beach (fifth column, second row) by Michael L. Baird; watermelon (first column, fifth row) by Patrick Feller.

The serpent has been a symbol of long life, healing, and knowledge among almost all cultures and religions since the beginning of recorded history. The serpent adopted as a logotype by the Institute of Medicine is a relief carving from ancient Greece, now held by the Staatliche Museen in Berlin.

Suggested citation: IOM (Institute of Medicine). 2012. *Accelerating Progress in Obesity Prevention: Solving the Weight of the Nation*. Washington, DC: The National Academies Press.

"Knowing is not enough; we must apply.
Willing is not enough; we must do."
—Goethe

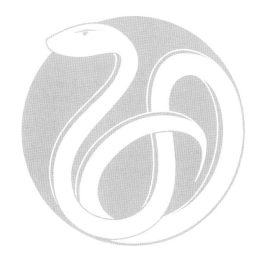

INSTITUTE OF MEDICINE
OF THE NATIONAL ACADEMIES

Advising the Nation. Improving Health.

THE NATIONAL ACADEMIES
Advisers to the Nation on Science, Engineering, and Medicine

The **National Academy of Sciences** is a private, nonprofit, self-perpetuating society of distinguished scholars engaged in scientific and engineering research, dedicated to the furtherance of science and technology and to their use for the general welfare. Upon the authority of the charter granted to it by the Congress in 1863, the Academy has a mandate that requires it to advise the federal government on scientific and technical matters. Dr. Ralph J. Cicerone is president of the National Academy of Sciences.

The **National Academy of Engineering** was established in 1964, under the charter of the National Academy of Sciences, as a parallel organization of outstanding engineers. It is autonomous in its administration and in the selection of its members, sharing with the National Academy of Sciences the responsibility for advising the federal government. The National Academy of Engineering also sponsors engineering programs aimed at meeting national needs, encourages education and research, and recognizes the superior achievements of engineers. Dr. Charles M. Vest is president of the National Academy of Engineering.

The **Institute of Medicine** was established in 1970 by the National Academy of Sciences to secure the services of eminent members of appropriate professions in the examination of policy matters pertaining to the health of the public. The Institute acts under the responsibility given to the National Academy of Sciences by its congressional charter to be an adviser to the federal government and, upon its own initiative, to identify issues of medical care, research, and education. Dr. Harvey V. Fineberg is president of the Institute of Medicine.

The **National Research Council** was organized by the National Academy of Sciences in 1916 to associate the broad community of science and technology with the Academy's purposes of furthering knowledge and advising the federal government. Functioning in accordance with general policies determined by the Academy, the Council has become the principal operating agency of both the National Academy of Sciences and the National Academy of Engineering in providing services to the government, the public, and the scientific and engineering communities. The Council is administered jointly by both Academies and the Institute of Medicine. Dr. Ralph J. Cicerone and Dr. Charles M. Vest are chair and vice chair, respectively, of the National Research Council.

www.national-academies.org

EDUARDO J. SANCHEZ, Vice President and Chief Medical Officer, Blue Cross and Blue Shield of Texas, Richardson

ELLEN WARTELLA, Al-thani Professor of Communication, Professor of Psychology and Professor of Human Development and Social Policy, Director of the Center on Media and Human Development at Northwestern University, Evanston, Illinois

Study Staff

LYNN PARKER, Scholar

LESLIE J. SIM, Senior Program Officer

HEATHER DEL VALLE COOK, Program Officer

EMILY ANN MILLER, Associate Program Officer

HEATHER BREINER, Research Associate

MATTHEW B. SPEAR, Program Associate (until July 2011)

ELENA OVAITT, Senior Program Assistant (from September 2011)

LAMIS JOMAA, Christine Mirzayan Science & Technology Policy Graduate Fellow (until December 2010)

ANTON L. BANDY, Financial Associate

GERALDINE KENNEDO, Administrative Assistant

LINDA D. MEYERS, Director, Food and Nutrition Board

Reviewers

This report has been reviewed in draft form by individuals chosen for their diverse perspectives and technical expertise, in accordance with procedures approved by the National Research Council's Report Review Committee. The purpose of this independent review is to provide candid and critical comments that will assist the institution in making its published report as sound as possible and to ensure that the report meets institutional standards for objectivity, evidence, and responsiveness to the study charge. The review comments and draft manuscript remain confidential to protect the integrity of the deliberative process. We wish to thank the following individuals for their review of this report:

Jenna Anding, Texas A&M University
Leann L. Birch, Pennsylvania State University
John C. Cawley, Cornell University
Lilian Cheung, Harvard University
Antonio Convit, New York University School of Medicine
Lori Dorfman, Berkeley Media Studies Group
John R. Finnegan, Jr., University of Minnesota School of Public Health
Vincent Fonseca, Texas Department of State Health Services
Wally Gomaa, ACAP Health
W. Philip T. James, International Association for the Study of Obesity
Christine M. Olson, Cornell University
Tom Robinson, Stanford University School of Medicine
Kate Rogers, H-E-B Stores
Robert Sege, Boston Medical Center
Dianne Stanton Ward, University of North Carolina at Chapel Hill
Derek Yach, PepsiCo., Inc.

Although the reviewers listed above have provided many constructive comments and suggestions, they were not asked to endorse the report's conclusions or recommendations, nor did they see the final draft of the report before its release. The review of this report was overseen by **Cutberto Garza,** Boston College and **Enriqueta C. Bond,** Burroughs Wellcome Fund. Appointed by the National Research Council and Institute of Medicine, they were responsible for making certain that an independent examination of this report was carried out in accordance with institutional procedures and that all review comments were carefully considered. Responsibility for the final content of this report rests entirely with the authoring committee and the institution.

Preface

Obesity is a public health issue of monumental importance to the nation. I would argue that it is the most significant public health challenge we face at this time, both because of the huge number of people it affects and because of the ripple effects it has and will have on the development of debilitating and costly chronic diseases. Obesity is a major contributor to the health care cost challenges we confront today in the United States. These costs have the potential to become catastrophic and unaffordable unless all sectors of society take the need for obesity prevention seriously and act responsibly. It is untenable to wait any longer until people are already sick, requiring that most of our efforts and funding be devoted to crisis intervention for diseases that could have been prevented or made less severe.

This report is part of a series of publications dedicated to providing accessible and useful information and analysis to policy makers and others working to turn the obesity epidemic around. Funded by the Robert Wood Johnson Foundation (and the Michael & Susan Dell Foundation for the committee's workshop and workshop report on measurement issues in obesity prevention), this report focuses on the areas of obesity prevention that are most important to pursue now to significantly accelerate progress against the epidemic. The committee reviewed the hundreds of recommendations that have been made related to obesity prevention, the evidence that supports them, and the progress that has been made in their implementation. I have become convinced through this process that the health of the nation and its children is inextricably linked to a complex web of influences on physical activity and diet. This truth must be communicated to individuals, families, communities, and the broader U.S. society so they can understand the nature of the threat and the multisector solutions that, working together, can make a real difference. We need to reach many different kinds of people with diverse interests and concerns—individuals moving through their daily lives unaware of these issues, policy makers and others who make decisions that control physical activity and food environments, health care providers, the education community, and the business community/private sector. We also must ensure that individuals, families, and communities are empowered to work for change so their environment will support them in their efforts to achieve and maintain a healthy weight. We all need to maintain our commitment to progress and acceleration in the areas that can make the most difference.

The committee has many people to thank for their support in developing this report and its recommendations. We begin by thanking in particular Laura Leviton and James Marks from the Robert Wood Johnson Foundation and Aliya Hussaini from the Michael & Susan Dell Foundation for their encouragement.

We appreciate the extensive contributions of Ross Hammond, who was commissioned to provide technical insight into integrating, developing, and using systems mapping techniques to inform our deliberations and decisions. His insight and expertise added to the quality of our decisions and helped visually communicate the dynamic nature of the relationships we were considering and how they fit within the greater societal context. We also thank Eric Olsen from Feeding America for his important input as an unpaid consultant.

In addition, we want to express our gratitude to Shari Cookson, Nick Doob, John Hoffman, Ali Moss, and Sarah Teale from Home Box Office (HBO) Documentary Films for their contributions as unpaid consultants. These film producers drew inspiration and guidance from our work and discussions for a series of documentaries on obesity prevention that, along with the release of the recommendations in this report, will serve as the foundation for a major national public health campaign on obesity prevention. This campaign will be coordinated by HBO and the Institute of Medicine (IOM) in association with the Centers for Disease Control and Prevention, Kaiser Permanente, the Michael & Susan Dell Foundation, and the National Institutes of Health.

The committee greatly benefited from the opportunity for discussion with the individuals who made presentations at and attended our workshops and meetings. (See Appendix C for a list of workshop and panel presentations.) We would also like to thank Preston Maring and Ray Baxter from Kaiser Permanente, as well as Martha Coven from the Domestic Policy Council and Rogan Kersh from Columbia University, for their presentations. The experience and insights of all these speakers contributed immeasurably to our deliberations.

I want to express my sincere appreciation and thanks to the committee members for their extraordinary volunteer efforts in the development of this report. A special thank you goes to Bill Purcell and M. R. C. Greenwood for their important role as vice chairs of the committee. Bill brought his immense experience as a public servant in government to the task and M. R. C. her vast knowledge of nutrition.

The committee could not have done its work without the outstanding guidance and support provided by the IOM staff: Lynn Parker and Leslie Sim, co-study directors; Heather Del Valle Cook, program officer; Emily Ann Miller, associate program officer; Heather Breiner, research associate; Elena Ovaitt, senior program assistant; and Lamis Jomaa, Christine Mirzayan Science & Technology Policy Fellow. Matthew Spear also provided highly skilled logistical support. Linda Meyers' guidance and counsel were invaluable throughout our deliberations. In addition, we are indebted to others throughout the IOM's office of reports and communications who patiently worked with us throughout external review, revisions of this report and report briefs, and the production process through final publication. They include Laura DeStefano, IOM report production manager; Vilija Teel, IOM report review manager; and Lauren Tobias, IOM communications director. And last but not least, the report greatly benefited from the copyediting skills of Rona Briere.

Daniel R. Glickman, *Chair*
Committee on Accelerating Progress in Obesity Prevention

Contents

Summary[1]

The United States continues to experience an epidemic of overweight and obesity. This national health condition constitutes a startling setback to major improvements achieved in other areas of health during the past century. The substantial and long-term human and societal costs of obesity, the great difficulty of treating this problem once it has developed, and the relatively slow progress made thus far in turning the national obesity numbers around underline the urgent need to develop a plan for accelerating progress in obesity prevention.

The Institute of Medicine's (IOM's) Committee on Accelerating Progress in Obesity Prevention was formed to address this challenge. The committee's overall charge was to develop a set of recommendations for accelerating progress toward obesity prevention over the next decade, as well as to recommend potential measures of progress toward this goal. Inherent in this charge was a recognition that, while a large number of promising individual programs and interventions currently are being supported, implemented, and evaluated, there is a growing need to identify a set of obesity prevention actions that, both individually and together, can accelerate meaningful change on a societal level.

Prior work by the nation's researchers to illuminate various aspects of the obesity problem has helped inform obesity prevention efforts. For example, there is a broad consensus that changes are necessary in the environments in which people live and the settings they frequent. Another major revelation has been that there are no simple or single-pronged solutions. Earlier work has helped researchers and health professionals understand the need for a "meta-strategy" for obesity prevention that includes a range of recommendations. Any one potential strategy can contribute to obesity prevention, but alone cannot solve this complex problem.

---

[1]This summary does not include references. Citations to support statements made herein are given in the body of the report.

THE CRITICAL IMPORTANCE OF OBESITY PREVENTION

Although the obesity epidemic in the United States has been instrumental in bringing worldwide attention to the problem, obesity also has become a problem worldwide. In the United States alone, one-third of adults are now obese, and the prevalence of obesity among children has risen from 5 to 17 percent in the past 30 years. Equally disturbing, these percentages generally are higher for ethnic minorities, for those who are low-income or less educated, and for rural populations. With obesity at these levels and with current trajectories suggesting the possibility of further increases, future health, social, and economic costs are likely to be devastating. Obesity is associated with major causes of death and disability, and its effect on predisposing individuals to the development of type 2 diabetes is so strong that the onset of this disease now is occurring in childhood.

In economic terms, the estimated annual cost of obesity-related illness based on data from the Medical Expenditure Panel Survey for 2000-2005 is $190.2 billion (in 2005 dollars), or nearly 21 percent of annual medical spending in the United States. Childhood obesity alone is responsible for $14.1 billion in direct medical costs. Many of these health-related obesity costs are absorbed by Medicare and Medicaid, important programs already under attack because of their national price tag. Moreover, obesity-related medical costs in general are expected to rise significantly, especially because today's obese children are likely to become tomorrow's obese adults. In fact, U.S. military leaders report that obesity has reduced their pool of potential recruits to the armed forces. As the U.S. economy struggles to stabilize and grow, obesity projections reveal that beyond the impact of growing medical costs attributable to obesity, the nation will incur higher costs for disability and unemployment benefits, and businesses will face the additional costs associated with obesity-related job absenteeism and lost productivity.

The causes of increased obesity in the United States—the influences that have led people to consume more calories (or energy) through food and beverages than they expend through physical activity—are multifactorial, ranging from cultural norms, to the availability of sidewalks and affordable foods, to what is seen on television. Many causes of obesity are the result of multiple changes in U.S. society that have affected various aspects of contemporary life, including physical activity and food consumption patterns. Exposure to these influences, both positive and negative, varies by subpopulation and can result in inequities in the prevalence of obesity. If a community has no safe places to walk or play, lacks food outlets offering affordable healthy foods, and is bombarded by advertisements for unhealthy foods and beverages, its residents will have less opportunity to engage in physical activity and eating behaviors that allow them to achieve and maintain a healthy weight. Successful obesity prevention thus involves reducing negative and increasing positive influences on a societal level. There also are genetically or biologically mediated influences on obesity in individuals. Taking a population approach to obesity prevention is not to deny the importance of these genetic or biological factors, but to recognize the difficulty of maintaining energy balance when sedentary lives are the norm and high-calorie foods are ubiquitous.

Tremendous strides have been made in addressing the epidemic over the past decade, measured by the sheer amount of attention to the problem, and by the number and coherence of efforts to address the problem and bolster the scientific underpinnings and policy basis for taking action. Evidence of stabilization in obesity prevalence in at least some demographic groups suggests that these deliberate initiatives to address the problem are on track, perhaps in concert with other, spontaneous countering forces. Given the scope and scale of what is needed and the inevitability of a time lag before true progress can be estimated, however, the developments to date create a unique opportunity to restate goals and refine targets and approaches in order to accelerate progress.

Broad positive societal changes that support and sustain individual and family behaviors will need to affect activity and eating environments for all ages. Prevention is critical to decreasing the prevalence of overweight and obesity among children, who are the focus of much of the prevention discussion. But obesity prevention in adults also is crucial to obesity prevention in children because adults are their role models, caregivers, and advocates. Moreover, prevention efforts can help reduce the gradual increase in weight that often occurs in adulthood and support the reduction of further excess weight gain among adults who are already overweight or obese.

STUDY APPROACH

In responding to its charge, the committee's main goal was to provide direction on what recommendations, strategies, and actions should be implemented in the short term to accelerate progress in obesity prevention over the next 10 years. The committee identified close to 800 previously published recommendations and associated strategies and actions related to obesity prevention and assessed the potential of each to help achieve this goal. To guide this assessment, the committee formulated a set of principles, summarized in Box S-1. The committee identified recommendations and associated strategies and actions with the broadest reach and the greatest potential to impact the development of obesity and prioritized

BOX S-1
Guiding Principles

The Committee on Accelerating Progress on Obesity Prevention formulated the following principles to guide the scope of its work and its decisions:

1. Bold, widespread, and sustained action will be necessary to accelerate progress in obesity prevention.

2. Priority and targeted actions must drive cultural and societal changes to improve environments that influence physical activity and food intake options.

3. Cultural and societal changes are needed to address obesity, and a systems approach must be taken when formulating obesity prevention recommendations so as to address the problem from all possible dimensions.

4. Solutions to the obesity epidemic must come from multiple sources, involve multiple levels and sectors, and take into account the synergy of multiple strategies.

5. Obesity prevention recommendations should be based on the best available scientific evidence as outlined in the Locate Evidence, Evaluate Evidence, Assemble Evidence, Inform Decisions (L.E.A.D.) framework.

6. The cost, feasibility, and practicality of implementing prior and further recommendations must be considered.

7. Unintended consequences of obesity prevention efforts must be considered.

8. Obesity prevention recommendations should incorporate ongoing evaluation of progress toward achieving benchmarks and of the need for any course corrections.

9. Recommendations to accelerate progress in obesity prevention must include an assessment of the potential for high impact, the reach and scope of potential effects, the timeliness of effects, the ability to reduce disparities and promote equity, and clearly measureable outcomes.

them using the best available scientific evidence. The committee also took into consideration progress made to date in implementing these recommendations, strategies, and actions; their ability to be evaluated or measured to assess their progress or impact; the timeliness of their effects; any unintended consequences; their potential to reduce disparities in the risk of obesity; and the feasibility and practicality of their implementation.

At the same time, the committee identified relationships among the recommendations and strategies and actions that could inform and strengthen their individual and overall impacts. This way of thinking—called a systems approach—allowed the committee to visualize and understand how recommendations and strategies on their own can be important to accelerate progress, and when implemented together with others, can interact and reinforce and sometimes inhibit impact on preventing obesity. This systems approach also helped the committee identify potential unintended effects (both positive and negative) that might not be apparent in considering individual solutions alone. Throughout this assessment, the committee looked as well for gaps in recommendations published to date.

The result of this work was the emergence of five critical areas—or environments for change: (1) environments for physical activity, (2) food and beverage environments, (3) message environments, (4) health care and work environments, and (5) school environments. These environments serve as the basis for the committee's recommendations and the respective strategies, actions, and outcome indicators.

TAKING A SYSTEMS PERSPECTIVE TO ACCELERATE PROGRESS

In this report, the committee presents five key interrelated recommendations whose implementation would have a substantial effect on accelerating obesity prevention over the next decade; an explanation of the kinds of engagement and leadership that can build capacity and mobilize action; and a call for monitoring progress in the implementation of the recommendations (see Figure S-1). While a Venn diagram such as that in Figure S-1 cannot illustrate the many and diverse interactions and feedback loops revealed by a systems map (as presented in Appendix B), it does reflect the critical areas of concern and their interrelationships. The committee's recommendations can have a profound impact on people in the environments with which they interact on a regular basis, including schools, places of employment, doctors' offices, child care settings, restaurants of all kinds, and everywhere food is sold. To implement these recommendations, the committee has identified strategies that individually have the greatest potential reach and

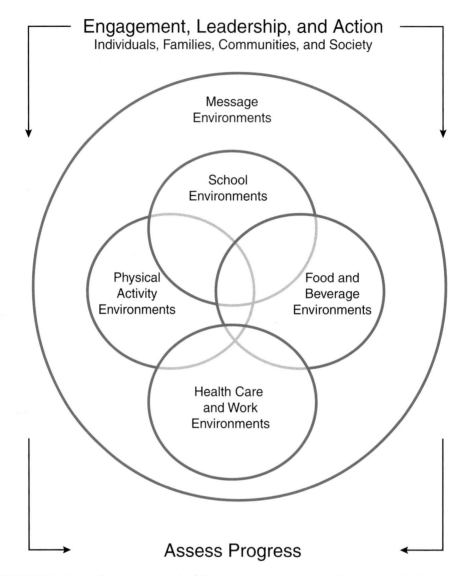

FIGURE S-1 Comprehensive approach of the Committee on Accelerating Progress in Obesity Prevention.

impact on preventing obesity, based on research evidence and the current level of progress in each area. For each strategy, the report also suggests a set of actions that are likely to make a positive contribution to that strategy's achievement based on research evidence or, where evidence is lacking or limited, have a logical connection with its achievement.

Each recommendation, strategy, and action has potential to accelerate obesity prevention. However, while the report necessarily presents the committee's recommendations individually, in linear form, the committee suggests that they be viewed by key stakeholders and sectors as unfolding simultaneously and influencing each others' success. This "systems perspective" helps to reveal, and create, the potential for combined impacts (or synergies) that can further accelerate progress in preventing obesity. This perspective also can assist in recognizing likely positive (i.e., supporting and accelerating success) and negative (i.e., acting as a barrier to success) interactions and feedback loops among the recommendations and strategies.

Engagement and Equity

It is essential to recognize that accelerating progress toward obesity prevention will need to occur at every level, from individual, to family, to community, to society as a whole. Acceleration will require engagement among all levels and all sectors in order to build capacity and achieve impact so that individuals and families can successfully manage and support healthy changes in lifestyle.

It is important to recognize as well that not all individuals, families, and communities are similarly situated. In many parts of the United States, low-income individuals and families live, learn, work, and play in neighborhoods that lack sufficient health-protective resources such as parks and open space, grocery stores, walkable streets, and high-quality schools. In any given community, the relative mix of community-level resources and risk factors is determined primarily through democratic local and regional decision-making processes; consequently, organized participation in these processes influences where these community resources and risks are located. Because of such factors as poverty, language barriers, and immigration status, low-income, minority, and other disadvantaged population groups often are underrepresented and their concerns marginalized in these decision-making processes. These groups are therefore less likely to benefit from access to health-protective resources. To change this situation, robust and long-term community engagement and civic participation among these disadvantaged populations become essential.

Leadership, Implementation, and Priorities

In presenting its recommendations throughout the report, the committee identifies leaders who are those individuals, agencies, organizations, or sectors traditionally seen as having the knowledge and control of and responsibility for the particular environments, policies, and practices that must change. The committee also introduces new ways to think about leadership, including identifying and calling on a broader set of individuals, families, communities, and society at large. A major premise of the committee's systems approach to leadership is that it is a shared responsibility across sectors and levels, and one that may not follow typical hierarchical or individual sector-based approaches. All individuals, organizations, agencies, and sectors that do or can influence physical activity and nutrition environments are called on to assess and begin to act on their potential roles as leaders in obesity prevention. Some traditional leaders may turn away from this responsibility, but many other less likely or unexpected leaders may step forward as willing actors.

Whether leaders are identified or self-identify, once awareness of the catastrophic nature of the obesity problem is understood and felt and the need for diverse and numerous leaders is recognized, all will share the moment of saying to themselves, "I can do something about this, and I want to play a role." From that point on, viewing their roles with a systems lens will guide them in new directions. They will act with new foresight—seeing how what they plan to do can or will intersect and interact with other actions that may be or have already been taken in their sector, other sectors, or across sectors. Funding for implementation is likely to become available as the seriousness of the obesity threat is understood, and calls and support for resources to combat a potential disaster emerge. In addition, the diversity of leaders throughout the system can bring existing assets to bear for use or redeployment and make available new resources, often from unexpected sources, that previously were not apparent or available.

Implicit in the committee's systems approach to leadership and implementation is the assumption that individual leaders will determine which recommendations, strategies, and potential actions are their priorities, or that those who choose to follow their lead will play a major role in determining these priorities. The committee did not give any recommended action or set of actions priority above any others, but rather saw leaders stepping up to implement different aspects of the five critical areas identified in Figure S-1. Leaders are called on to start from where they have the most influence and likelihood of success, a decision resulting from their unique assessment of a range of community-specific or local-level factors.

Assessment

The changes recommended by the committee should begin now and, once implemented, continue for a sustained period. Much of this work has already begun in a number of sectors at the local, state, and national levels. It will be essential to monitor and track progress in the implementation of the committee's recommendations, as well as to conduct sustained research on the magnitude and nature of their impact, both individually and in tandem. While the confluence of all the recommendations will likely have the most impact, each step toward acceleration of progress will be significant and cumulative in its impact.

The Vision

The committee's recommendations, strategies, and actions can be seen as a system of large-scale transformative approaches that is urgently needed to accelerate progress in obesity prevention. This system comprises major reforms in access to and opportunities for physical activity; widespread reductions in the availability of unhealthy food and beverage options and increases in access to healthier options at affordable, competitive prices; an overhaul of messages that surround Americans (through marketing and education) with respect to physical activity and food consumption; expansion of the obesity prevention support structure provided by health care providers, insurers, and employers that interfaces with the U.S. population in every workplace and health care setting; and schools being made a major national focal point for obesity prevention. By viewing the committee's recommendations from a systems perspective, one can see that as individual changes are achieved in each of these environments, these changes also have the potential to support and accelerate the progress of other recommended changes within each environment and in other environments as well.

To gain a better sense of the potentially transformational nature of this system of reforms, it is helpful to imagine a United States in which they have been fully implemented in ways that take into account the potential positive and negative aspects of their interaction. For example, physical activity would be an integral and routine part of most people's lives, and adults and children would have access to places and opportunities for enjoyable movement everywhere they spend their time. Healthy foods would be the most visible, attractive, and easy to obtain options in all places that sell or serve food. Education about food would involve every child in hands-on skill-building experiences with making food choices in stores and restaurants and preparing foods at home, and children and their parents would hear more from television and digital media about activity and healthy foods than about sedentary pursuits and unhealthy foods. Patients would leave every health care provider visit with more knowledge about obesity prevention that they could put into action, supported by their immediate environment, and workplaces would play a major role in increasing the physical activity and healthy foods available to their employees. And schools would be nutrition and wellness centers for children and their families in every community.

RECOMMENDATIONS AND STRATEGIES

The committee offers five recommendations, along with strategies for their implementation, under five respective overarching goals. Specific actions associated with each strategy, a detailed systems map illustrating the interactions among the recommendations and strategies, and indicators that can serve as measures of progress are presented in the body of the report. The committee firmly believes that implementing its recommendations is essential to improve and maintain the nation's health. Without focused and sustained effort in these areas, the obesity epidemic will lead to more increases in the costs of being less well and less productive, including reduced ability for the nation and its citizens to compete in life and in the workplace. If these issues are important to each of the sectors with the potential to contribute to obesity prevention, it is their obligation to act promptly and in a sustained manner in the interests of the nation's health and security.

Goal 1: Make physical activity an integral and routine part of life.

Recommendation 1: Communities, transportation officials, community planners, health professionals, and governments should make promotion of physical activity a priority by substantially increasing access to places and opportunities for such activity.[2]

Strategy 1-1: Enhance the physical and built environment. Communities, organizations, community planners, and public health professionals should encourage physical activity by enhancing the physical and built environment, rethinking community design, and ensuring access to places for such activity.

---

[2]Note that physical education and opportunities for physical activity in schools are covered in Recommendation 5, on school environments.

Strategy 1-2: Provide and support community programs designed to increase physical activity. Communities and organizations should encourage physical activity by providing and supporting programs designed to increase such activity.

Strategy 1-3: Adopt physical activity requirements for licensed child care providers. State and local child care and early childhood education regulators should establish requirements for each program to improve its current physical activity standards.

Strategy 1-4: Provide support for the science and practice of physical activity. Federal, state, and local government agencies should make physical activity a national health priority through support for the translation of scientific evidence into best-practice applications.

Goal 2: Create food and beverage environments that ensure that healthy food and beverage options are the routine, easy choice.

Recommendation 2: Governments and decision makers in the business community/private sector[3] should make a concerted effort to reduce unhealthy food and beverage options[4] and substantially increase healthier food and beverage options at affordable, competitive prices.

Strategy 2-1: Adopt policies and implement practices to reduce overconsumption of sugar-sweetened beverages. Decision makers in the business community/private sector, in nongovernmental organizations, and at all levels of government should adopt comprehensive strategies to reduce overconsumption of sugar-sweetened beverages.[5]

---

[3]The business community/private sector includes private employers and privately owned and/or operated locations frequented by the public, such as movie theaters, shopping centers, sporting and entertainment venues, bowling alleys, and other recreational/entertainment facilities.

[4]Although there is no consensus on the definition of "unhealthy" foods/beverages, the term refers in this report to foods and beverages that are calorie-dense and low in naturally occurring nutrients. Such foods and beverages contribute little fiber and few essential nutrients and phytochemicals, but contain added fats, sweeteners, sodium, and other ingredients. Unhealthy foods and beverages displace the consumption of foods recommended in the Dietary Guidelines for Americans and may lead to the development of obesity.

[5]Sugar-sweetened beverages are defined to include all beverages containing added caloric sweeteners, including, but not limited to, sugar- or otherwise calorically sweetened regular sodas, less than 100 percent fruit drinks, energy drinks, sports drinks, and ready-to-drink teas and coffees.

Strategy 2-2: Increase the availability of lower-calorie and healthier food and beverage options for children in restaurants. Chain and quick-service restaurants should substantially reduce the number of calories served to children and substantially expand the number of affordable and competitively priced healthier options available for parents to choose from in their facilities.

Strategy 2-3: Utilize strong nutritional standards for all foods and beverages sold or provided through the government, and ensure that these healthy options are available in all places frequented by the public. Government agencies (federal, state, local, and school district) should ensure that all foods and beverages sold or provided through the government are aligned with the age-specific recommendations in the current Dietary Guidelines for Americans. The business community and the private sector operating venues frequented by the public should ensure that a variety of foods and beverages, including those recommended by the Dietary Guidelines for Americans, are sold or served at all times.

Strategy 2-4: Introduce, modify, and utilize health-promoting food and beverage retailing and distribution policies. States and localities should utilize financial incentives such as flexible financing or tax credits, streamlined permitting processes, and zoning strategies, as well as cross-sectoral collaborations (e.g., among industry, philanthropic organizations, government, and the community) to enhance the quality of local food environments, particularly in low-income communities. These efforts should include encouraging or attracting retailers and distributors of healthy food (e.g., supermarkets) to locate in underserved areas and limiting the concentration of unhealthy food venues (e.g., fast-food restaurants, convenience stores). Incentives should be linked to public health goals in ways that give priority to stores that also commit to health-promoting retail strategies (e.g., through placement, promotion, and pricing).

Strategy 2-5: Broaden the examination and development of U.S. agriculture policy and research to include implications for the American diet. Congress, the Administration, and federal agencies should examine the implications of U.S. agriculture policy for obesity, and should ensure that such policy includes understanding and implementing, as appropriate, an optimal mix of crops and farming methods for meeting the Dietary Guidelines for Americans.

Goal 3: Transform messages about physical activity and nutrition.

Recommendation 3: Industry, educators, and governments should act quickly, aggressively, and in a sustained manner on many levels to transform the environment that surrounds Americans with messages about physical activity, food, and nutrition.[6]

Strategy 3-1: Develop and support a sustained, targeted physical activity and nutrition social marketing program. Congress, the Administration, other federal policy makers, and foundations should dedicate substantial funding and support to the development and implementation of a robust and sustained social marketing program on physical activity and nutrition. This program should encompass carefully targeted, culturally appropriate messages aimed at specific audiences (e.g., tweens, new parents, mothers); clear behavior-change goals (e.g., take a daily walk, reduce consumption of sugar-sweetened beverages among adolescents, introduce infants to vegetables, make use of the new front-of-package nutrition labels); and related environmental change goals (e.g., improve physical environments, offer better food choices in public places, increase the availability of healthy food retailing).

Strategy 3-2: Implement common standards for marketing foods and beverages to children and adolescents. The food, beverage, restaurant, and media industries should take broad, common, and urgent voluntary action to make substantial improvements in their marketing aimed directly at children and adolescents aged 2-17. All foods and beverages marketed to this age group should support a diet that accords with the Dietary Guidelines for Americans in order to prevent obesity and risk factors associated with chronic disease risk. Children and adolescents should be encouraged to avoid calories from foods that they generally overconsume (e.g., products high in sugar, fat, and sodium) and to replace them with foods they generally underconsume (e.g., fruits, vegetables, and whole grains). The standards set for foods and beverages marketed to children and adolescents should be widely publicized and easily available to parents and other consumers. They should cover foods and beverages marketed to children and adolescents aged 2-17 and should apply to a broad range of marketing and advertising practices, including digital marketing and the use of licensed characters and toy premiums. If such marketing standards have not been adopted within 2 years by a substantial

---

[6]Note that instruction in food and nutrition for children and adolescents in schools is covered in Recommendation 5, on school environments.

majority of food, beverage, restaurant, and media companies that market foods and beverages to children and adolescents, policy makers at the local, state, and federal levels should consider setting mandatory nutritional standards for marketing to this age group to ensure that such standards are implemented.

Strategy 3-3: Ensure consistent nutrition labeling for the front of packages, retail store shelves, and menus and menu boards that encourages healthier food choices. The Food and Drug Administration (FDA) and the U.S. Department of Agriculture should implement a standard system of nutrition labeling for the front of packages and retail store shelves that is harmonious with the Nutrition Facts panel, and restaurants should provide calorie labeling on all menus and menu boards.

Strategy 3-4: Adopt consistent nutrition education policies for federal programs with nutrition education components. USDA should update the policies for Supplemental Nutrition Assistance Program Education and the policies for other federal programs with nutrition education components to explicitly encourage the provision of advice about types of foods to reduce in the diet, consistent with the Dietary Guidelines for Americans.

Goal 4: Expand the role of health care providers, insurers, and employers in obesity prevention.

Recommendation 4: Health care and health service providers, employers, and insurers should increase the support structure for achieving better population health and obesity prevention.

Strategy 4-1: Provide standardized care and advocate for healthy community environments. All health care providers should adopt standards of practice (evidence-based or consensus guidelines) for prevention, screening, diagnosis, and treatment of overweight and obesity to help children, adolescents, and adults achieve and maintain a healthy weight, avoid obesity-related complications, and reduce the psychosocial consequences of obesity. Health care providers also should advocate, on behalf of their patients, for improved physical activity and diet opportunities in their patients' communities.

Strategy 4-2: Ensure coverage of, access to, and incentives for routine obesity prevention, screening, diagnosis, and treatment. Insurers (both public and private) should ensure that health insurance coverage and access provisions address obesity prevention, screening, diagnosis, and treatment.

Strategy 4-3: Encourage active living and healthy eating at work. Worksites should create, or expand, healthy environments by establishing, implementing, and monitoring policy initiatives that support wellness.

Strategy 4-4: Encourage healthy weight gain during pregnancy and breastfeeding, and promote breastfeeding-friendly environments. Health service providers and employers should adopt, implement, and monitor policies that support healthy weight gain during pregnancy and the initiation and continuation of breastfeeding. Population disparities in breastfeeding should be specifically addressed at the federal, state, and local levels to remove barriers and promote targeted increases in breastfeeding initiation and continuation.

Goal 5: Make schools a national focal point for obesity prevention.

Recommendation 5: Federal, state, and local government and education authorities, with support from parents, teachers, and the business community and the private sector, should make schools a focal point for obesity prevention.

Strategy 5-1: Require quality physical education and opportunities for physical activity in schools. Through support from federal and state governments, state and local education agencies and local school districts should ensure that all students in grades K-12 have adequate opportunities to engage in 60 minutes of physical activity per school day. This 60-minute goal includes access to and participation in quality physical education.

Strategy 5-2: Ensure strong nutritional standards for all foods and beverages sold or provided through schools. All government agencies (federal, state, local, and school district) providing foods and beverages to children and adolescents have a responsibility to provide those in their care with foods and beverages that promote health and learning. The Dietary Guidelines for Americans provide specific science-based recommendations for optimizing dietary intake to prevent disease and promote health. Implementation of these guidelines would shift children's and adolescents' dietary intake to prevent obesity and risk factors associated with chronic disease risk by increasing the amounts of fruits, vegetables, and high-fiber grains they consume; decreasing their consumption of sugar-sweetened beverages, dietary fat in general, solid fats, and added sugars; and ensuring age-appropriate portion sizes of meals and other foods and beverages. Federal, state, and local decision makers are responsible for ensuring that nutrition standards based on the Dietary Guidelines are adopted by schools; these decision makers, in partnership with regulatory agencies, parents, teachers, and food manufacturers, also are responsible for ensuring that these standards are implemented fully and that adherence is monitored so as to protect the health of the nation's children and adolescents.

Strategy 5-3: Ensure food literacy, including skill development, in schools.
Through leadership and guidance from federal and state governments, state and local education agencies should ensure the implementation and monitoring of sequential food literacy and nutrition science education, spanning grades K-12, based on the food and nutrition recommendations in the Dietary Guidelines for Americans.

1

The Vision

Key Messages

- The Institute of Medicine's (IOM's) Committee on Accelerating Progress in Obesity Prevention was charged with charting pathways to a timely resolution of the obesity epidemic in the U.S. population.

- The committee's vision is for a successful, sustainable society that supports obesity prevention and offers broad opportunities for everyone to lead a healthy, productive life.

- Taking a systems perspective will accelerate the realization of this vision.

- Achieving this vision will involve mobilizing the population through engagement and leadership at all levels—individuals, families, communities, and society—and in all sectors.

- Targeted actions are needed to reduce the inequitable distribution of health promotion resources and risk factors that contribute to health disparities in low-income, minority, and other disadvantaged populations.

The epidemic of obesity in the United States has major human and societal costs, both now and for future generations. Obesity affects the entire childhood experience, predisposes adolescents to obesity in adulthood, and increases the risk of chronic illness and reduced quality of life and success in adulthood. Currently, a majority of U.S. adults and a substantial proportion of children and adolescents have weight levels in the overweight or obese range (Flegal et al., 2010; Ogden et al., 2010a). The percentage of people who are already obese translates to an estimated total of nearly 73 million adults and 12 million children and adolescents (Ogden et al., 2010b,c), and those overweight are likely to become obese if they gain weight over time. The United States is far from alone in facing the challenges of this epidemic. Many aspects of the epidemic and its causes reach across the globe. An estimated 1.5 billion adults worldwide are overweight or obese (Finucane et al., 2011), and the World Health Organization estimates that 35 million preschool children in developing countries and 43 million preschool children worldwide are overweight or obese (de Onis et al., 2010). However, the nature of the factors causing this epidemic is such that the search for effective solutions must focus on specific drivers as they exist and operate within countries, regions, and localities.

The purpose of this report, developed by the Institute of Medicine's (IOM's) Committee on Accelerating Progress in Obesity Prevention, is to chart the pathways to a timely resolution of the obesity epidemic in the U.S. population. The committee was tasked with formulating a coherent set of recommendations that, if implemented, would be likely to *significantly accelerate progress toward preventing obesity over the next decade,* taking advantage, where possible, of favorable emerging developments. The committee was tasked further with recommending tangible, practical indicators with which to measure progress toward this goal. Specifically, the committee's charge was to review prior obesity-related recommendations; consider relevant information on progress toward their implementation; develop principles to guide the selection of recommendations fundamental to achieving progress in obesity prevention; and recommend potential indicators that can act as markers of progress and can be readily evaluated through the use of current databases and/or relatively simple measures or surveys. This report responds to the challenges of this charge. The audience for the report includes public policy makers at all levels; private-sector decision makers; leaders in other institutions, including foundations, the education system, and professional and community-based organizations and health agencies; and the public in general.

This chapter sets the stage by articulating the committee's vision for success (Box 1-1) and introducing concepts of a systems perspective and of engagement and leadership as essential elements for achieving this vision. A clear vision is essential to guard against thinking about obesity prevention in isolation from the complex social and economic systems within which the determinants of obesity—physical activity and eating patterns—are embedded. The committee's vision imagines what society would look like if obesity prevention were achieved effectively, equitably, and sustainably. It allows for the identification of socially desirable pathways for change and indicators for assessing whether initiatives undertaken are on the right track before their longer-term effects can be fully evaluated. Inherent in the committee's vision is the belief that children and adults should be able to satisfy their needs, be productive, and lead high-quality lives. Another critical common value expressed in the committee's development of this vision is the need for safeguards to ensure equity so that children and adults in communities affected by social and economic disparities have opportunities to achieve a healthy weight in the environments where they live, learn, work, and play.

The underlying logic of the committee's vision is illustrated in Figure 1-1. Favorable environments and behavioral settings positively influence individual, family, and population expectations, norms, and behaviors related to physical activity and healthy eating. Outcomes for individuals and society reflect decreased obesity rates with commensurate improvements in the health and societal outcomes highlighted in Chapter 2. Strategies and actions that drive overall environments in a health-promoting direction will be at the core of efforts to accelerate progress in preventing obesity. The cross-cutting factors listed at the bottom of the figure are a reminder that particular strategies and actions will affect individuals and populations differently depending on their circumstances, resources, and outlooks (IOM, 2007).

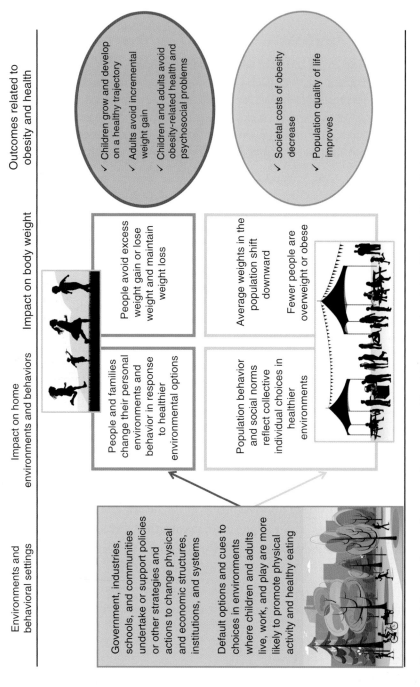

Environments and behavioral settings

Government, industries, schools, and communities undertake or support policies or other strategies and actions to change physical and economic structures, institutions, and systems

Default options and cues to choices in environments where children and adults live, work, and play are more likely to promote physical activity and healthy eating

Impact on home environments and behaviors

People and families change their personal environments and behavior in response to healthier environmental options

Population behavior and social norms reflect collective individual choices in healthier environments

Impact on body weight

People avoid excess weight gain or lose weight and maintain weight loss

Average weights in the population shift downward

Fewer people are overweight or obese

Outcomes related to obesity and health

✓ Children grow and develop on a healthy trajectory
✓ Adults avoid incremental weight gain
✓ Children and adults avoid obesity-related health and psychosocial problems

✓ Societal costs of obesity decrease
✓ Population quality of life improves

Race/ethnicity; gender; socioeconomic status; residential area; and social, political, and historical contexts that influence the baseline, opportunities, and responses to changes in environments for physical activity and eating.

FIGURE 1-1 The logic of populationwide obesity prevention.

A SYSTEMS PERSPECTIVE

Several IOM reports and other prior analyses of potential solutions to the obesity epidemic, relevant both to the United States and globally, have established the inherent complexity of the problem (IOM, 2010). An impressive body of evidence confirms that the drivers of the epidemic involve interactions among several complex, ever-changing systems, including the food system, transportation systems, community infrastructure, school systems, health care systems, and the intricate behavioral and physiological systems that influence individual physical activity and eating behaviors and body weight. Reflecting this complexity, a prior IOM report calls for taking a systems approach to obesity prevention (IOM, 2010). Specifically, that report explains how a systems approach is an evolution of and expansion upon strategies already proposed or currently in use to prevent obesity. It is an approach that focuses on the whole picture and not just a single element, awareness of the wider context of any action, and an appreciation for interactions among different components of the problem. Further details on how the current committee took a systems approach can be found in Chapter 4 and Appendix B.

Building a society of healthy children, families, and communities will require coordinated change at multiple levels—from individuals, to families, to communities, to society as a whole. Pathways for change to curb and then reverse the epidemic of obesity involve core elements of the social fabric. The current environments in which eating and physical activity take place are the cumulative result of decisions that have been made over several decades, in numerous societal sectors. Many of those decisions have led—often inadvertently—to environments that run counter to the achievement or maintenance of healthy weight (Huang and Glass, 2008; Popkin et al., 2005). Americans have adjusted to these current ways of life and may strongly value many of the conveniences and pleasures they afford. Approaches that are inconsistent with fundamental values and principles will be undesirable and, ultimately, untenable.

Many initiatives needed for success in obesity prevention must occur through changes in societal sectors or institutions that influence health, including ones that are beyond the traditional health sector. Strategies must be carefully crafted to ensure that they will align with the goals and processes of these other sectors. Acceleration of obesity prevention will require reaching and engaging with multiple stakeholder groups. This need for action across a broad spectrum of society, together with the evolution of the problem over several decades, suggests that some time will be needed before solutions can be put in place and show effects.

The committee's focus was on how the process of change that is needed—and is in many respects already under way—can be accelerated.

Two other elements are crucial for successful implementation of the committee's recommendations to accelerate progress in obesity prevention utilizing a systems perspective: (1) the engagement of individuals, families, communities, and society and (2) the identification of leaders who can mobilize the changes needed while reducing disparities in the risk for obesity.

LEVELS OF ENGAGEMENT TO MOBILIZE CHANGE

The concept of "engagement" conveys the importance of collaborative approaches, "working with and through groups of people affiliated by geographic proximity, special interest, or similar situations" (CDC, 1997, p. 9)—that is, involving those affected by issues to address the issues that affect them. As described in this section, engagement is required at all levels of the population and across levels—individuals, families, communities, and the larger society—in order to build capacity, accelerate progress in obesity prevention, and reduce disparities in resources to ensure equity of impact in relation to the risk of obesity. The levels are interdependent, and all are necessary to achieve impact. Although its deliberations focused on strategies at the community and societal levels (see Chapter 3 for more detail), the committee recognizes the interdependence of these broader levels with the engagement of individuals and families. Every level of the population must play an active role in the system. Their engagement, as detailed below, could motivate a successful social movement for positive change.

Societal-Level Engagement

Prevention of obesity at the societal level requires supports for child health and development, including food, education, and family life. The health of the public is ultimately a collective responsibility, and the fear of engendering political opposition through bold and widespread action can stand in the way of positive change in the nation's current physical activity, food, and other environments that influence individual behavior and choice. Awareness, will, and action on the part of the public and the business community/private sector, as well as government at all levels, must increase if the necessary changes are to occur.

Population behavior is influenced by several societal subsystems, including the economy, the political system, social institutions, and culture (de Silva-Sanigorski and Economos, 2010). To influence behavior on a broad societal level, multiple subsystems must be targeted, and communities can be seen as important social forces in the process of change. As the broader society develops strategies to tackle the obesity epidemic, it will be able to draw on lessons learned from a range of successful social change efforts, such as those designed to increase breastfeeding rates, seat belt use, smoking cessation, and recycling (Economos et al., 2001). As described by de Silva-Sanigorski and Economos (2010, pp. 57-58) "key elements identified from these past successes include

- recognition that there was a crisis;
- major economic implications associated with the crisis;
- a science base including research, data, and evidence;
- sparkplugs, or leaders who can work for their cause through their knowledge, competence, talents, skills, and even charisma;
- coalitions to move the agenda forward and a strategic, integrated media advocacy campaign;
- involvement of the government at the state level to apply regulatory and fiscal authority, and at the local level to implement change;
- mass communication that includes consistent positive messages supported by scientific consensus and repeated in a variety of venues;
- policy and environmental changes that promote healthy lifestyle behaviors; and
- a plan that includes many components which work synergistically."

Community-Level Engagement

Community engagement is a powerful vehicle for bringing about environmental and behavioral changes that will improve the health of the community and its members. It often involves partnerships and coalitions that help mobilize resources and influence systems, change relationships among partners, and serve as catalysts for changing policies, programs, and practices (CDC, 1997). As described later in this report, the recognition of social, cultural, and environmental factors influencing obesity has motivated a shift to community-level strategies for health promotion, with the understanding that change at this level will encourage and sustain individual-level behavior change. There is no consistent definition of a "community"; however, experience suggests that it may be defined as "a group of people sharing a common goal, interest, or identity—for example, culture, social, political, health, economic interests or a particular geographic association" (Bell et al., 2010, p. 233). Within the field of community health, this broad definition gives way to two subclassifications of community: "communities of identity" (shared ethnicity, religion, illness) and "communities of location" (towns, cities, distinct neighborhoods) (Campbell and Murray, 2004; Israel et al., 2003).

Geographically defined communities hold diverse resources, ranging from the institutional (including worksites, places of worship, schools, and service and information providers), to the interpersonal (including peer networks, coalitions, and task forces), to community leaders and policy makers. Communities have their own history, social norms, traditions, and knowledge. These assets contribute points of leverage and resistance, intersections that spark strongly positive or negative reactions. Community-based interventions aim to apply community assets purposefully and efficiently to address an issue the community would like to resolve (Issel, 2009). Communities differ in their readiness or pre-existing capacity to address a given issue, such as obesity prevention, and those seeking to catalyze change in a community must employ different strategies for different readiness levels.

Community coalitions can be developed and supported to encourage the deep and meaningful engagement and organization of community members to realize systemic change at the local level (National Opinion Research Center, 2011). When people create or are involved in developing programs or policies, they value them more (Huang and Story, 2010). The formation of local, community-based coalitions can improve the reach and rate of information exchange nationally or at the societal level (Butterfoss et al., 1993).

Family/Household- and Individual-Level Engagement

The need for a major emphasis on change at the societal and community levels stems from the fact that many determinants of both voluntary and routine eating and physical activity behaviors are outside of the direct control of individuals and families. However, the ultimate success of changes at these levels depends on the extent to which the changes reach and are adopted and sustained by individuals and families. As described by Finegood (2011, p. 228), "given the heterogeneous nature of individuals and their environments, it is impossible to take individuals out of the solution equation." This suggests it is important to consider the relationship between individuals/families and their environment to find effective solutions to obesity (Brownell et al., 2010). Engagement with individuals is foundational for achieving broad social action on obesity prevention in many ways. Children and adults, particularly caregivers, make decisions about their own physical activity and eating behaviors on a daily basis; they may also make decisions that affect other people's physical activity and food choices and environments, have responsibility for organizing the context in which people make such decisions (Finegood et al., 2010; Thaler and Sunstein, 2009), and take civic actions that influence policy makers. If individuals are engaged in the effort to accelerate obesity prevention, success is more likely to be achieved (Bar-Yam, 2004).

Building the awareness and will within households to influence the home environment and family dynamics positively with respect to physical activity and food choices is an essential part of changing the overall system. The reasons to foster will and action within households across the United States are especially clear in relation to prevention of obesity in children. Children learn to assimilate their parents' health-related behaviors at a young age (Perryman, 2011). Furthermore, parents act as decision makers for their children in the areas of physical activity and nutrition. An estimated 66 percent of the caloric intake of children and adolescents occurs within the home (Poti and Popkin, 2011). Parents also serve as role models for their children, helping to shape physical activity values and behaviors, providing a sense of portion control and nutrient balance, and building related skills. For example, limiting children's television time, using parental controls, and disallowing television in the bedroom can help reduce exposure to the marketing of unhealthy food products and reduce sedentary behavior.

Society benefits if all families have the social and material resources to raise their children to be healthy, educated, and productive members of their communities and nation. A healthy home environment can begin before conception with strong maternal nutrition, supported by other family members (IOM, 2005). It can prevent rapid early infant weight gain from ages 0 to 4 months, which has been shown to be a risk factor for childhood obesity (Birch and Davison, 2001; Stettler et al., 2003). And a healthy home environment can reach parents, grandparents, and extended family members, supporting a life-course perspective on obesity prevention.

The skill base for healthy living has eroded, however, and many people need support on parenting, cooking, and media use (Golan and Crow, 2004). Moreover, the resources available to parents to meet their children's needs vary considerably. While the value of creating the optimal healthy environment for children is clear, society has largely left this responsibility to individual families, even though the financial or political resources to affect changes in major corporate interests, government programs, or policy generally are not available to individuals or individual families (Prilleltensky, 2010). For families to be able to raise healthy, well-educated children, communities and societal structures must assist in providing access to opportunities for physical activity, healthy food, and adequate health care and other social services that support health (Scarr, 1996).

Reducing Disparities: Equity of Impact in Relation to Risk

Not all individuals, families, and communities are similarly situated with respect to environments that influence food and physical activity. A variety of characteristics historically linked to social exclusion or discrimination, such as race or ethnicity, religion, socioeconomic status, gender, age, mental health, disability, sexual orientation or gender identity, geographic location, and immigration status, are known to influence health status. In its 2011 *Action Plan to Reduce Racial and Ethnic Health Disparities,* the Department of Health and Human Services (HHS) highlights that health disparities "are closely linked with social, economic, and environmental disadvantage" and "are often driven by the social conditions in which individuals live, learn, work and play" (HHS, 2011, p. 1).

As described in Chapter 2, the burden of obesity is notably greater in racial/ethnic minority and low-income populations. A high level of community engagement and carefully targeted approaches will be particularly important to accelerate obesity prevention in such communities. In many parts of the United States, racial/ethnic minority and low-income individuals and families live, learn, work, and play in neighborhoods that lack sufficient health-protective resources, such as parks and open space, grocery stores, walkable streets, and high-quality schools (Adler et al., 2007; Iton et al., 2008). Additionally, community-level risk factors, including freeways, incinerators, ports, heavy industry, and other sources of noxious pollution, often are concentrated in these same places (Adler et al., 2007). This relative absence of health-promoting resources and disproportionate concentration of unhealthy risk factors contributes to increased levels of chronic stress among individuals experiencing these conditions (Iton et al., 2008), and this chronic stress is in turn associated with increased levels of sedentary activity and increased calorie consumption (Adler et al., 2007).

The persistence of concentrated health disparities in many American communities is strongly influenced by the relative paucity of community-based health improvement strategies focused on creating robust local participatory decision-making processes. In any given community, the relative mix of these community-level resources and risk factors is determined primarily through democratic local and regional land use decision-making processes; consequently, organized participation in these processes influences where these community resources and risks are located. Because of such factors as poverty, language barriers, and immigration status, low-income, minority, and other disadvantaged population groups often are underrepresented and their concerns marginalized in these land use decision-making processes (Iton et al., 2008). These groups are therefore less likely to benefit from access to health-protective resources and more likely to live in proximity to noxious land uses. To change this inequitable resource and risk distribution, robust and long-term community engagement and civic participation among these disadvantaged populations must occur.

LEADERSHIP

Responsibility for leading efforts to make the changes needed to prevent obesity potentially rests with everyone that can influence physical activity and food environments. There are obvious leaders that have traditionally been seen as having the responsibility for making environmental and policy changes to influence societal change, but the engagement of all individuals, families, communities, and society, as described in the previous section, may identify another set of willing and capable leaders whose actions will be necessary to achieve impact. Chapter 10 further details how taking a systems perspective helps define and identify leaders and how these leaders should approach implementing the necessary changes.

THE ISSUE OF RESPONSIBILITY

The committee's vision, its decision to take a systems perspective, and its belief in the need for engagement and leadership at multiple levels and across multiple sectors help inform the issue of who is responsible for addressing the epidemic of obesity. Traditionally, obesity has been blamed on the failure of individuals to exercise personal responsibility (Brownell et al., 2010; Leichter, 2003). In addition, this view has been used as the basis for resisting government efforts—legislative and regulatory—to address the problem. Recently, the discourse has been reframed by Brownell and colleagues (2010) as a constructive approach to a controversial issue. They assert that "personal responsibility can be embraced as a value" (p. 378) by expanding its meaning to include such actions as improved school nutrition, menu labeling, changes in industry marketing practices, and even such controversial measures as taxes on foods and beverages that lead to the choice of healthier items. Such an approach could bridge the divide between views based on individual versus collective responsibility (Brownell et al., 2010). This train of thought argues for making obesity prevention a political priority that reestablishes the responsibility of the country—both the public and private sectors—to nurture and protect children, and to support the health priorities of the adults and families who influence them and make the decisions that determine the overall physical activity and food environments.

The committee's recommendations (outlined in Chapters 5-9) have the potential to accelerate progress in obesity prevention by identifying changes that are needed across all levels and sectors of society, but it is also important to view them as a whole—an interrelated system of critical areas in which changes are needed. The responsibility for implementing these changes is one that must be shared. Engagement and leadership across all levels and sectors of the population will be powerful vehicles for bringing about environmental and behavioral changes that can improve the health of the population.

OVERVIEW OF THE REPORT

The next two chapters provide background on and fundamentals of the problem of obesity, including an assessment of the current problem and how, in general, the problem is addressed at a population level. Chapter 2 describes the consequences of obesity; reviews current trends of overweight and obesity and societal trends that are drivers of excess weight gain at a population level; and outlines advances in and barriers to implementing environmental and policy changes that can help accelerate progress in obesity prevention. Chapter 3 describes the logic of obesity prevention, including goals and key pathways and targets for change, and explains the importance of taking a systems perspective on the problem. Chapters 2 and 3 are particularly geared toward audiences unfamiliar with the current situation regarding obesity and obesity prevention approaches from a societal perspective, but they also highlight several current issues that required the committee's careful consideration in determining which strategies and actions to recommend. Chapter 4 then presents the methodology used by the committee in developing its recommendations. This chapter explains how the committee defined the concept of accelerating progress in obesity prevention in order to screen and evaluate the numerous interventions recommended in prior reports and to enhance or choose among these interventions, and highlights the importance of viewing the committee's recommendations as an interrelated, synergistic system.

The remainder of the report presents the committee's recommendations for accelerating progress in obesity prevention. The committee identified five critical action arenas—environments for change—for making progress in obesity prevention. Chapters 5 through 9 present recommendations under five respective goals, together with specific strategies, actions, and outcome indicators, in relation to these five environments: environments for physical activity (Chapter 5); food and beverage environments (Chapter 6); message environments with respect to physical activity and healthy eating (Chapter 7); health care and work environments (Chapter 8); and school environments (Chapter 9). Chapter 10 concludes the report by addressing leadership and implementation, prioritization, and assessment of the committee's recommendations in the context of a systems perspective.

REFERENCES

Adler, N. E., J. Stewart, S. Cohen, M. Cullen, A. Diez Roux, W. Dow, G. Evans, I. Kawachi, M. Marmot, K. Matthews, B. McEwen, J. Schwartz, T. Seeman, and D. Williams. 2007. *Reaching for a healthier life: Facts on socioeconomic status and health in the US*. San Francisco, CA: The John D. and Catherine T. MacArthur Foundation Research Network on Socioeconomic Status and Health.

Bar-Yam, Y. 2004. *Making things work: Solving complex problems in a complex world*, edited by C. Ramalingam, L. Burlingame, and C. Ogata. Cambridge, MA: NECSI-Knowledge Press.

Bell, C., E. Elliott, and A. Simmons. 2010. Community capacity building. In *Preventing childhood obesity. Evidence policy and practice*, edited by E. Waters, J. C. Seidell, B. A. Swinburn, and R. Uauy. Hoboken, NJ: Wiley-Blackwell. Pp. 232-242.

Birch, L. L., and K. K. Davison. 2001. Family environmental factors influencing the developing behavioral controls of food intake and childhood overweight. *Pediatric Clinics of North America* 48(4):893-907.

Brownell, K. D., R. Kersh, D. S. Ludwig, R. C. Post, R. M. Puhl, M. B. Schwartz, and W. C. Willett. 2010. Personal responsibility and obesity: A constructive approach to a controversial issue. *Health Affairs* 29(3):379-387.

Butterfoss, F. D., R. M. Goodman, and A. Wandersman. 1993. Community coalitions for prevention and health promotion. *Health Education Research* 8(3):315-330.

Campbell, C., and M. Murray. 2004. Community health psychology: Promoting analysis and action for social change. *Journal of Health Psychology* 9(2):187-195.

CDC (Centers for Disease Control and Prevention). 1997. *Principles of community engagement*. Atlanta, GA: CDC/ATSDR Committee on Community Engagement.

de Onis, M., M. Blossner, and E. Borghi. 2010. Global prevalence and trends of overweight and obesity among preschool children. *American Journal of Clinical Nutrition* 92(5):1257-1264.

de Silva-Sanigorski, A. M., and C. Economos. 2010. Evidence of multi-setting approaches for obesity prevention: Translation to best practice. In *Preventing childhood obesity: Evidence, policy, and practice*, edited by E. Waters, J. C. Seidell, B. A. Swinburn, and R. Uauy. Hoboken, NJ: Wiley-Blackwell. Pp. 57-63.

Economos, C. D., R. C. Brownson, M. A. DeAngelis, P. Novelli, S. B. Foerster, C. T. Foreman, J. Gregson, S. K. Kumanyika, and R. R. Pate. 2001. What lessons have been learned from other attempts to guide social change? *Nutrition Reviews* 59(3 Pt. 2):S40-S56; discussion S57-S65.

Finegood, D. T. 2011. The complex systems science of obesity. In *The Oxford handbook of the social science of obesity*, edited by J. H. Cawley. New York: Oxford University Press. Pp. 208-236.

Finegood, D. T., T. D. N. Merth, and H. Rutter. 2010. Implications of the foresight obesity system map for solutions to childhood obesity. *Obesity* 18(Suppl. 1):S13-S16.

Finucane, M. M., G. A. Stevens, M. J. Cowan, G. Danaei, J. K. Lin, C. J. Paciorek, G. M. Singh, H. R. Gutierrez, Y. Lu, A. N. Bahalim, F. Farzadfar, L. M. Riley, and M. Ezzati. 2011. National, regional, and global trends in body-mass index since 1980: Systematic analysis of health examination surveys and epidemiological studies with 960 country-years and 9.1 million participants. *Lancet* 377(9765):557-567.

Flegal, K. M., M. D. Carroll, C. L. Ogden, and L. R. Curtin. 2010. Prevalence and trends in obesity among US adults, 1999-2008. *Journal of the American Medical Association* 303(3):235-241.

Golan, M., and S. Crow. 2004. Parents are key players in the prevention and treatment of weight-related problems. *Nutrition Reviews* 62(1):39-50.

HHS (U.S. Department of Health and Human Services). 2011. *Action plan to reduce racial and ethnic health disparities.* http://minorityhealth.hhs.gov/npa/files/Plans/HHS/HHS_Plan_complete.pdf (accessed October 25, 2011).

Huang, T. T., and T. A. Glass. 2008. Transforming research strategies for understanding and preventing obesity. *Journal of the American Medical Association* 300(15):1811-1813.

Huang, T. T. K., and M. T. Story. 2010. A journey just started: Renewing efforts to address childhood obesity. *Obesity* 18(Suppl. 1):S1-S3.

IOM (Institute of Medicine). 2005. *Preventing childhood obesity: Health in the balance.* Washington, DC: The National Academies Press.

IOM. 2007. *Progress in preventing childhood obesity: How do we measure up?* Washington, DC: The National Academies Press.

IOM. 2010. *Bridging the evidence gap in obesity prevention: A framework to inform decision making.* Washington, DC: The National Academies Press.

Israel, B. A., A. J. Schulz, E. A. Parker, A. B. Becker, A. J. I. Allen, and J. R. Guzman. 2003. Critical issues in developing and following community based participatory research principles. In *Community-based participatory research for health*, edited by M. Minkler and N. Wallerstein. San Francisco, CA: John Wiley & Sons. Pp. 53-76.

Issel, L. M. 2009. *Health program planning and evaluation. A practical, systematic approach for community health.* 2nd ed. Boston, MA: Jones and Bartlett Publishers.

Iton, T., S. Witt, and D. Kears. 2008. *Life and death from unnatural causes. Health and social inequity in Alameda County.* Oakland, CA: Alameda County Public Health Department.

Leichter, H. M. 2003. "Evil habits" and "personal choices": Assigning responsibility for health in the 20th century. *Milbank Quarterly* 81(4):603-626.

National Opinion Research Center. 2011. *Developing a conceptual framework to assess the sustainability of community coalitions post-federal funding.* http://aspe.hhs.gov/health/reports/2010/sustainlit/report.shtml (accessed November 17, 2011).

Ogden, C. L., M. D. Carroll, L. R. Curtin, M. M. Lamb, and K. M. Flegal. 2010a. Prevalence of high body mass index in US children and adolescents, 2007-2008. *Journal of the American Medical Association* 303(3):242-249.

Ogden, C. L., M. M. Lamb, M. D. Carroll, and K. M. Flegal. 2010b. Obesity and socioeconomic status in children and adolescents: United States, 2005-2008. *NCHS Data Brief* (51):1-8.

Ogden, C. L., M. M. Lamb, M. D. Carroll, and K. M. Flegal. 2010c. Obesity and socio-economic status in adults: United States, 2005-2008. *NCHS Data Brief* (50):1-8.

Perryman, M. L. 2011. Ethical family interventions for childhood obesity. *Preventing Chronic Disease* 8(5):A99.

Popkin, B. M., K. Duffey, and P. Gordon-Larsen. 2005. Environmental influences on food choice, physical activity and energy balance. *Physiology and Behavior* 86(5):603-613.

Poti, J. M., and B. M. Popkin. 2011. Trends in energy intake among US children by eating location and food source, 1977-2006. *Journal of the American Dietetic Association* 111(8):1156-1164.

Prilleltensky, I. 2010. Child wellness and social inclusion: Values for action. *American Journal of Community Psychology* 46(1-2):238-249.

Scarr, S. 1996. How people make their own environments: Implications for parents and policymakers. *Psychology, Public Policy, and Law* 2(2):204-228.

Stettler, N., S. K. Kumanyika, S. H. Katz, B. S. Zemel, and V.A. Stallings. 2003. Rapid weight gain during infancy and obesity in young adulthood in a cohort of African Americans. *American Journal of Clinical Nutrition* 77:1374-1378.

Thaler, R. H., and C. R. Sunstein. 2009. *Nudge: Improving decisions about health, wealth and happiness.* New York: Penguin Books.

2

Assessing the Current Situation

Key Messages

- Populationwide obesity has serious health, economic, and social consequences for individuals and for society at large.

- Almost one-third of children and two-thirds of adults in the United States are overweight or obese.

- Although the vast majority of people who are obese are not poor or racial/ethnic minorities, the percentage of people within poor and ethnic minority populations who are affected by obesity is relatively higher, sometimes markedly so, for one or both sexes compared with the nonpoor or whites. Particular attention to these high-risk groups is essential in obesity prevention efforts.

- Causes of the high rates of obesity can be traced to trends in environmental influences on physical activity and food intake.

- Important advances have occurred in national guidance, policy, research directions, and partnership initiatives, as well as consensus on the need for a broad, prevention-oriented approach to the obesity epidemic. However, direct opposition to some potential obesity prevention strategies impedes their acceptance and implementation.

- Evidence that levels of obesity may be stabilizing may be an important sign that these advances are having a positive effect. However, complex realities associated with the obesity epidemic give rise to several considerations—including some that can serve as major roadblocks—that must be addressed when measures are taken to accelerate preventive efforts.

The process of developing strategies to accelerate obesity prevention begins with a situation assessment. This chapter provides such an assessment by presenting data on the consequences the nation faces if the epidemic persists; the starting point for acceleration of preventive efforts with respect to obesity prevalence in the general population and in populations at particularly high risk; contributory trends related to physical activity, food intake, and media use and other factors relevant to sedentary behavior; and positive steps that have already been taken and have momentum, along with the roadblocks that could limit further advances. The nature of change trajectories needed to track progress toward the goal of seeing obesity levels decline is also discussed.

HUMAN AND SOCIETAL CONSEQUENCES OF THE OBESITY EPIDEMIC

The consequences of today's high rates of obesity have two broad dimensions. The first is the direct and sometimes devastating health and social consequences to individuals—the potential for illness or disability, social ostracism, discrimination, depression, and poor quality of life. The second dimension encompasses the indirect effects of obesity on society, reflected in population fitness, health care costs, and other aspects of the economy.

Human Costs

As shown in Table 2-1, obesity is associated with major causes of death and disability, as well as with psychosocial consequences that impair functioning and quality of life. The effect of obesity in predisposing to the development of type 2 diabetes is particularly strong, so much so that the onset of this disease—formerly observed only in adults—also now occurs during childhood (CDC, 2011). Adverse effects are observed throughout the life course and may be transmitted from mother to child through the characteristics of the gestational environment (IOM, 2009). According to current estimates, one-third of all children born today (and one-half of Latino and black children) will develop type 2 diabetes in their lifetime (Narayan et al., 2003). One dire projection is that obesity may lead to a generation with a shorter life span than that of their parents (American Heart Association, 2010; Olshansky et al., 2005).

The highest prevalence of obesity-related conditions occurs in middle-aged and older adults, with direct effects on quality of life and on rates of disease, disability, and death at an early age. High blood pressure is the most prevalent of these con-

TABLE 2-1 Physical Health, Psychosocial, and Functional Consequences of Obesity Over the Life Course

Physical Health	Psychosocial	Functional
• Cardiovascular disease	• Stigma	• Unemployment
• Cancer	• Negative stereotyping	• Mobility limitations
• Glucose intolerance and insulin resistance	• Discrimination	• Disability
	• Teasing and bullying	• Low physical fitness
• Type 2 diabetes	• Social marginalization	• Absenteeism from school or work
• Hypertension	• Low self-esteem	
• Dyslipidemia	• Negative body image	• Disqualification from active service in the military and fire/police services
• Hepatic steatosis	• Depression	
• Choleslitasis		
• Sleep apnea		• Reduced productivity
• Reduction of cerebral blood flow		• Reduced academic performance
• Menstrual abnormalities		
• Orthopedic problems		
• Gallbladder disease		
• Hyperuricemia and gout		

SOURCE: Adapted from IOM, 2010a.

ditions, and is a major risk factor for cardiovascular diseases. High blood pressure affects a third of U.S. adults aged 20 and over and more than half of adults aged 55 and older. Together high blood pressure, coronary heart disease, heart failure, and stroke affect 37 to 39 percent of women and men aged 40 to 59 and 72 to 73 percent of women and men aged 60 to 79. Eight percent of adults have a diagnosis of type 2 diabetes, another 3 percent are undiagnosed, and an additional 37 percent have prediabetes (Roger et al., 2011). Both high blood pressure and diabetes (diagnosed and undiagnosed) increased between 1988-1994 and 2005-2008 at the same time that increases in obesity were observed (see below). And a growing literature suggests various types of reductions in brain structural integrity (due to low blood flow to the brain) among both obese adolescents and adults (Gunstad et al., 2006; Maayan et al., 2011; Willeumier et al., 2011). In addition to these physical risks, obese adults face discrimination in employment settings and are subjected to inappropriate slurs and humor (Puhl and Heuer, 2001; Wear et al., 2006).

Obese children and adolescents also suffer an array of obesity-related comorbidities, ranging from sleep apnea, to type 2 diabetes, to hypertension, to liver disease, to orthopedic problems. These conditions over time may contribute to shorter lifespans for obese children and adolescents. Poor health-related quality of life—physical, psychosocial, emotional, social, and school functioning—is 5.5 times greater in obese children and adolescents than in their normal-weight peers (Schwimmer et al., 2003). Childhood obesity is a major contributor to chronic illness and accounts for increased use of medication and physician visits and associated loss of school time (Van Cleave et al., 2010). Data suggest that obese children and adolescents miss more school days than their normal-weight peers regardless of age, ethnicity, sex, and school attended (Geier et al., 2007). And overweight or obese children and adolescents in every grade experience poorer academic outcomes than their normal-weight peers (Taras and Potts-Datema, 2005).

Box 2-1 puts a human face on a day in the life of obese children and adolescents. A study of adolescents found that nearly 30 percent of girls and 25 percent of boys were teased by peers about their weight, and 29 percent of girls and 16 percent of boys were teased by family members (Eisenberg et al., 2003). Teasing about weight is associated with depression, low self-esteem and body satisfaction, and suicidal thoughts and attempts (Eisenberg et al., 2003). Obesity associates individuals with "different" negative stereotypes, which can encourage others to stigmatize them and discount their worth (Gray et al., 2011; Vander Wal and Mitchell, 2011; Williams et al., 2008).

Economic and Societal Costs

Economic and societal costs (see Table 2-2) are linked to the impact of the outcomes shown previously in Table 2-1 on health care costs and productivity. Many health care expenditures are both a direct and indirect result of the current epidemic of overweight and obesity (Wolf, 1998; Wolf and Colditz, 1998). Direct costs include preventive, diagnostic, and treatment services related to obesity; indirect costs are those associated with morbidity and mortality. The estimated annual cost of obesity-related illness based on data from the Medical Expenditure Panel Survey for 2000-2005 is $190 billion (in 2005 dollars), which represents 20.6 percent of annual health care spending in the United States (Cawley and Meyerhoefer, 2011). Childhood obesity alone is responsible for $14.1 billion in direct medical costs (Trasande and Chatterjee, 2009).

Recent studies have modeled the economic benefits of reducing obesity prevalence in the U.S. population. Obesity is the major modifiable risk factor for the development of diabetes and also increases the risk of developing hypertension. It is estimated that reducing the prevalence of diabetes and hypertension by 5 percent would save approximately $9 billion annually in the near term; with resulting

BOX 2-1
Childhood Days: Stories from Life*

For many children and adolescents who are overweight or obese, childhood is a gauntlet of disappointment, depression, and disease. For example:

- Mark and Kathy bring their 3-year-old child to a health clinic. Both parents are obese. They are adamant: "We do not want our child to go through what we did as children."

- Jonathan is 9 years old. He has sleep apnea, and must wear a heavy device on his face at night. This means he must take his "machine" for overnight visits with friends and relatives and try to explain why he is "different."

- Kelly is 10 years old. She is depressed and has suicidal thoughts. She reports, "The teasing starts on the bus to school, continues through the school day, and all the way home." She has changed schools, but the teasing has only started again.

- Tasha is an obese 15-year-old who loves soccer. She did well on the school team last year, but worries constantly that she won't make the team next fall because of her weight.

- Marco is 17 years old, with obesity and hypertension. Asked about his plans for the future, he responds with emotion, "I've always wanted to become a firefighter, but I know I won't be able to because of my weight."

Similar stories about the challenges of living with obesity as an adult would remind us of the day-to-day burdens of living with hypertension, diabetes, or knee pain; the trips to doctors' offices; and the costs and side effects of medication. Too often, the immediate response to life stories such as these can be, "Why don't they just lose weight?" Yet data show that contemporary culture, economics, and society pose many barriers to the types of healthy diets that prevent obesity from occurring and to the difficult tasks of losing excess weight and sustaining lower weight levels.

---

*The individuals described in these illustrative examples are real pediatric patients; names have been changed for confidentiality.

TABLE 2-2 The Key Costs Identified from Research on the Economic Impact of Obesity

Cost Category	Subcategories	Key Results, and Range of Estimates
Direct medical spending		Relative medical costs for overweight (vs. normal weight)
		Relative medical costs for obese (vs. normal weight)
		Annual direct costs of childhood obesity
		U.S.-wide annual cost of "excess" medical spending attributable to overweight/obesity
Productivity costs	Absenteeism	Excess days of work lost due to obesity
		Relative risk ratio of having "high absenteeism"
		National costs of annual absenteeism from obesity
	Presenteeism	National annual costs of presenteeism obesity
		Relative productivity loss due to obesity
	Disability	Relative risk ratio of receiving disability income support
	Premature mortality	Years of life lost due to obesity
		QALYs lost due to obesity
	Total	National annual indirect costs of obesity

Relative Costs	Total Costs	Total Nondollar Amounts
10-20% higher[a,b]		
36-100% higher[a-d]		
	$14.3 billion[e,f]	
	$86-147 billion (total)[c]	
	$640 billion (women 40-65 only)[g]	
		1.02-4.72 days[h-i]
1.24-1.53 times higher[j,k]		
	$3.38-6.38 billion, or $79-132 per obese person[j,l]	
	$57,000 per employee[l] (1998 USD)	
	$8 billion[m] (2002 USD)	
1.5% higher[j]		
5.64-6.92 percentage points higher[n]		
		1-13 years per obese person[o]
		2.93 million QALYs total in U.S. in 2004[p]
	$5 (1994 USD)-$66 billion[m,q]	

continued

TABLE 2-2 Continued

Cost Category	Subcategories	Key Results, and Range of Estimates
Transportation costs	Fuel costs	Annual excess jet fuel use attributable to obesity
		Annual excess fuel use by noncommercial passenger highway vehicles
		Additional fuel required in noncommercial passenger highway sector per lb of average passenger weight increase
	Environmental costs	OECD-wide CO_2 emissions from transportation per 5 kg average weight per person
Human capital accumulation costs		Highest grade completed
		Days absent from school

NOTES: OECD = Organisation for Economic Co-operation and Development; QALY = quality-adjusted life-years.

[a]Thompson et al., 1999; [b]Thompson et al., 2001; [c]Finkelstein et al., 2009; [d]Thorpe et al., 2004; [e]Cawley, 2010; [f]Trasande and Chatterjee, 2009; [g]Gorsky et al., 1996; [h]Pronk et al., 1999; [i]Tsai et al., 2008; [j]Trogdon et al., 2008; [k]Serxner et al., 2001; [l]Durden et al., 2008; [m]Ricci and Chee, 2005; [n]Burkhauser and Cawley, 2004; [o]Fontaine et al., 2003; [p]Groessl et al., 2004; [q]Thompson et al., 1998; [r]Dannenberg et al., 2004; [s]Jacobson and King, 2009; [t]Jacobson and McLay, 2006; [u]Michaelowa and Dransfield, 2008; [v]Gortmaker et al., 1993; [w]Kaestner et al., 2009; [x]Geier et al., 2007.

SOURCE: Reprinted with permission from *Diabetes, Metabolic Syndrome and Obesity: Targets and Therapy*, volume 3, Hammond, R. A., and R. Levine, The economic impact of obesity in the United States, pages 285-295, Copyright 2010, with permission from Dove Medical Press Ltd.

reductions in comorbidities and related conditions, savings could rise to approximately $24.7 billion annually in the medium term (Ormond et al., 2011).

Many of these obesity-related health care costs are paid with public dollars. For example, it is estimated that total Medicare and Medicaid spending would be 8.5 percent and 11.8 percent lower, respectively, in the absence of obesity (Finklestein et al., 2009). Moreover, these health care costs are expected to rise significantly, since today's increased rates of childhood obesity predict further increases in adult obesity and concomitant increases in hypertension, stroke, dyslipidemia, cancers (endometrial, breast, and colon), osteoarthritis, sleep apnea, liver and gall bladder disease, respiratory problems, and type 2 diabetes.

Relative Costs	Total Costs	Total Nondollar Amounts
	$742 million (2010 USD)	350 million gallons[r]
	$2.53-2.7 billion (2010 USD)	938 million-1 billion gallons[s,t]
	$105 million per lb (2010 USD)	39 million gallons[t]
		10 million tons[u]
0.1-0.3 fewer grades completed[v,w]		
1.2-2.1 more days absent from school[x]		

The U.S. economy struggles today to cope with health care spending; this struggle will grow progressively more difficult as today's obese children mature. Beyond growing medical costs attributed to obesity, the nation will incur higher costs for disability and unemployment benefits. Businesses currently suffer because of obesity-related job absenteeism ($4.3 billion annually) (Cawley et al., 2007); these costs also will continue to grow. Societal expenses add to the effects of the reduced standard of living and quality of life experienced by affected individuals and their families.

Obesity has economic implications even in the absence of health detriments. For example, employers are less likely to hire obese than normal-weight individuals with the same qualifications; when hired, obese individuals are likely to report being paid lower wages and suffering other additional discrimination (Giel et al., 2010; Han et al., 2011). The result is underutilization of available skills at a cost to both society and individuals. The economic repercussions of discrimination affect families as well. Because decreased fitness in obese people may lead to increased health problems (IOM, 2010a) and reduced household income (Cawley, 2004; Puhl and Brownell, 2001), the additional struggles due to loss of health and income may in turn lead to an erosion of family cohesiveness and strength. Rising rates of obesity also affect national security; U.S. military leaders have recently described the role of obesity in reducing the pool of potential recruits to the armed services (Christeson et al., 2010).

These human and societal consequences clearly justify action. Agreement is now widespread that priority should be given to population-oriented preventive approaches that can curb the development or exacerbation of excess weight gain and obesity rather than to individual case finding and treatment. This applies not only to children and adolescents, so that lifelong prevention can begin as early as possible, but also to adults, among whom the health burdens of obesity are greatest. Even without further growth in current levels of overweight and obesity, future burdens of obesity-related illness, poor health, and quality of life will continue to grow significantly, as will the financial costs of health care for families, employers, health care institutions, and the public.

OBESITY PREVALENCE AND TRENDS

The United States continues to experience an epidemic of overweight and obesity that compels timely and effective action. Although obesity is not a new problem, the percentage of people affected was relatively stable until the 1980s, when it began to rise (NCHS, 2010). By adulthood, the prevalence of obesity is approximately twice that observed during childhood, reflecting both the tracking of child and adolescent obesity into adult years and the new onset of obesity as many adults experience gradual, progressive weight gain in their 20s, 30s, and 40s. Currently, a majority of U.S. adults and a substantial proportion of children and adolescents have weight levels in the overweight or obese range.

Definitions of Overweight and Obesity

Definitions of overweight and obesity for children, adolescents, and adults are provided in Box 2-2. According to these definitions, two-thirds of adult

Adults

Overweight is defined as a body mass index (BMI) (a ratio of weight in kilograms to the square of height in meters) of 25-29.9. Adults with a BMI of 30 or greater are considered obese. Among those who are obese, the increasing health risks at higher levels of weight are sometimes indicated by further classification into grades of increasing severity: grade 1 obesity is defined as a BMI of 30 to 34.9, grade 2 is a BMI of 35.0 to 39.9, and grade 3 is a BMI of 40 or greater.

Children and Adolescents

Overweight and obesity are defined by cutoffs on sex- and age-specific Centers for Disease Control and Prevention (CDC) BMI reference curves to account for growth and maturation: overweight, including obesity, is defined as a BMI at or above the 85th percentile; obesity is defined as a BMI at or above the 95th percentile.

Americans are overweight or obese, and the proportion who are obese has more than doubled since 1976-1980, when it was 15 percent (NCHS, 2011). Even more stunning is the parallel phenomenon in adolescents aged 12 to 19, among whom the 5 percent obesity prevalence of 1976-1980 has now more than tripled (NCHS, 2011). Figure 2-1 shows the consistent proportion of men and women in the overweight range (reflecting fewer people in the healthy weight range) but continuing trends of increasing obesity during the most recent two decades. In men, the prevalence of obesity increased by 13 percentage points from 1988 to 2008—from 19 percent to 32 percent—and doubled (from 5 percent to 11 percent) within the grade 2 obesity category. In women, obesity prevalence increased by 10 percentage points during the same period—from 25 percent to 35 percent—with a 7 percentage point increase in the grade 2 obesity category (from 11 percent to 18 percent) (NCHS, 2011). Figure 2-2 shows the steady gradient of increasing obesity preva-

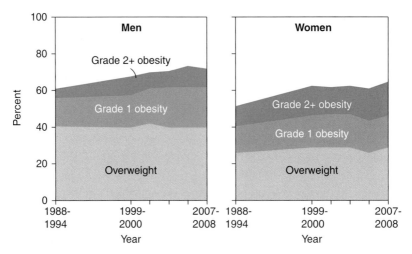

FIGURE 2-1 Overweight and obesity among adults aged 20 and over.
SOURCE: NCHS, 2011.

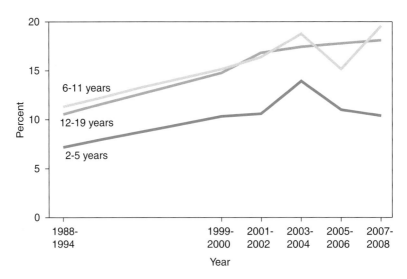

FIGURE 2-2 Obesity among U.S. children and adolescents by age, 1988-1994 through 2007-2008.
SOURCE: NCHS, 2011.

lence in children and adolescents in the 1990s—from 7 percent to 10 percent at ages 2 to 5, and from 11 percent to 15 percent at ages 6 to 11 and 12 to 19 (NCHS, 2011). Data for adults, children, and adolescents indicate flattening of trends in the most recent periods (Ogden et al., 2012).

The combined prevalence of overweight and obesity in children and adolescents aged 2 to 19 (i.e., at or above the 85th age-sex body mass index [BMI] percentile) in 2007-2008 was 32 percent for boys and 31 percent for girls (not shown in Figure 2-2) (Ogden et al., 2010a). Overweight and obesity affected 21 percent of both boys and girls aged 2 to 5 and 35 percent and 34 percent, respectively, of boys and girls aged 6 to 19 (Ogden et al., 2010a).

Data for the overall U.S. population do not reveal the particularly high obesity rates in some racial/ethnic minority populations and socioeconomic status groups. Adults, particularly women, children, and adolescents in the black and Mexican American populations, as well as people living below or near the poverty level, are at particularly high risk of obesity (Freedman, 2011). That is, although the vast majority of people who are obese are not minorities or poor, the percentage of people within racial/ethnic minority and poor populations who are affected by obesity is relatively higher, sometimes markedly so, for one or both sexes compared with whites or the nonpoor; higher obesity prevalence also is observed more in rural than in urban populations (Flegal et al., 2010; Liu et al., 2008; Ogden et al., 2010a,b,c; Patterson et al., 2004). In most cases, these demographic differences were observed before the obesity epidemic was evident in the general population, but obesity prevalence in these high-risk groups has tracked upward with increases in obesity affecting the population at large.

Figures 2-3 and 2-4 illustrate income-related differences in obesity prevalence in adults and children and adolescents, respectively, in the U.S. population overall and the increases in prevalence over time. The data are stratified by income categories using the poverty income ratio (PIR). The PIR adjusts income level for family size and farm-nonfarm income and expresses it as a ratio of the federal poverty threshold. It is used for determining eligibility for federal assistance programs such as the Supplemental Nutrition Assistance Program (SNAP, formerly known as the Food Stamp Program) and free or reduced-price school meals. For example, the cutoff for participation in SNAP is 130 percent of the PIR. Obesity is more prevalent in women and in children and adolescents of both sexes with incomes below 130 percent of the poverty level and least prevalent in those with incomes 350 percent or more above the poverty level (Ogden et al., 2010b,c). For example, obesity prevalence in 2005-2008 was 42 percent, 39 percent, and 29 percent in women in the low, middle, and high PIR categories, respectively (Ogden et al., 2010c). In children and adolescents (Figure 2-4), obesity prevalence in 2005-2008 was 21 percent versus 12 percent in boys in the low versus high PIR categories, and 19 percent versus 12 percent in girls in the low versus high PIR

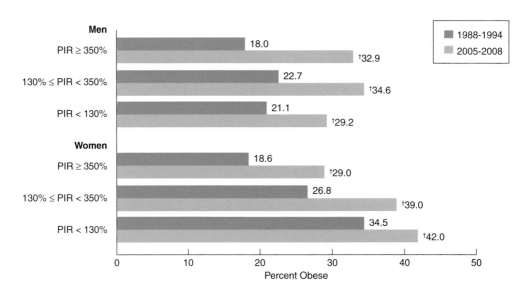

FIGURE 2-3 Prevalence of obesity among adults aged 20 and over by poverty income ratio and sex, United States, 1988-1994 to 2005-2008.

NOTES: PIR = poverty income ratio; † = significant increase.

SOURCE: Ogden et al., 2010c.

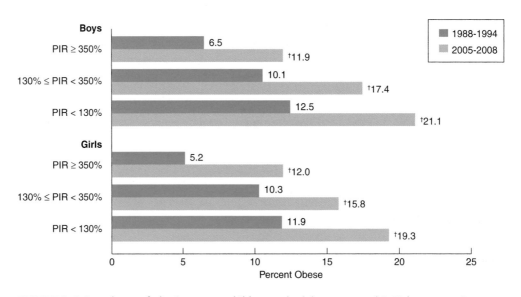

FIGURE 2-4 Prevalence of obesity among children and adolescents aged 2-19 by poverty income ratio and sex, United States, 1988-1994 to 2005-2008.

NOTES: PIR = poverty income ratio; † = significant increase.

SOURCE: Ogden et al., 2010b.

Accelerating Progress in Obesity Prevention

categories (Ogden et al., 2010b). As illustrated by Figures 2-5 and 2-6 later in this section, some of the higher risk among women and children and adolescents in the low-income categories relates to the relatively higher proportions of blacks and Mexican Americans with incomes below or near the poverty level (NCHS, 2011).

Comparison of the light and dark green bars within each income category in Figures 2-3 and 2-4 shows the substantial increases in obesity prevalence over time. For example, in 1988-1994, the prevalence of obesity among men with incomes at or above 350 percent of the poverty level was 18 percent; in 2005-2008 this figure had increased to 33 percent (Ogden et al., 2010c). The corresponding figures for those with incomes below 130 percent of the poverty level were 21 and 29 percent. Similar increases occurred among women (Ogden et al., 2010c). In children and adolescents, the prevalence of obesity increased from 7 to 12 percent between 1988-1994 and 2005-2008 among boys living at or above 350 percent of the poverty level (Ogden et al., 2010b); among boys with incomes below 130 percent of the poverty level, the prevalence of obesity increased from 13 to 21 percent during this period (Ogden et al., 2010b).

In Figures 2-5 and 2-6, obesity prevalence for non-Hispanic blacks and Mexican American adults and children and adolescents, respectively, are shown alongside data for non-Hispanic whites to illustrate racial/ethnic disparities. The data are stratified by PIR to allow assessment of income differences in obesity prevalence within racial/ethnic categories. Figure 2-5 shows that black and Mexican American women—particularly black women—have higher obesity prevalence in all income categories, and that black and Mexican American men have higher obesity prevalence than white men in the highest income category. Figure 2-6 shows that Mexican American boys and black girls have higher obesity prevalence than others in all income categories with the exception of Mexican American girls in families with incomes 130 percent or more below the poverty level.

Taken together, these prevalence data emphasize the overall proportion of U.S. children and adults who are overweight or obese, the general trends of increase over time with some early signs that increases are abating, and the high risks in populations defined by poverty, race/ethnicity, or both poverty and race/ethnicity—indicating the need for particular attention to acceleration of obesity prevention efforts in these groups (also discussed in Chapter 3).

CONTRIBUTORY TRENDS

As noted in Chapter 1, the obesity epidemic in the general population and in pockets of high risk is attributable to changes in the environments in which

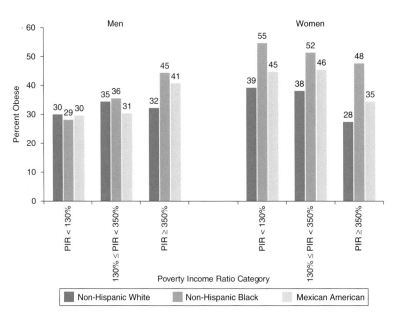

FIGURE 2-5 Obesity prevalence among adults aged 20 and older by sex and race/ethnicity within poverty income ratio categories, 2005-2008.
NOTE: PIR = poverty income ratio.
SOURCE: Ogden et al., 2010c.

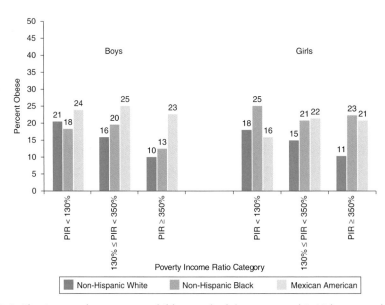

FIGURE 2-6 Obesity prevalence among children and adolescents aged 2-19 by sex and race/ethnicity within poverty income ratio categories, 2005-2008.
NOTE: PIR = poverty income ratio.
SOURCE: Ogden et al., 2010b.

Americans live that shape physical activity patterns and food consumption in people's daily lives. In brief, children, families, and people in general are at every turn surrounded—even bombarded—by inducements that discourage physical activity and encourage overeating. People's physiological systems are designed to eat whenever possible and to store energy as fat or muscle as a defense against the possibility of food scarcity. The physiological target for obesity prevention is balancing energy intake with the energy needed for bodily functions and physical activity to prevent the accumulation of excess body fat. Evidence of upward trends in weight levels indicates positive energy balance at a population level: on average, people are consuming energy in excess of their energy expenditure. There is no way for people to precisely monitor their energy balance on a day-to-day basis.

From an evolutionary perspective, people's ability to metabolize food and their underlying genetic predispositions related to food do not change within a few decades. Although genes do influence individual differences in susceptibility to obesity, trends have increased; therefore, populationwide obesity can be explained only by changes in environments that have fostered changes in behaviors related to energy balance—that is, have led the average person to be less active, eat more, or both. Educating individuals about their physical activity and food environments and motivating them to behave in different ways is a key aspect of obesity prevention, but cannot be effective unless the environment is supportive.

Following an approach used in the 2005 Institute of Medicine (IOM) report on childhood obesity, several trends related to physical activity, sedentary behavior, and food consumption that potentially contribute to increased obesity prevalence are highlighted in Tables 2-3 through 2-5. Inferences about the role of these specific influences in causing obesity are based on correlations rather than direct evidence of causation, in part because no single trend is responsible.

Table 2-3 shows that, although both adults and children and adolescents reported increased leisure-time physical activity over time, recommended levels of physical activity were not being achieved. A barrier to engaging in physical activity that is often cited is the lack of time; at least for adults, however, the availability of leisure time has increased over time. Because recommended levels of physical activity still are not being met, low levels of or decreases in physical activity among adults or children and adolescents can reasonably be attributed to decreases in active transportation (walking or biking), decreases in the availability of physical education classes, and increased and heavy use of television and other electronic media. In current work and school environments, physical activity is not given priority; thus, people must try to fit physical activity into available leisure

TABLE 2-3 Trends in Physical Activity in U.S. Adults or the Overall Population and Children and Adolescents Over Time

Variable	Changes in Adults or Overall Population Over Time	Changes in Children and Adolescents Over Time
Availability of leisure time	*Increased* (18-64 years of age) • 1965 = 34.6 hr/week[a] • 1985 = 39.4 hr/week[a] *Increased* (15+ years of age) • 2003 = 5.11 hr/day[b] • 2009 = 5.25 hr/day[b]	*Decreased* (6-12 years of age)[c] • 1981 = ~57 hr/week • 1997 = ~50 hr/week • 2003 = ~48 hr/week
Physical education classes attended daily	Not applicable	*Decreased* (high school students)[d] • 1991 = 41.6% • 1995 = 25.4% • 2009 = 33.3%
Leisure-time physical activity	*Increased* (18+ years of age)[e] participating in leisure-time aerobic and muscle-strengthening activities that meet physical activity guidelines • 1999 = 15.0% • 2009 = 19.1%	*Increased* (high school students participating in ≥1 sport)[f] • 1999 = 55.1% • 2009 = 58.3%
No leisure-time physical activity	*Decreased* (18+ years of age)[g] • 1988 = 30.5% • 2008 = 25.1%	Not reported
Meet physical activity guidelines	*Increased* (18+ years of age)[g] • 1999 = 15.0% • 2009 = 19.1%	2009 = Only 18.4% of high school[d] students meeting guidelines
Active transport	*Decreased* (employed individuals who walk to work)[b] • 1977 = 4.1% • 2009 = 2.8%	*Decreased*[i] (walk to school [5-15 years of age]) • 1977 = 20.2% of school trips • 2001 = 12.5% of school trips

SOURCES: [a]Robinson and Godbey, 1997; [b]Bureau of Labor Statistics, 2004, 2010; [c]Hofferth, 2009; [d]CDC, 2010b; [e]CDC/NCHS, 2011; [f]CDC, 2000, 2010b; [g]CDC, 2010a; [h]Santos et al., 2011; [i]Sturm, 2005.

time, where it competes with other pursuits. Table 2-4 provides a look at those key trends in media use that contribute to sedentary behavior.

Table 2-5 shows that trends of increased consumption of calories and foods in most categories were observed concurrently with increases in food availability, food portion sizes, and food consumption away from home. Consumption of dietary sweeteners and sweetened beverages, which has been directly associated with poor dietary quality and weight gain (DGAC, 2010; Woodward-Lopez et al., 2010) increased, while consumption of milk, which is more nutritious, decreased (Ogden et al., 2011; Woodward-Lopez et al., 2010). While increased consumption of fruits and vegetables and grains (not shown in Table 2-5) appears to be a positive trend, the increases were due largely to increased intake of high-caloric-density foods such as french fries and snack foods (Johnston et al., 2000; Lorson et al., 2009; USDA, 2003). Also not shown in Table 2-5 but clearly identified as a driver of caloric intake is increased marketing of high-calorie foods and beverages (Harris et al., 2010; Healthy Eating Research, 2011). The high availability of these foods and their heavy marketing compared with lower-calorie alternatives work in combination.

Trends illustrate that, for both children and adolescents and adults, requirements for physical activity have decreased while inducements to be inactive have increased, and food availability and consumption have increased. The challenges arise from the fact that these changes in environments for activity and eating reflect technological advances related to transportation or food manufacturing and to labor-saving devices in both home and work settings, communication patterns, and both occupational and recreational use of digital media. Impacts of these changes on the development of obesity are largely unintended consequences of changes in societal processes designed to achieve otherwise desirable economic and social goals (e.g., decrease in time allocated for physical education to increase time for academic work) or incidental to business imperatives within the profit-making sector (e.g., the food industry, the media industry, or employers in general). To prevent obesity, these trends must be considered to identify socially constructive ways to reverse or work around them. Addressing the obesity epidemic requires approaches that can disentangle societal development and technological progress from impacts on physical activity, eating, and related health outcomes (Uusitalo et al., 2002) and that make physical activity and healthy eating an individual and societal priority.

TABLE 2-4 Trends in Media Use That Influence Sedentary Behavior in U.S. Adults or Overall Population and Children and Adolescents Over Time

Variable	Changes in Adults or Overall Population Over Time	Changes in Children and Adolescents Over Time
Hours of media use	Not reported	*Increased* (8-18 years of age)[a] • 1999 = 6:19 hr/day • 2004 = 6:21 hr/day • 2009 = 7:38 hr/day
Hours of television viewing	*Increased* (15+ years of age)[b] • 2003 = 2.57 hr/day • 2009 = 2.82 hr/day	*Decreased* (3-12 years of age)[c] • 1981 = 17:35 hr/week • 1997 = 13:29 hr/week *Increased* (8-18 years of age)[a] • 1999 = 3:47 hr/day • 2004 = 3:51 hr/day • 2009 = 4:29 hr/day
Internet adoption	*Increased* (18+ years of age)[d] • 1995 = 14% use among U.S. adults • 2011 = 78% use among U.S. adults	*Increased* (12-17 years of age)[e] • 2000 = 73% use among U.S. teens • 2009 = 93% use among U.S. teens
Home Internet access	*Increased* (U.S. households)[f] • 1997 = 18% • 2009 = 68.7%	*Increased* (8-18 years of age)[a] • 1999 = 47% • 2004 = 74% • 2009 = 84%
Hours of computer use	Not reported	*Increased* (8-18 years of age)[a] • 1999 = 0:27 hr/day • 2004 = 1:02 hr/day • 2009 = 1:29 hr/day
Hours of video game use	Not reported	*Increased* (8-18 years of age)[a] • 1999 = 0:26 hr/day • 2004 = 0:49 hr/day • 2009 = 1:13 hr/day
Social networking site use	*Increased* (18+ years or age)[g] • 2005 = 8% use among U.S. adults • 2011 = 65% use among U.S. adults	*Increased* (12-17 years of age)[h] • 2006 = 55% use among teens • 2009 = 73% use among teens

SOURCES: [a]Rideout et al., 2010; [b]Bureau of Labor Statistics, 2004, 2010; [c]Hofferth and Sandberg, 2001; [d]Pew Research Center, 2011a; [e]Pew Research Center, 2011b; [f]U.S. Census Bureau, 2009; [g]Madden and Zickuhr, 2011; [h]Lenhart et al., 2010.

TABLE 2-5 Trends in U.S. Food Supply and Consumption Relevant to Obesity Prevention Over Time

Variable	Changes in Adult or Overall Population Over Time	Changes in Children and Adolescents Over Time
Portion size	*Increased from 1977-1978 to 1994-1996* (2+ years of age)[a] • Soft drinks +49 kcal/day • Fruit drinks +50 kcal/day • Hamburgers +97 kcal/day • Cheeseburgers +136 kcal/day • Mexican fast food +133 kcal/day	*Increased from 1977-1978 to 2003-2006* (2-18 years of age)[b] • Soft drinks increased ~100 mL • Fruit drinks increased ~43 mL • Hamburgers increased 31 g/portion (+90 kcal/day) • Cheeseburgers increased 22 g/portion (+90 kcal/day) • Pizza increased 41 g/portion (+131 kcal/day) • Mexican fast food increased 48 g/portion (+149 kcal/day)
Daily total energy intake	*Increased*[c] Males (20+ years of age) • 1971-1974 = 2,450 kcal/day • 2005-2008 = 2,656 kcal/day *Increased* Females (20+ years of age) • 1971-1974 = 1,542 kcal/day • 2005-2008 = 1,811 kcal/day	*Increased*[d] (2-18 years of age) • 1977-1978 = 1,842 kcal/day • 1989-1991 = 1,802 kcal/day • 1994-1998 = 1,947 kcal/day • 2003-2006 = 2,022 kcal/day
Energy from carbohydrates	*Increased*[c] Males (20+ years of age) • 1971-1974 = 42.4% • 2005-2008 = 47.4% *Increased*[c] Females (20+ years of age) • 1971-1974 = 45.4% • 2005-2008 = 49.5%	*Increased*[e] Boys (6-11 years of age) • 1977-1978 = 46.8% • 2007-2008 = 55.0% *Increased*[e] Girls (6-11 years of age) • 1977-1978 = 47.4% • 2007-2008 = 54.0%

continued

TABLE 2-5 Continued

Variable	Changes in Adult or Overall Population Over Time	Changes in Children and Adolescents Over Time
Energy from fat	*Decreased[c]* Males (20+ years of age) • 1971-1974 = 36.9% • 2005-2008 = 33.6% *Decreased[c]* Females (20+ years of age) • 1971-1974 = 36.1% • 2005-2008 = 33.8%	*Decreased[e]* Boys (6-11 years of age) • 1977-1978 = 38.5% • 2007-2008 = 33.0% *Decreased[e]* Girls (6-11 years of age) • 1977-1978 = 38.2% • 2007-2008 = 33.0%
Energy from protein	*Decreased[c]* Males (20+ years of age) • 1971-1974 = 16.5% • 2005-2008 = 15.6% *Decreased[c]* Females (20+ years of age) • 1971-1974 = 16.9% • 2005-2008 = 15.8%	*Decreased[e]* Boys and girls (6-11 years of age) • 1977-1978 = 15.6% • 2007-2008 = 14.0%
Percentage of sugar-sweetened beverage consumption	*Increased* (20+ years of age)[f] • 1988-1994 = 58% • 1999-2004 = 63%	*Increased* (2-19 years of age)[g] • 1988-1994 = 79% • 1999-2004 = 81%
Percentage of daily energy eaten away from home	Not available	*Increased* (2-18 years of age)[d] • 1994-1998 = 32.7% • 2003-2006 = 33.9%
Percentage of fast food consumed at home versus in store	Not available	*Increased* (2-18 years of age)[d] • 1994-1998 = 38% • 2003-2006 = 49%

SOURCES: [a]Nielson and Popkin, 2003; [b]Piernas and Popkin, 2011; [c]CDC/NCHS, 2011; [d]Poti and Popkin, 2011; [e]Enns et al., 2002; USDA, 2010; [f]Bleich et al., 2009; [g]Wang et al., 2008.

ADVANCES DURING THE PAST DECADE AND BARRIERS TO FURTHER PROGRESS

Awareness of the obesity epidemic in the United States, first in adults and then in children and adolescents, emerged in the mid-1990s (Kuczmarski et al., 1994; Troiano et al., 1995). Since then we have come to realize not only that obesity causes multiple social and economic problems as described above, but also that it results from multiple changes in society that have affected many aspects of contemporary life, including activity patterns and food consumption. In 2001 *The Surgeon General's Call to Action to Prevent and Decrease Overweight and Obesity* was issued (HHS, 2001). This call constituted official recognition of the obesity epidemic as a priority within the Department of Health and Human Services. It set forth principles for a nationwide public health response that would address the problem at multiple levels and involve multiple sectors of society and a broad array of public and private entities. The importance of facilitating individual weight management was emphasized, but there was also a strong emphasis on changing aspects of the environment viewed as contributory. In 2003, Dr. Elias Zerhouni, then Director of the National Institutes of Health, formed an organizationwide task force to develop a related research strategy. In 2004, this task force released a strategic plan that called for research across a spectrum of obesity-related topics and approaches and drew attention to the need for studies focusing on special populations at high risk of obesity. This plan was updated in 2011. These and several subsequent milestones and both public- and private-sector initiatives are highlighted in Table 2-6 and Box 2-3.

Included in Table 2-6 are several IOM reports that have provided a foundation for many of the policy and other initiatives that have been undertaken and that continue to inform the process of obesity-related policy and program development. These include *Progress in Preventing Childhood Obesity: How Do We Measure Up?* (IOM, 2007b), which offers specific guidance for foundations, industry, and government, and *Local Government Actions to Prevent Childhood Obesity* (IOM, 2009), which provides several examples of ways in which local government officials have promoted healthier lifestyles in their communities and recommends starting points that could help officials initiate childhood obesity prevention plans tailored to their jurisdictions' resources and needs.

The committee highlights these milestones and initiatives to demonstrate that many of society's stakeholders are acknowledging their responsibility to address obesity and are moving to respond. Although children have been a primary focus

TABLE 2-6 Selected Milestones in Obesity Prevention from the Past Decade

	2001-2003[a]	2004-2006[b]	2007-2009[c]	2010-2012[d]
Federal guidance	*Surgeon General's Call to Action to Prevent and Decrease Overweight and Obesity* Formation of NIH Obesity Research Task Force	*Strategic Plan for NIH Obesity Research*	CDC's first Weight of the Nation Conference 2008 Physical Activity Guidelines for Americans IWG in Food Marketing to Children—Tentative Proposed Nutrition Standards	Launch of the First Lady's Let's Move Campaign White House Task Force Report on Childhood Obesity Prevention 2010 Dietary Guidelines for Americans *Strategic Plan for NIH Obesity Research*
Federal policy		*Child Nutrition and WIC Reauthorization,* Public Law 108-265, 108th Cong., 2d sess. (June 30, 2004), 118, 729 Safe Routes to School Program. *Safe Accountable, Flexible, and Efficient Transportation Equity Act: A Legacy for Users,* Public Law 109-59, 109th Cong., 1st sess. (August 10, 2005), 119, 1404[d]	ARRA funding for CDC's "Communities Putting Prevention to Work" USDA interim rule to modify WIC food package	*Healthy, Hunger-Free Kids Act,* Public Law 111-296, 111th Cong., 2d sess. (December 13, 2010), 124, 3183

TABLE 2-6 Continued

	2001-2003[a]	2004-2006[b]	2007-2009[c]	2010-2012[d]
Nonprofit and private sector		Convergence Partnership for Healthy Eating and Active Living AHA and William J. Clinton Foundation Alliance for a Healthier Generation Children's Food and Beverage Advertising Initiative	RWJF commitment to reverse the childhood obesity epidemic by 2015 National Collaborative on Childhood Obesity Research (NCCOR)	Partnership for a Healthier America (Let's Move) Healthy Weight Commitment— food manufacturers commit to removing calories from the food supply
IOM guidance		*Preventing Childhood Obesity: Health in the Balance* *Food Marketing to Children and Youth: Threat or Opportunity*	*Progress in Preventing Childhood Obesity: How Do We Measure Up?* *Nutrition Standards for Foods in Schools: Leading the Way Toward Healthier Youth* *Local Government Actions to Prevent Childhood Obesity*	*School Meals: Building Blocks for Healthy Children* *Bridging the Evidence Gap in Obesity Prevention: A Framework to Inform Decision Making* *Early Childhood Obesity Prevention Policies*

NOTES: AHA = American Heart Association; ARRA = American Recovery and Reinvestment Act of 2009; CDC = Centers for Disease Control and Prevention; IOM = Institute of Medicine; IWG = Interagency Working Group; NIH = National Institutes of Health; RWJF = Robert Wood Johnson Foundation; USDA = U.S. Department of Agriculture; WIC = Special Supplemental Nutrition Program for Women, Infants, and Children.

SOURCE: [a]HHS, 2001; NIH, 2004; [b]Alliance for a Healthier Generation, 2005; Bell and Dorfman, 2008; Better Business Bureau, 2006; IOM, 2005, 2006b; NIH, 2004; [c]CDC, 2009a; FTC, 2009; HHS, 2008, 2009; IOM, 2007a,b, 2009; NCCOR, 2012; RWJF, 2007; USDA, 2007; [d]Healthy Weight Commitment Foundation, 2010; IOM, 2010a,b, 2011; Let's Move Campaign, 2010; NIH, 2011; USDA/HHS, 2010; White House, 2010a,b.

BOX 2-3
National Initiatives to Address Obesity

- The **2004 Child Nutrition and WIC Reauthorization Act** (Public Law 108-265, 108th Cong., 2d sess. [June 30, 2004], 118, 729) required that all local education authorities (i.e., school districts) receiving federal support for school meals create **school wellness policies**. These policies were to be developed with broad participation of parents, students, and school food providers and administrators. They were to specify goals for nutrition education, physical activity, and other school-based wellness activities, as well as standards for foods available on the school campus. The **Healthy, Hunger-Free Kids Act of 2010** (Public Law 111-296, 111th Cong., 2d sess. [December 13, 2010], 124, 3183), which renewed the 2004 act, included several enhancements to this policy.

- The transportation bill of 2005 established the national **Safe Routes to School** (SRTS) program to allow and encourage more children to walk and bicycle safely to school. SRTS funding supports infrastructure changes to build roads, sidewalks, and bike lanes and pathways and also includes funding to support educational, promotional, and traffic enforcement activities (Public Law 109-59, 109th Cong., 1st sess. [August 10, 2005], 119, 1404).

- The **Alliance for a Healthier Generation**, a major public health campaign to address childhood obesity, was founded in 2005 as a partnership between the American Heart Association and the William J. Clinton Foundation. Alliance programs focus on children directly, as well as on school environments, health care institutions, and industry (Alliance for a Healthier Generation, 2005).

- The **Convergence Partnership** was formed in 2006 to "strengthen and accelerate multi-field, equity-focused efforts among practitioners, policymakers, funders, and advocates to create environments that support healthy eating and active living." The partnership is a coalition of several foundations with an interest in this area: the California Endowment, Kaiser Permanente, Kresge Foundation, Nemours, the Robert Wood Johnson Foundation, and the W.K. Kellogg Foundation, as well as advisors from the Centers for Disease Control and Prevention (CDC) (Bell and Dorfman, 2008).

- Also in 2006, in response to an Institute of Medicine (IOM) report on food marketing to children (IOM, 2006a) and calls from the Federal Trade Commission for better regulation of marketing to children, the **Children's Food and Beverage Advertising Initiative** was formed by several major food companies together with the Council of Better Business Bureaus. The stated purpose of this initiative was to shift child-oriented advertising to a healthier mix of products (Better Business Bureau, 2006).

- In 2007, the **Robert Wood Johnson Foundation**, the nation's largest health philanthropy, announced a $500 million commitment to reverse the epidemic of childhood obesity by 2015, to be implemented through a variety of research and programmatic funding activities nationwide (RWJF, 2007).

- The American Recovery and Reinvestment Act included $650 million in federal funding to support community-based prevention programs, leading to **Communities Putting Prevention to Work** initiatives in localities throughout the United States. More than half of these funds were awarded to projects that included a focus on obesity (HHS, 2009).

- In 2009, CDC convened an inaugural national **Weight of the Nation** conference to focus attention on obesity prevention efforts and share knowledge of promising or effective approaches from communities throughout the United States. A second conference will be held in 2012 (CDC, 2009b).

- The **National Collaborative on Childhood Obesity Research** (NCCOR) was created in 2009 as a collaborative among several components of the National Institutes of Health, CDC, and the Robert Wood Johnson Foundation, later joined by the U.S. Department of Agriculture. NCCOR leverages the diverse resources of these entities to create innovative funding initiatives and tools to support research and practice related to childhood obesity (NCCOR, 2012).

- The U.S. Department of Agriculture issued an interim rule to modify the **Special Supplemental Nutrition Program for Women, Infants, and Children** (WIC) food package along lines recommended in an IOM report on this topic (IOM, 2006b), focused in particular on improving the appropriateness of the package for obesity prevention and control. The interim rule was implemented program-wide and is pending finalization (USDA, 2007).

- First Lady Michelle Obama came forward as a champion for the childhood obesity prevention effort, launching a multicomponent **Let's Move** campaign to promote healthier environments and behaviors related to physical activity and eating in schools, homes, and communities (White House, 2010a).

continued

BOX 2-3
Continued

- In conjunction with the launch of Let's Move, President Obama formed a **White House Task Force on Childhood Obesity** (2010) under the leadership of the White House Domestic Policy advisor, with a mandate to develop an interagency plan for solving the childhood obesity problem within a generation. Task force members include senior-level representation from across government, including the Departments of Agriculture, Health and Human Services, Education, and the Interior; the Office of Management and Budget; the First Lady's Office; and the Assistant to the President for Economic Policy. A few months later, the task force issued the requested report, which included 79 recommendations (White House, 2010b; White House Task Force on Childhood Obesity, 2010).

- Also in conjunction with Let's Move, a new foundation—the **Partnership for a Healthier America**—was formed with the First Lady as honorary chair and two prominent policy makers as honorary vice chairs. The foundation is intended to serve as an independent, transparent mechanism for developing and tracking major private-sector commitments to facilitating the reduction of childhood obesity (Let's Move Campaign, 2010).

- A large coalition of food and beverage manufacturers—the **Healthy Weight Commitment Foundation**—announced a pledge to the Let's Move campaign to remove 1.5 trillion calories from the food supply by 2015 (Healthy Weight Commitment Foundation, 2010).

- In response to a congressional mandate, CDC, the Federal Trade Commission, the Food and Drug Administration, and the U.S. Department of Agriculture formed an **Interagency Working Group** to develop guidelines for food and beverage advertising to children and adolescents aged 2 to 17. The preliminary standards were released for public comment in December 2010 (FTC, 2010).

- The 2010 revision of the **Dietary Guidelines for Americans** was framed with particular reference to the importance of avoiding obesity. The guidelines include explicit advice related to foods that should be reduced in the diet as well as those that should be increased to achieve a better overall balance within calorie limits (USDA/HHS, 2010).

of these efforts, changes in society aimed at preventing child obesity will impact adults as well.

Figures 2-7 and 2-8, which display counts of media reports related to obesity generally or childhood obesity specifically, demonstrate the tremendous increase in public awareness that has led to or accompanied widespread efforts to address obesity, both in the United States and globally. Similar counts have been made of increases in the development of state and local policies designed to improve information available to parents and consumers, improve opportunities for physical activity, and introduce incentives to support better availability of healthy foods and discourage consumption of unhealthy foods and beverages. For example, the Trust for America's Health (TFAH) publishes an annual compilation of the current status of each state's obesity and related health profiles, as well as legislative actions aimed at obesity reduction (Trust for America's Health and RWJF, 2011). Highlights of TFAH's 2011 report are presented in Box 2-4. In reflecting on the data 10 years after his 2001 *Call to Action* (HHS, 2001), former Surgeon General Dr. David Satcher concluded that important progress has been made, but that much more remains to be done (Trust for America's Health and RWJF, 2011). He also concluded that even though individuals bear responsibility for their own health, the public and private sectors must get involved to enable an environment that fosters healthy living.

Both public and private employers are offering health and wellness programs to workers (Claxton et al., 2010), including policies that support breastfeeding mothers (see the discussion in Chapter 8). Such policies are important as breastfeeding may be beneficial for obesity prevention in both children and their mothers (IOM, 2009, 2011; Moreno et al., 2011).

Clearly, however, not all developments during this period have been favorable. Indeed, many countering forces act as barriers to further progress. Some relate to competing priorities and limited resources. For example, the most frequently cited barriers to offering physical activity opportunities for students during the school day are priority given to time for academic work and limited resources and staff capacity for physical education programs (Agron et al., 2010; Young et al., 2007). Other barriers reflect more deliberate opposition to change from commercial vested interests. In particular, food and beverage companies are strongly opposed to statutory regulations on advertising or other aspects of marketing, preferring that any changes be voluntary. Chapter 10 provides a broader discussion of the challenges related to opposing views of what should be done to address obesity and who should take responsibility for doing it.

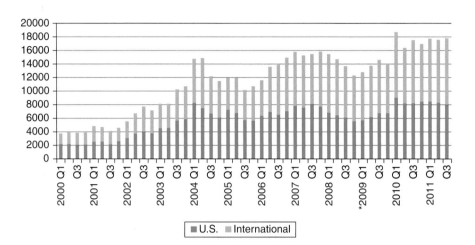

FIGURE 2-7 Global trends in obesity-related media coverage from the first quarter of 2000 through the third quarter of 2011.
NOTE: Figures retrieved from Lexis-Nexis searches on "obesity or obese" in U.S. and international newspapers and newswires, and beginning in the first quarter of 2009 (as indicated by *), online news sources.
SOURCE: Reprinted from IFIC, 2011.

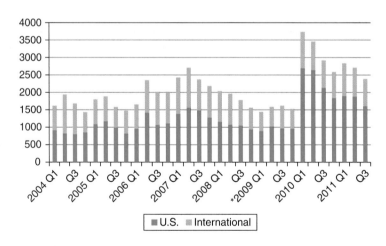

FIGURE 2-8 Global trends in childhood obesity-related media coverage from the first quarter of 2004 through the third quarter of 2011.
NOTE: Figures retrieved from Lexis-Nexis searches on "childhood obesity" in U.S. and international newspapers and newswires, and beginning in the first quarter of 2009 (as indicated by *), online news sources.
SOURCE: Reprinted from IFIC, 2011.

BOX 2-4
Major State Legislative Efforts Identified in the 2011 Fat as in Fat report

- Twenty states and Washington, DC, have stricter school meal standards than the U.S. Department of Agriculture (USDA). Seven years ago, only four states had standards that were stricter than USDA requirements.

- Thirty-five states and Washington, DC, have nutritional standards for competitive foods. Seven years ago, only six states had nutritional standards for competitive foods.

- Twenty-nine states and Washington, DC, limit when and where competitive foods may be sold beyond federal requirements. Seven years ago, 17 states had laws regarding when and where competitive foods can be sold that were stricter than federal requirements.

- Every state has some physical education requirements for students. However, these requirements often are limited or not enforced, and many programs are inadequate.

- Twenty-one states have legislation that requires body mass index (BMI) screening or weight-related assessments other than BMI for children and adolescents in school. Seven years ago, only four states required BMI screening or other weight-related assessments for children and adolescents in school.

- Twenty-six states and Washington, DC, currently have farm-to-school programs. Five years ago, only New York had a law that established a farm-to-school program.

- Sixteen states have passed complete streets laws. Seven years ago, only five states had complete streets laws.

- Thirty-four states and Washington, DC, have sales taxes on sodas.

- Four states have laws requiring the posting of nutrition information on menus and menu boards in chain restaurants with 20 or more in-state locations.

SOURCE: Trust for America's Health and RWJF, 2011. Adapted with permission of Trust for America's Health (TFAH), Washington, DC.

Partly because of the combination of facilitating and countering influences, outcomes of efforts to address obesity have yet to yield a clear picture showing that obesity levels are on the decline. Given increased public awareness and the continually growing number and diversity of positive initiatives, however, there are many indications that the time is ripe for responding to recommendations for mounting a more aggressive and comprehensive obesity prevention effort.

TRACKING PROGRESS ON OUTCOMES

It is generally understood that even when promising interventions are identified, the effects of social and economic phenomena that have evolved over decades cannot be turned around overnight. Nevertheless, given that substantive efforts to address the obesity epidemic have now been in place for at least a decade (e.g., since the 2001 U.S. Surgeon General's *Call to Action* [HHS, 2001]), it is reasonable to ask whether there are signs of progress. The ability to track changes in population weight status depends on the collection of weight and height measurements (or self-reported data, with recognition of the substantial potential for error in such data) in community settings and at the state and federal levels for use in assessing average BMI and the percentage of children, adolescents, and adults who are overweight or obese. Particularly salient will be evidence of reduced incidence of new cases of obesity and favorable shifts in the overall BMI distribution such that the percentage of the population in the healthy weight range increases, with attention to other goals as appropriate to ensure the overall quality of the way in which BMI changes are being achieved. Data with which to assess overweight and obesity levels and BMI distributions in the United States are collected on an ongoing basis through the National Health and Nutrition Examination Survey (NHANES) and reported regularly by the National Center for Health Statistics (NCHS, 2011), and are also collected in some states (Flegal et al., 2010; Ogden et al., 2010a, 2012). Analyses of these data include assessment of changes in prevalence trends and in recent years have indicated changes that may signify the beginnings of a leveling off of the epidemic, but without downward movement.

At the national level, obesity prevalence data for both children and adolescents and adults suggest that although high levels persist, trends of increase are absent or variable, depending on the population subgroup examined (Flegal et al., 2010; Ogden et al., 2010a,b,c, 2012). No statistically significant trend of increase in obesity among women was observed during the 10 years prior to 2009-2010, both overall and by racial/ethnic subgroups (non-Hispanic whites, non-Hispanic blacks, and Mexican Americans). However, significant increases in obesity prevalence were apparent in men for at least the first part of this time period, overall and for non-Hispanic white and non-Hispanic black men (Flegal et al., 2010; Ogden et al., 2012). Findings were similar in children and adolescents: BMI distributions in the 10-year period before 2009-2010 were stable in girls in all racial/ethnic groups; in boys, a significant increase in BMI was observed only at ages 6 to 19 and only in the highest BMI category (at or above the 97th percentile) (Ogden et al., 2010a, 2012). The Pediatric Nutrition Surveillance System, which reports data on children aged 0-5 from low-income families participating in federal nutrition programs, reported this phenomenon based on data obtained from 2003 to 2008 (CDC, 2009b); the self-report data from youth in grades 9 through 12 that were collected between 2005 and 2007 yielded a similar picture (CDC, 2010b; Eaton et al., 2008).

The possibility that obesity prevalence trends are stabilizing was supported by a comparative analysis of the trends in several countries that have also been undertaking initiatives to curb rising obesity levels. Data from nine countries (Australia, China, England, France, the Netherlands, New Zealand, Sweden, Switzerland, and the United States) suggest that among children and adolescents aged 2-19, the mean (SD) unweighted rate of change in the prevalence of overweight and obesity was +0.00 (0.49) percent per year between 1995 and 2008 (+0.01 [0.56] percent for overweight alone and −0.01 [0.24] percent for obesity alone) (Olds et al., 2011). It is unclear why prevalence appears to be flattening. Olds and colleagues (2011) hypothesize that stabilization may be occurring as a result of the numerous public health campaigns and interventions that have been aimed at childhood obesity for the past several years beginning to have a cumulative effect and the rates of childhood overweight and obesity reaching a saturation point of equilibrium. However, self-selection bias in the available data cannot be ruled out (because of increased awareness of childhood obesity and perceived stigmatization, parents have declined participation in later measurement years compared with the baseline). Moreover, while rates, which still remain high, appear to be stabilizing, it is unclear whether this stabilization will continue over the long term or merely represents a temporary lull (Olds et al., 2011).

There is also evidence of improvements in obesity trends at the state level. Measured BMI data were collected in Arkansas from approximately 400,000 students in all K-12 grades for 2003-2007 and for nearly 180,000 students in grades K, 2, 4, 6, 8, and 10 during 2008-2010. The prevalence of overweight vacillated only slightly over the 7-year period, beginning at 21 percent in school year 2003-2004 and ending at 17 percent in 2009-2010 (ACHI, 2011). Similarly, rates of obesity were 20.9 percent in 2003-2004 and 21.0 percent in 2009-2010. Thus while the rates in Arkansas were higher than the national rates, the change in rates over the 7-year period mirrored the phenomenon of leveling observed in the national data. The Obesity and School BMI Measurement Initiative is but one part of a multipronged statewide effort to improve the health of Arkansas children that is being spearheaded by the Arkansas Center for Health Improvement (Raczynski et al., 2009). Hence, the potential for analyses linking observed BMI changes to effects of interventions may exist.

Two reports chronicle changes in BMI among children and adolescents in California between 2001 and 2008. Unlike Arkansas, California mandated measuring students at only three grade levels: grades 5, 7, and 9. Given the size of the state, the BMI data set over this 8-year time period contains more than 8 million student height and weight records. The analysis of this data set by Sanchez-Vaznaugh and colleagues (2010) reveals a lessening of the BMI upward slope between the years prior to versus the years after the 2004-2005 school year. The authors postulate that statewide policies limiting competitive foods and beverages in K-12 schools may have been associated with this observed leveling of the BMI slope. While the overall pattern of change in overweight and obesity in California children and adolescents mirrored that of the nation, with only a slight change between 2001 and 2008 (overweight rates were 38.3 percent in 2001 and 38.0 percent in 2008, while obesity in the same cohort was 20.3 percent in 2001 and 19.8 percent in 2008), the data reveal distinctly different patterns of BMI change by race/ethnicity (Madsen et al., 2010). A population-based decline in the prevalence of high BMI after 2005 was observed among most boys and for white girls. Even rates for Hispanic boys, a group with a high prevalence of obesity, declined during this period. The rates for Hispanic girls leveled, while the rates for black and American Indian girls continued to climb during the 8-year period. The leveling phenomenon that is documented by the NHANES analyses also may reflect a combination of patterns unique to different racial/ethnic groups, with some rates declining, some leveling, and others continuing to rise. Thus while obesity rates may appear to be improving slightly, the disparities in rates may actually be widening. Interpretation of these trends is complicated because these are cross-sectional data and because it is difficult to know over what time period changes in trends can be considered to signify probable future patterns of stabilization and eventually decreases. Complementary analyses would include examination of longitudinal data to track weight changes over time and determine whether the percentage of children, adolescents, or adults becoming obese at any given age is decreasing. If so, this would suggest promising future trends, particularly if it were to be observed in the youngest children. Regardless, any sign of a flattening of trends of increase is potentially favorable and warrants close attention to potential contributors.

The possible effects of the economic recession on trends in obesity are unclear. Ludwig and Pollack (2009) have raised the possibility that an increase in obesity is associated with the economic recession because limited incomes may increase reliance on low-cost, high-calorie foods (although the authors note that this situation also may provide opportunities for new initiatives to address obesity). In contrast, an analysis in *The Economist* suggests that trends in consumer spending may have positive health effects, including more spending on fruits and vegetables and less spending on sugar and sweets (*The Economist*, 2011). Effects could differ for different population groups. In any case, secular trends reflecting population responsiveness to economic constraints would not represent a desirable or sustainable long-term context for achieving and maintaining healthy population weights.

CONCLUSION

Prior to the late 20th century, overweight and obesity were not considered a populationwide health risk. Instead, food scarcity and hunger were the primary food-related public policy issues. An assessment of the current situation highlights the pressing need for populationwide efforts to address obesity among adults and children and adolescents, with a particular emphasis on high-risk groups for whom the general efforts may be insufficient to close gaps. Even today, many people may regard "baby fat" and childhood "chubbiness" as indicators of good health and/or economic security, and fail to recognize the relationship of obesity to many serious chronic diseases and economic and societal costs. Asserting that people should simply eat less or that parents should simply feed their children better ignores these historical perspectives and the complex societal influences at work. A strategy that assumes that parents or others have or should have an inherent skill set to bear the sole responsibility for preventing obesity for their children or for themselves is unlikely to be successful. Instead, obesity prevention approaches require modifying factors that shape individual choices and incidental behaviors (Kumanyika, 2008).

The committee's vision for obesity prevention rests on the ability to modify factors that shape individual choices, as well as behaviors that are natural and unconscious responses to environmental cues and situations. These factors are varied, complex, and interrelated, and numerous small changes may contribute collectively to influencing population shifts. Some evidence indicates that trends of continuing increases in obesity prevalence may be leveling off, although this observation does not apply evenly across all population subgroups and also may not be sustained or lead to a lessening of the current high rate. Contributors to these potential precursors of success must be identified and translated into approaches for permanent change. Of greatest importance in this respect is that early signs of success, even if real, not be misunderstood to *be* success. Success will occur once population weight levels are in a healthy range. All of the adverse consequences—human and economic—of the obesity epidemic described here are entrenched and will continue to increase as children and adolescents on a course to become obese mature. The next chapter of this report describes specific goals and strategies for addressing obesity and examines practical and policy considerations relevant to their implementation.

REFERENCES

ACHI (Arkansas Center for Health Improvement). 2011. *Combating childhood obesity*. http://www.achi.net/ChildObDocs/2004%20Statewide%20BMI%20Report.pdf (accessed October 14, 2011).

Agron, P., V. Berends, K. Ellis, and M. Gonzalez. 2010. School wellness policies: Perceptions, barriers, and needs among school leaders and wellness advocates. *Journal of School Health* 80(11):527-535.

Alliance for a Healthier Generation. 2005. *Clinton Foundation and American Heart Association form alliance to create a healthier generation*. http://www.healthiergeneration.org/uploadedFiles/For_Media/afhg_nr_alliance_formation_5-3-05.pdf (accessed January 4, 2012).

American Heart Association. 2010. *Understanding childhood obesity*. http://www.heart.org/idc/groups/heart-public/@wcm/@fc/documents/downloadable/ucm_304175.pdf (accessed December 29, 2011).

Bell, J., and L. Dorfman. 2008. *Introducing the healthy eating active living convergence partnership*. http://www.convergencepartnership.org/atf/cf/%7B245A9B44-6DED-4ABD-A392-AE583809E350%7D/CP_Introduction_printed.pdf (accessed January 4, 2012).

Better Business Bureau. 2006. *New food, beverage initiative to focus kids' ads on healthy choices; revised guidelines strengthen CARU's guidance to food advertisers*. http://www.bbb.org/us/article/new-food-beverage-initiative-to-focus-kids-ads-on-healthy-choices-revised-guidelines-strengthen-carus-guidance-to-food-advertisers-672 (accessed January 4, 2012).

Bleich, S. N., Y. C. Wang, Y. Wang, and S. L. Gortmaker. 2009. Increasing consumption of sugar-sweetened beverages among US adults: 1988-1994 to 1999-2004. *The American Journal of Clinical Nutrition* 89(1):372.

Bureau of Labor Statistics. 2004. *Time use survey—first results announced by BLS.* Washington, DC: U.S. Department of Labor.

Bureau of Labor Statistics. 2010. *American time use survey—2009 results.* Washington, DC: U.S. Department of Labor.

Burkhauser, R. V., and J. Cawley. 2004. *Obesity, disability, and movement onto the disability insurance rolls.* http://www.mrrc.isr.umich.edu/publications/Papers/pdf/wp089.pdf (accessed December 29, 2011).

Cawley, J. 2004. The impact of obesity on wages. *Journal of Human Resources* 39(2):451-474.

Cawley, J. 2010. The economics of childhood obesity. *Health Affairs* 29(3):364-371.

Cawley, J., and C. Meyerhoefer. 2011. The medical care costs of obesity: An instrumental variables approach. *Journal of Health Economics* 31(1):219-230.

Cawley, J., J. A. Rizzo, and K. Haas. 2007. Occupation-specific absenteeism costs associated with obesity and morbid obesity. *Journal of Occupational and Environmental Medicine* 49(12):1317-1324.

CDC (Centers for Disease Control and Prevention). 2000. Youth Risk Behavior Surveillance—United States, 1999. *Morbidity and Mortality Weekly Report Surveillance Summaries* 49(SS-5):1-95.

CDC. 2009a. Obesity prevalence among low-income, preschool-aged children—United States, 1998-2008. *Morbidity and Mortality Weekly Report* 58(28):769-773.

CDC. 2009b. *Weight of the Nation conference.* http://www.cdc.gov/nccdphp/DNPAO/news/conferences/won.html (accessed January 4, 2012).

CDC. 2010a. *1988-2008 no leisure-time physical activity trend chart.* http://www.cdc.gov/nccdphp/dnpa/physical/stats/leisure_time.htm (accessed December 14, 2011).

CDC. 2010b. *1991-2009 High School Youth Risk Behavior Survey data.* http://apps.nccd.cdc.gov/youthonline. (accessed November 11, 2011).

CDC. 2011. *Diabetes public health resource.* http://www.cdc.gov/diabetes/projects/cda2.htm (accessed September 21, 2011).

CDC/NCHS (National Center for Health Statistics). 2011. *Health, United States, 2010: With special feature on death and dying.* http://www.cdc.gov/nchs/data/hus/hus10.pdf (accessed December 15, 2011).

Christeson, W., A. D. Taggart, and S. Messner-Zidell. 2010. *Too fat to fight: Retired military leaders want junk food out of America's schools.* Washington, DC: Mission: Readiness.

Claxton, G., B. DiJulio, H. Whitmore, J. D. Pickreign, M. McHugh, A. Osei-Anto, and B. Finder. 2010. Health benefits in 2010: Premiums rise modestly, workers pay more toward coverage. *Health Affairs* 29(10):1942-1950.

Dannenberg, A. L., D. C. Burton, and R. J. Jackson. 2004. Economic and environmental costs of obesity: The impact on airlines. *American Journal of Preventive Medicine* 27(3):264.

DGAC (Dietary Guidelines Advisory Committee). 2010. *Report of the Dietary Guidelines Advisory Committee on the Dietary Guidelines for Americans, 2010, to the Secretary of Agriculture and the Secretary of Health and Human Services.* Washington, DC: U.S. Department of Agriculture, Agricultural Research Service.

Durden, E. D., D. Huse, R. Ben-Joseph, and B. C. Chu. 2008. Economic costs of obesity to self-insured employers. *Journal of Occupational and Environmental Medicine* 50(9):991-997.

Eaton, D. K., L. Kann, S. Kinchen, S. Shanklin, J. Ross, J. Hawkins, W. A. Harris, R. Lowry, T. McManus, D. Chyen, C. Lim, N. D. Brener, and H. Wechsler. 2008. Youth risk behavior surveillance—United States, 2007. *Morbidity and Mortality Weekly Report Surveillance Summaries* 57(4):1-131.

Eisenberg, M. E., D. Neumark-Sztainer, and M. Story. 2003. Associations of weight-based teasing and emotional well-being among adolescents. *Archives of Pediatrics and Adolescent Medicine* 157(8):733-738.

Enns, C. W., S. J. Mickle, and J. D. Goldman. 2002. Trends in food and nutrient intakes by children in the United States. *Family Economics and Nutrition Review* 14(2):56-68.

Finkelstein, E. A., J. G. Trogdon, J. W. Cohen, and W. Dietz. 2009. Annual medical spending attributable to obesity: Payer- and service-specific estimates. *Health Affairs* 28(5):w822-w831.

Flegal, K. M., M. D. Carroll, C. L. Ogden, and L. R. Curtin. 2010. Prevalence and trends in obesity among US adults, 1999-2008. *Journal of the American Medical Association* 303(3):235-241.

Fontaine, K. R., D. T. Redden, C. Wang, A. O. Westfall, and D. B. Allison. 2003. Years of life lost due to obesity. *Journal of the American Medical Association* 289(2):187-193.

Freedman, D. S. 2011. Obesity—United States, 1988-2008. *Morbidity and Mortality Weekly Report Surveillance Summaries* 60(Suppl.):73-77.

FTC (Federal Trade Commission). 2009. *Interagency working group in food marketing to children—tentative proposed nutrition standards.* http://www.ftc.gov/bcp/workshops/sizingup/SNAC_PAC.pdf (accessed December 1, 2011).

FTC. 2010. *Interagency working group on food marketed to children preliminary proposed nutrition principles to guide industry self-regulatory efforts: Request for comments.* http://www.ftc.gov/os/2011/04/110428foodmarketproposedguide.pdf (accessed September 21, 2011).

Geier, A. B., G. D. Foster, L. G. Womble, J. McLaughlin, K. E. Borradaile, J. Nachmani, S. Sherman, S. Kumanyika, and J. Shults. 2007. The relationship between relative weight and school attendance among elementary schoolchildren. *Obesity (Silver Spring)* 15(8):2157-2161.

Giel, K. E., A. Thiel, M. Teufel, J. Mayer, and S. Zipfel. 2010. Weight bias in work settings—a qualitative review. *Obesity Facts* 3(1):33-40.

Gorsky, R. D., E. Pamuk, D. F. Williamson, P. A. Shaffer, and J. P. Koplan. 1996. The 25-year health care costs of women who remain overweight after 40 years of age. *American Journal of Preventive Medicine* 12(5):388-394.

Gortmaker, S. L., A. Must, J. M. Perrin, A. M. Sobol, and W. H. Dietz. 1993. Social and economic consequences of overweight in adolescence and young adulthood. *New England Journal of Medicine* 329(14):1008-1012.

Gray, W. N., S. L. Simon, D. M. Janicke, and M. Dumont-Driscoll. 2011. Moderators of weight-based stigmatization among youth who are overweight and non-overweight: The role of gender, race, and body dissatisfaction. *Journal of Developmental and Behavioral Pediatrics* 32(2):110-116.

Groessl, E. J., R. M. Kaplan, E. Barrett-Connor, and T. G. Ganiats. 2004. Body mass index and quality of well-being in a community of older adults. *American Journal of Preventive Medicine* 26(2):126-129.

Gunstad, J., R. H. Paul, R. A. Cohen, D. F. Tate, and E. Gordon. 2006. Obesity is associated with memory deficits in young and middle-aged adults. *Eating and Weight Disorders* 11(1):e15-e19.

Hammond, R. A., and R. Levine. 2010. The economic impact of obesity in the United States. *Diabetes, Metabolic Syndrome and Obesity: Targets and Therapy* 3:285-295.

Han, E., E. C. Norton, and L. M. Powell. 2011. Direct and indirect effects of body weight on adult wages. *Economics and Human Biology* 9(4):381-392.

Harris, J. L., M. E. Weinberg, M.B. Schwartz, C. Ross, J. Ostroffa, and K. D. Brownell. 2010. *Trends in television food advertising. Progress in reducing unhealthy marketing to young people?* New Haven, CT: Rudd Center for Food Policy and Obesity.

Healthy Eating Research. 2011. *Food and beverage marketing to children and adolescents: An environment at odds with good health. A research synthesis, April 2011.* http://www.healthyeatingresearch.org/publications-mainmenu-111/research-briefs-and-syntheses-mainmenu-114/287 (accessed January 3, 2012).

Healthy Weight Commitment Foundation. 2010. *Fighting obesity by balancing calories in with calories out-good health is good business: New website promotes healthy workforce culture.* http://www.healthyweightcommit.org/news/Good_Health/ (accessed January 4, 2012).

HHS (U.S. Department of Health and Human Services). 2001. *The Surgeon General's call to action to prevent and decrease overweight and obesity*, edited by HHS, Public Health Service and Office of the Surgeon General. Rockville, MD: Government Printing Office.

HHS. 2008. *2008 Physical Activity Guidelines for Americans*. http://www.health.gov/paguidelines/guidelines/default.aspx (accessed January 4, 2012).

HHS. 2009. *ARRA prevention and wellness: Communities putting prevention to work funding opportunities announcement (FOA)*. https://www.cfda.gov/index?s= program&mode=form&tab=step1&id=a95be544fa1fddcece3663dade4b9e35 (accessed January 4, 2012).

Hofferth, S. L. 2009. Changes in American children's time-1997 to 2003. *Electronic International Journal of Time Use Research* 6(1):26.

Hofferth, S. L., and J. F. Sandberg. 2001. Changes in American children's time— 1981-1997. In *Children at the millennium: Where have we come from, where are we going*. The Netherlands. Pp. 193-229.

IFIC (International Food Information Council). 2011. *Global trends in childhood obesity-related media coverage from Q1 2004 through Q3 2011*. Washington, DC: IFIC.

IOM (Institute of Medicine). 2005. *Preventing childhood obesity: Health in the balance*. Washington, DC: The National Academies Press.

IOM. 2006a. *Food marketing to children and youth: Threat or opportunity?* Washington, DC: The National Academies Press.

IOM. 2006b. *WIC food packages: Time for a change*. Washington, DC: The National Academies Press.

IOM. 2007a. *Nutrition standards for foods in schools: Leading the way toward healthier youth*. Washington, DC: The National Academies Press.

IOM. 2007b. *Progress in preventing childhood obesity: How do we measure up?* Washington, DC: The National Academies Press.

IOM. 2009. *Local government actions to prevent childhood obesity*. Washington, DC: The National Academies Press.

IOM. 2010a. *Bridging the evidence gap in obesity prevention: A framework to inform decision making*. Washington, DC: The National Academies Press.

IOM. 2010b. *School meals: Building blocks for healthy children*. Washington, DC: The National Academies Press.

IOM. 2011. *Early childhood obesity prevention policies*. Washington, DC: The National Academies Press.

Jacobson, S. H., and D. M. King. 2009. Measuring the potential for automobile fuel savings in the US: The impact of obesity. *Transportation Research Part D: Transport and Environment* 14(1):6-13.

Jacobson, S. H., and L. A. McLay. 2006. The economic impact of obesity on automobile fuel consumption. *The Engineering Economist* 51(4):307-323.

Johnston, C. S., C. A. Taylor, and J. S. Hampl. 2000. More Americans are eating "5 a day" but intakes of dark green and cruciferous vegetables remain low. *Journal of Nutrition* 130(12):3063-3067.

Kaestner, R., M. Grossman, and B. Yarnoff. 2009. *Effects of weight on adolescent educational attainment*. http://www.nber.org/papers/w14994.pdf (accessed December 28, 2011).

Kuczmarski, R. J., K. M. Flegal, S. M. Campbell, and C. L. Johnson. 1994. Increasing prevalence of overweight among U.S. Adults. The National Health and Nutrition Examination Surveys, 1960 to 1991. *Journal of the American Medical Association* 272(3):205-211.

Kumanyika, S. K. 2008. Environmental influences on childhood obesity: Ethnic and cultural influences in context. *Physiology and Behavior* 94(1):61-70.

Lenhart, A., K. Purcell, A. Smith, and K. Zickuhr. 2010. *Social media & mobile Internet use among teens and young adults*. http://pewinternet.org/~/media//Files/Reports/2010/PIP_Social_Media_and_Young_Adults_Report_Final_with_toplines.pdf (accessed December 29, 2011).

Let's Move Campaign. 2010. *The Partnership for a Healthier America: Supporting America's move to raise a healthier generation of kids*. http://www.letsmove.gov/partnership-healthier-america (accessed January 4, 2012).

Liu, J., K. J. Bennett, N. Harun, and J. C. Probst. 2008. Urban-rural differences in overweight status and physical inactivity among US children aged 10-17 years. *Journal of Rural Health* 24(4):407-415.

Lorson, B. A., H. R. Melgar-Quinonez, and C. A. Taylor. 2009. Correlates of fruit and vegetable intakes in US children. *Journal of the American Dietetic Association* 109(3):474-478.

Ludwig, D. S., and H. A. Pollack. 2009. Obesity and the economy: From crisis to opportunity. *Journal of the American Medical Association* 301(5):533-535.

Maayan, L., C. Hoogendoorn, V. Sweat, and A. Convit. 2011. Disinhibited eating in obese adolescents is associated with orbitofrontal volume reductions and executive dysfunction. *Obesity (Silver Spring)* 19(7):1382-1387.

Madden, M., and K. Zickuhr. 2011. *65% of online adults use social networking sites*. http://pewinternet.org/~/media//Files/Reports/2011/PIP-SNS-Update-2011.pdf (accessed December 29, 2011).

Madsen, K. A., A. E. Weedn, and P. B. Crawford. 2010. Disparities in peaks, plateaus, and declines in prevalence of high BMI among adolescents. *Pediatrics* 126(3):434-442.

Michaelowa, A., and B. Dransfield. 2008. Greenhouse gas benefits of fighting obesity. *Ecological Economics* 66(2-3):298-308.

Moreno, M. A., F. Furtner, and F. P. Rivara. 2011. Breastfeeding as obesity prevention. *Archives of Pediatrics and Adolescent Medicine* 165(8):772.

Narayan, K. M., J. P. Boyle, T. J. Thompson, S. W. Sorensen, and D. F. Williamson. 2003. Lifetime risk for diabetes mellitus in the United States. *Journal of the American Medical Association* 290(14):1884-1890.

NCCOR (National Collaborative on Childhood Obesity Research). 2012. *NCCOR: National Collaborative on Childhood Obesity Research*. http://nccor.org/ (accessed January 4, 2012).

NCHS (National Center for Health Statistics). 2010. *Health, United States, 2009. With special feature on medical technology*. Hyattsville, MD: NCHS.

NCHS. 2011. *Health, United States, 2010: With special feature on death and dying*. Hyattsville, MD: NCHS.

Nielsen, S. J., and B. M. Popkin. 2003. Patterns and trends in food portion sizes, 1977-1998. *Journal of the American Medical Association* 289(4):450.

NIH (National Institutes of Health). 2004. *Strategic plan for NIH obesity research*. Bethesda, MD: National Institute of Diabetes and Digestive and Kidney Diseases/National Heart, Lung, and Blood Institute.

NIH. 2011. *Strategic plan for NIH obesity research: A report of the NIH Obesity Research Task Force*. NIH publication no. 11-5493. Washington, DC: HHS.

Ogden, C. L., M. D. Carroll, L. R. Curtin, M. M. Lamb, and K. M. Flegal. 2010a. Prevalence of high body mass index in US children and adolescents, 2007-2008. *Journal of the American Medical Association* 303(3):242-249.

Ogden, C. L., M. M. Lamb, M. D. Carroll, and K. M. Flegal. 2010b. Obesity and socioeconomic status in children and adolescents: United States, 2005-2008. *NCHS Data Brief* (51):1-8.

Ogden, C. L., M. M. Lamb, M. D. Carroll, and K. M. Flegal. 2010c. Obesity and socio-economic status in adults: United States, 2005-2008. *NCHS Data Brief* (50):1-8.

Ogden, C. L., B. K. Kit, M. D. Carroll, and S. Park. 2011. Consumption of sugar drinks in the United States, 2005-2008. *NCHS Data Brief* (71):1-7.

Ogden C. L., M. D. Carroll, B. K. Kit, and and K. M. Flegal. 2012. Prevalence of obesity in the United States, 2009-2010. *NCHS Data Brief* (82):1-7.

Olds, T., C. Maher, S. Zumin, S. Peneau, S. Lioret, K. Castetbon, Bellisle, J. de Wilde, M. Hohepa, R. Maddison, L. Lissner, A. Sjoberg, M. Zimmermann, I. Aeberli, C. Ogden, K. Flegal, and C. Summerbell. 2011. Evidence that the prevalence of childhood overweight is plateauing: Data from nine countries. *International Journal of Pediatric Obesity* 6(5-6):342-360.

Olshansky, S. J., D. J. Passaro, R. C. Hershow, J. Layden, B. A. Carnes, J. Brody, L. Hayflick, R. N. Butler, D. B. Allison, and D. S. Ludwig. 2005. A potential decline in life expectancy in the United States in the 21st century. *New England Journal of Medicine* 352(11):1138-1145.

Ormond, B. A., B. C. Spillman, T. A. Waidmann, K. J. Caswell, and B. Tereshchenko. 2011. Potential national and state medical care savings from primary disease prevention. *American Journal of Public Health* 101(1):157-164.

Patterson, P. D., C. G. Moore, J. C. Probst, and J. A. Shinogle. 2004. Obesity and physical inactivity in rural America. *Journal of Rural Health* 20(2):151-159.

Piernas, C., and B. M. Popkin. 2011. Food portion patterns and trends among US children and the relationship to total eating occasion size, 1977-2006. *The Journal of Nutrition* 141(6):1159-1164.

Pew Research Center (Pew Internet and American Life Project). 2011a. *Internet adoption, 1995-2011.* http://pewinternet.org/Static-Pages/Trend-Data/Internet-Adoption.aspx (accessed December 20, 2011).

Pew Research Center. 2011b. *Tech usage over time.* http://pewinternet.org/Trend-Data-for-Teens/Usage-Over-Time.aspx (accessed December 20, 2011).

Poti, J. M., and B. M. Popkin. 2011. Trends in energy intake among US children by eating location and food source, 1977-2006. *Journal of the American Dietetic Association* 111(8):1156-1164.

Pronk, N. P., M. J. Goodman, P. J. O'Connor, and B. C. Martinson. 1999. Relationship between modifiable health risks and short-term health care charges. *Journal of the American Medical Association* 282(23):2235-2239.

Puhl, R., and K. D. Brownell. 2001. Bias, discrimination, and obesity. *Obesity* 9(12):788-805.

Puhl, R. M., and C. A. Heuer. 2009. The stigma of obesity: A review and update. *Obesity (Silver Spring)* 17(5):941-964.

Raczynski, J. M., J. W. Thompson, M. M. Phillips, K. W. Ryan, and H. W. Cleveland. 2009. Arkansas act 1220 of 2003 to reduce childhood obesity: Its implementation and impact on child and adolescent body mass index. *Journal of Public Health Policy* 30(Suppl. 1):S124-S140.

Ricci, J. A., and E. Chee. 2005. Lost productive time associated with excess weight in the U.S. workforce. *Journal of Occupational and Environmental Medicine* 47(12):1227-1234.

Rideout, V., U. G. Foehr, and D. F. Roberts. 2010. *Generation m2: Media in the lives of 8-18 year olds.* Washington, DC: Kaiser Family Foundation.

Robinson, J. P., and G. Godbey. 1997. *Time for life: The surprising ways Americans use their time.* University Park, PA: Pennsylvania State University Press.

Roger, V. L., A. S. Go, D. M. Lloyd-Jones, R. J. Adams, J. D. Berry, T. M. Brown, M. R. Carnethon, S. Dai, G. de Simone, E. S. Ford, C. S. Fox, H. J. Fullerton, C. Gillespie, K. J. Greenlund, S. M. Hailpern, J. A. Heit, P. M. Ho, V. J. Howard, B. M. Kissela, S. J. Kittner, D. T. Lackland, J. H. Lichtman, L. D. Lisabeth, D. M. Makuc, G. M. Marcus, A. Marelli, D. B. Matchar, M. M. McDermott, J. B. Meigs, C. S. Moy, D. Mozaffarian, M. E. Mussolino, G. Nichol, N. P. Paynter, W. D. Rosamond, P. D. Sorlie, R. S. Stafford, T. N. Turan, M. B. Turner, N. D. Wong, and J. Wylie-Rosett. 2011. Heart disease and stroke statistics—2011 update: A report from the American Heart Association. *Circulation* 123(4):e18-e209.

RWJF (The Robert Wood Johnson Foundation). 2007. *Robert Wood Johnson Foundation announces $500 million commitment to reverse childhood obesity in U.S.* http://www.rwjf.org/childhoodobesity/product.jsp?id=21938 (accessed January 4, 2012).

Sanchez-Vaznaugh, E. V., B. N. Sanchez, J. Baek, and P. B. Crawford. 2010. "Competitive" food and beverage policies: Are they influencing childhood overweight trends? *Health Affairs* 29(3):436-446.

Santos, A., N. McGuckin, H. Y. Nakamoto, D. Gray, and L. Liss. 2011. *Summary of travel trends: 2009 National Household Travel Survey.* Washington, DC: U.S. Department of Transportation and Federal Highway Administration.

Schwimmer, J. B., T. M. Burwinkle, and J. W. Varni. 2003. Health-related quality of life of severely obese children and adolescents. *Journal of the American Medical Association* 289(14):1813-1819.

Serxner, S. A., D. B. Gold, and K. K. Bultman. 2001. The impact of behavioral health risks on worker absenteeism. *Journal of Occupational and Environmental Medicine* 43(4):347-354.

Sturm, R. 2005. Childhood obesity—what we can learn from existing data on societal trends, part 2. *Preventing Chronic Disease* 2(2).

Taras, H., and W. Potts-Datema. 2005. Obesity and student performance at school. *Journal of School Health* 75(8):291-295.

The Economist. 2011. US consumer spending: How the economic slowdown has changed consumer spending in America. http://www.economist.com/blogs/dailychart/2011/10/us-consumer-spending (accessed November 11, 2011).

Thompson, D., J. Edelsberg, K. L. Kinsey, and G. Oster. 1998. Estimated economic costs of obesity to U.S. business. *American Journal of Health Promotion* 13(2):120-127.

Thompson, D., J. Edelsberg, G. A. Colditz, A. P. Bird, and G. Oster. 1999. Lifetime health and economic consequences of obesity. *Archives of Internal Medicine* 159(18):2177-2183.

Thompson, D., J. B. Brown, G. A. Nichols, P. J. Elmer, and G. Oster. 2001. Body mass index and future healthcare costs: A retrospective cohort study. *Obesity Research* 9(3):210-218.

Thorpe, K. E., C. S. Florence, D. H. Howard, and P. Joski. 2004. The impact of obesity on rising medical spending. *Health Affairs* Suppl. Web Exclusives:W4-480-486.

Trasande, L., and S. Chatterjee. 2009. The impact of obesity on health service utilization and costs in childhood. *Obesity (Silver Spring)* 17(9):1749-1754.

Trogdon, J. G., E. A. Finkelstein, T. Hylands, P. S. Dellea, and S. J. Kamal-Bahl. 2008. Indirect costs of obesity: A review of the current literature. *Obesity Reviews* 9(5):489-500.

Troiano, R. P., K. M. Flegal, R. J. Kuczmarski, S. M. Campbell, and C. L. Johnson. 1995. Overweight prevalence and trends for children and adolescents. The National Health and Nutrition Examination Surveys, 1963 to 1991. *Archives of Pediatrics and Adolescent Medicine* 149(10):1085-1091.

Trust for America's Health and RWJF. 2011. *F as in fat: How obesity threatens America's future*. Washington, DC: Trust for America's Health.

Tsai, S. P., F. S. Ahmed, J. K. Wendt, F. Bhojani, and R. P. Donnelly. 2008. The impact of obesity on illness absence and productivity in an industrial population of petrochemical workers. *Annals of Epidemiology* 18(1):8-14.

U.S. Census Bureau. 2009. *Households with a computer and Internet use: 1984 to 2009*. http://www.census.gov/hhes/computer/publications/index.html (accessed December 20, 2011).

USDA (U.S. Department of Agriculture). 2003. *Agriculture fact book 2001-2002*. Washington, DC: Government Printing Office.

USDA. 2007. *Special Supplemental Nutrition Program for Women, Infants and Children (WIC): Revisions in the WIC food packages—interim rule*. http://www.fns.usda.gov/wic/regspublished/foodpackages-interimrule.htm (accessed January 12, 2012).

USDA. 2010. *What we eat in America NHANES 2007-2008 data: Percentages of energy from protein, carbohydrate, fat and alcohol by gender and age in the United States*. http://www.ars.usda.gov/SP2UserFiles/Place/12355000/pdf/0708/Table_6_EIN_RAC_07.pdf (accessed December 19, 2011).

USDA/HHS. 2010. *Dietary Guidelines for Americans, 2010. 7th ed*. Washington, DC: U.S. Government Printing Office.

Uusitalo, U., P. Pietinen, and P. Puska. 2002. Dietary transition in developing countries: Challenges for chronic disease prevention. In *Globalization, diets and noncommunicable diseases*. Geneva, Switzerland: World Health Organization. Pp. 6-31.

Van Cleave, J., S. L. Gortmaker, and J. M. Perrin. 2010. Dynamics of obesity and chronic health conditions among children and youth. *Journal of the American Medical Association* 303(7):623-630.

Vander Wal, J. S., and E. R. Mitchell. 2011. Psychological complications of pediatric obesity. *Pediatric Clinics of North America* 58(6):1393-1401.

Wang, Y. C., S. N. Bleich, and S. L. Gortmaker. 2008. Increasing caloric contribution from sugar-sweetened beverages and 100% fruit juices among US children and adolescents, 1988-2004. *Pediatrics* 121(6):e1604-e1614.

Wear, D., J. M. Aultman, J. D. Varley, and J. Zarconi. 2006. Making fun of patients: Medical students' perceptions and use of derogatory and cynical humor in clinical settings. *Academic Medicine* 81(5):454-462.

White House. 2010a. *First Lady Michelle Obama launches Let's Move: America's move to raise a healthier generation of kids.* http://www.whitehouse.gov/the-press-office/first-lady-michelle-obama-launches-lets-move-americas-move-raise-a-healthier-genera (accessed January 4, 2012).

White House. 2010b. *Presidential memorandum—establishing a task force on childhood obesity.* http://www.whitehouse.gov/the-press-office/presidential-memorandum-establishing-a-task-force-childhood-obesity (accessed January 4, 2012).

White House Task Force on Childhood Obesity. 2010. *Solving the problem of childhood obesity within a generation: White House Task Force on Childhood Obesity report to the President.* Washington, DC: Executive Office of the President of the United States.

Willeumier, K. C., D. V. Taylor, and D. G. Amen. 2011. Elevated BMI is associated with decreased blood flow in the prefrontal cortex using SPECT imaging in healthy adults. *Obesity (Silver Spring)* 19(5):1095-1097.

Williams, K. J., C. A. Taylor, K. N. Wolf, R. F. Lawson, and R. Crespo. 2008. Cultural perceptions of healthy weight in rural Appalachian youth. *Rural Remote Health* 8(2):932.

Wolf, A. M. 1998. What is the economic case for treating obesity? *Obesity Research* 6(Suppl. 1):2S-7S.

Wolf, A. M., and G. A. Colditz. 1998. Current estimates of the economic cost of obesity in the United States. *Obesity Research* 6(2):97-106.

Woodward-Lopez, G., J. Kao, and L. Ritchie. 2010. To what extent have sweetened beverages contributed to the obesity epidemic? *Public Health Nutrition* 1-11.

Young, D. R., G. M. Felton, M. Grieser, J. P. Elder, C. Johnson, J. S. Lee, and M. Y. Kubik. 2007. Policies and opportunities for physical activity in middle school environments. *Journal of School Health* 77(1):41-47.

3

Goals, Targets, and Strategies for Change

Key Messages

- Now that obesity prevention efforts have some momentum, clarification of goals and targets for change going forward is essential.

- Goals for children, adolescents, and adults focus on prevention, with identification of specific behavioral targets and key outcomes for individuals and populations.

- An ecological model can be used to identify behavioral settings and sectors of influence in which and by which actions can be taken to improve environments for physical activity and healthful eating. Strategies for taking action are multifaceted and interrelated and include policy and legislative approaches, approaches that change organizational policies and practices and environments in communities and neighborhoods, health communication and social marketing approaches, and interventions in health care settings.

- Although there is not yet agreement on the set of specific strategies that will be effective, existing frameworks and successful models of social change can offer guidance on how to tackle the obesity epidemic utilizing a systems approach.

- Several major practical and policy considerations require close attention during the planning of strategies to accelerate obesity prevention, including the realities of the way Americans live, issues related to freedom of choice, food marketing to children and adolescents, potential adverse effects for

people who are obese, and effects on high-risk racial/ethnic minority and
low-income populations.

- Measures with which to track progress are critical. Progress in achieving
  obesity prevention can be assessed in the short term by indicators of change
  in the environments that influence physical activity and eating.

It is clear from the preceding chapters that tremendous strides have been made
in addressing the obesity epidemic, given the sheer amount of attention to the
problem and the number and coherence of efforts to address the epidemic and
bolster the scientific underpinnings and policy basis for taking action. Evidence
of the stabilization of obesity prevalence in at least some demographic groups
suggests that these deliberate initiatives to address the epidemic are on track, perhaps in concert with other, spontaneous countering forces. Given the scope and
scale of what is needed and the inevitability of a time lag before true progress can
be estimated, however, the developments to date create a unique opportunity to
restate goals and refine targets and approaches in order to accelerate progress. As
reviewed in this chapter, the goals themselves are clear with respect to the desired
outcomes, as well as the types of behavioral changes that are relevant. There is
not yet agreement on what specific set of strategies and actions will best curb and
ultimately reverse the trends of increasing obesity prevalence. However, existing
frameworks and successful models of social change can offer guidance on how
to tackle the obesity epidemic and strongly indicate the need to take a systems
approach, as described in Chapter 4.

GOALS OF OBESITY PREVENTION

The overall goal of obesity prevention is to create, through directed societal
change, an environmental-behavioral synergy to foster the achievement and maintenance of healthy weight among individuals and in the population at large (IOM,
2005). This goal reflects a focus on prevention of obesity development, that is,
primary prevention. Primary prevention emphasizes strategies that increase the

likelihood of shifting physical activity, eating, and weight management toward energy balance in the population as a whole, including those groups and individuals at high risk of becoming obese. In this report, primary prevention is viewed as relevant to the continuum of excess weight—prevention of the progression from normal weight to overweight, from overweight to obesity, and from mild or moderate to more severe obesity.

The logic of beginning obesity prevention during childhood is self-evident. At every life stage, from infancy onward, sustained excess weight and obesity increase the risk of longer-term obesity. In adults, obesity prevention targets those who enter adulthood with weight in the normal range, as well as those who may already be somewhat overweight or obese, to limit the severity of obesity and obesity-related health and social consequences. The need for effective preventive strategies is heightened by the seemingly intractable nature of established obesity, making the reduction of *incidence*—new cases of obesity—a priority. Effective treatments for established obesity continue to be elusive despite decades of research on treatment strategies, an active commercial weight loss industry, and a majority of U.S. adults trying to lose or maintain their weight at any given time. However, the need for prevention would persist even if effective treatments were available. In the absence of prevention, there would be a continual influx of people needing treatment (i.e., a majority of the population) such that the demand for treatment would exceed the supply.

Goals for Children and Adolescents

Goals for children and adolescents outlined in the Institute of Medicine (IOM) report *Preventing Childhood Obesity: Health in the Balance* (IOM, 2005) continue to inform actions at the national and community levels (see Box 3-1). For children and adolescents, obesity prevention means maintaining a healthy weight trajectory and preventing excess weight gain while growing, developing, and maturing (IOM, 2010). Goals include prevention of obesity and its adverse consequences during childhood, as well as longer-term prevention of obesity in adulthood, because children who are obese may remain so throughout life. Given the general increase in media attention to obesity as a result of the epidemic (see Chapter 2, Figures 2-7 and 2-8) and the potential for an increased focus on body size to foster inappropriate weight concern or dieting (Davison et al., 2003; Ikeda et al., 2006), an explicit goal has been added to those originally stated by the IOM (2005) to highlight the importance of maintaining a positive body image and avoiding excessive weight concern.

BOX 3-1

BOX 3-1
Goals of Obesity Prevention in Children and Adolescents

Individual Children and Adolescents

- A healthy weight trajectory, as defined by the Centers for Disease Control and Prevention body mass index (BMI) charts

- A healthful diet (quality and quantity)

- Appropriate amounts and types of physical activity

- Achievement of physical, psychosocial, and cognitive growth and developmental goals

- A healthy body image and the absence of potentially adverse weight concern or restrictive eating behaviors

Population of Children and Adolescents

- Reduction in the incidence of childhood and adolescent obesity

- Reduction in the prevalence of childhood and adolescent obesity

- Reduction of mean population BMI levels

- Improvement in the proportion of children and adolescents with dietary quality meeting the Dietary Guidelines for Americans

- Improvement in the proportion of children and adolescents meeting physical activity guidelines

- Achievement of physical, psychological, and cognitive growth and developmental goals

Examples of Possible Intermediate Indexes of Progress Toward Obesity Prevention in Children and Adolescents

- Increased number of children and adolescents who walk and bike to school safely

- Improved access to and affordability of fruits and vegetables for low-income populations

- Increased availability and use of community recreational facilities

- Increased play and physical activity opportunities

- Increased number of new industry products and advertising messages that promote energy balance at a healthy weight

- Increased availability and affordability of healthful foods and beverages at supermarkets, grocery stores, and farmers' markets located within walking distance of the communities they serve

- Changes in institutional and environmental policies that promote energy balance

SOURCE: Adapted from IOM, 2005, 2007.

Goals for Adults

As noted in Chapter 2, the major human and societal consequences of obesity culminate during the adult years, and these consequences can be mitigated by stabilization of weight in the adult population. The payoff for intervening during adulthood is immediate in reducing both human and societal costs by limiting the development or exacerbation of obesity-related diseases during adulthood. There is a payoff as well in the direct and indirect effects on the familial context for the development of childhood obesity (Seidell et al., 2005).

Gradual weight gain during adulthood is typical and is commonly, although erroneously, viewed as a part of normal aging (Lewis et al., 2000; Williamson et al., 1990). A gradual weight gain of 1 or 2 pounds per year means a gain of 10 or 20 pounds in 10 years and twice that in a 20-year period. For example, adults recruited from four geographic areas in the United States for the longitudinal Coronary Artery Risk Development in Young Adults (CARDIA) study at ages 18 to 30 gained an estimated average of 1 to 2 pounds annually during the 10-year period from 1985-1986 to 1995-1996 (Lewis et al., 2000). This weight gain shifted many people from the healthy weight range into the overweight range, from the overweight range into the obese range, or from a moderate to an extreme level of obesity. As shown in Figure 3-1, this weight gain was associated with substantial increases in the prevalence of overweight and obesity (body mass index [BMI] of 25 or greater) in both blacks and whites and both men and women: 52 percent to 76 percent of adults in these race/sex subgroups were in the healthy weight range (BMI 18.5 to 24.9) at the start of this period, but only 28 percent to 58 percent were in this range 10 years later; the prevalence of extreme obesity (BMI of 40 or more) at least doubled in all subgroups (Lewis et al., 2000).

Goals of obesity prevention in adults are shown in Box 3-2. They are similar in concept to those for children and adolescents but focus on the weight trajectories and related behaviors associated with aging and, in women, reproduction. Weight levels of adults and of children and adolescents are interrelated in that parents and other adults are role models for children and adolescents. Moreover, maternal obesity may have direct effects on the risk of obesity in children and adolescents through gestational factors (IOM, 2009; Norman and Reynolds, 2011).

TARGETS FOR BEHAVIORAL AND ENVIRONMENTAL CHANGE

The available evidence points to a specific set of widely agreed-upon behavioral changes that are likely to promote energy balance. These behaviors are identified

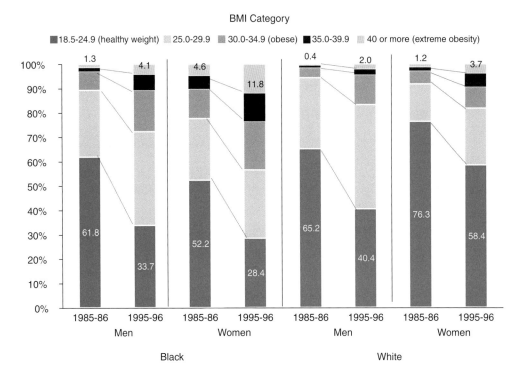

BMI Category

■ 18.5-24.9 (healthy weight)   25.0-29.9   ■ 30.0-34.9 (obese)   ■ 35.0-39.9   40 or more (extreme obesity)

FIGURE 3-1 Ten-year changes in the distribution of body mass index in the Coronary Artery Risk Development in Young Adults (CARDIA) study.
SOURCE: Lewis et al., 2000.

as essential elements in obesity prevention for children, adolescents, and adults, as appropriate to life stage (Box 3-3). For physical activity, targeted behaviors relate to specified amounts of physical activity following guidelines for children, adolescents, and adults and decreases in television viewing—a major form of physical *in*activity. For eating behaviors, the focus is on overall dietary quality as well as appropriate caloric consumption, achieved by increasing plant-based dietary components; reducing the consumption of sugar-sweetened beverages and of high-calorie, energy-dense foods; increasing breastfeeding and responsive child feeding; and ensuring the intake of nutrients needed to promote optimal linear growth.

In general terms, the types of environmental changes needed to motivate and support the indicated changes in individual behavior are directly related to the types of changes identified in the preceding chapters as having led to population-wide increases in weight gain and obesity and listed in Boxes 3-1 and 3-2 as

BOX 3-2
Goals of Obesity Prevention in Adults

Individual Adults

- Maintenance of weight during adult years, i.e., avoiding gradual incremental weight gain with increasing age

- Maintenance of waist size during adult years, i.e., avoiding gradual accumulation of fat around the abdomen

- Avoidance of weight regain after voluntary weight loss

- A high-quality diet with appropriate caloric intake (quality and quantity)

- Appropriate amounts and types of physical activity

- Appropriate prepregnancy weight, pregnancy weight gain, and subsequent post-partum weight loss

- A healthy body image and the absence of potentially adverse weight concern or restrictive eating behaviors

Population of Adults

- Reduction in the incidence of adult obesity

- Reduction in the prevalence of adult obesity

- Reduction of mean population body mass index (BMI) levels

- Improvement in the proportion of adults with dietary quality meeting the Dietary Guidelines for Americans

- Improvement in the proportion of adults meeting physical activity guidelines

- A population with weight and fitness levels conducive to a productive society

Examples of Possible Intermediate Indexes of Progress Toward Obesity Prevention in Adults

- Increased number of adults who routinely use active means of transportation, e.g., walking or cycling

- Improved access to and affordability of fruits and vegetables for low-income populations

- Increased availability, affordability, and use of community recreational facilities

- Increased opportunities to be physically active at work

- Increased number of new industry products and advertising messages that promote energy balance at a healthy weight

- Increased availability and affordability of healthful foods and beverages at supermarkets, grocery stores, and farmers' markets located within walking distance of the communities they serve

- Community designs and social characteristics that encourage being physically active outdoors

- Changes in institutional and environmental policies that promote energy balance

SOURCES: IOM, 1995; USDA/HHS, 2010.

BOX 3-3
Target Individual Behaviors for Obesity Prevention

Activity-related

- Increase physical activity/promote an active lifestyle.

- Children and adolescents get at least 60 minutes of physical activity per day.

- Adults aim for 150 minutes of moderate-intensity or 75 minutes of vigorous-intensity physical activity per week.

- Decrease television viewing.

Diet-related

- Increase the consumption of fruits and vegetables and legumes, whole grains, and nuts.

- Limit calories from added sugars, solid fats, and alcohol.

- Decrease the consumption of sugar-sweetened beverages/soft drinks.

- Increase breastfeeding initiation, duration, and exclusivity.

- Reduce the consumption of high-calorie, energy-dense foods.

- Parents accept their child's ability to regulate energy intake instead of eating until the plate is empty.

- Ensure appropriate micronutrient intake to promote optimal linear growth.

SOURCE: IOM, 2010.

potential intermediate indicators of progress. Thus, the needed changes relate to options for physical activity, factors that predispose to sedentary behavior, the food supply, and food availability and promotion. Potential strategies for effecting such changes are the focus of the remainder of this chapter.

A COMPREHENSIVE AND INTEGRATED APPROACH TO PREVENTING AND ADDRESSING OBESITY

Identification of the behavioral and environmental variables that contribute to the populationwide obesity epidemic and how they influence and interact with each other is needed to determine which prevention efforts are the most promising. Both the 2005 IOM report and the follow-up report, *Progress in Preventing Childhood Obesity: How Do We Measure Up?* (IOM, 2007) use an ecological approach to identify leverage points for developing effective intervention strategies to promote energy balance, and specifically address individual factors, behavioral settings, sectors of society, and social norms and values that may constrain or reinforce regular physical activity and healthful eating as the accepted and encouraged standard. Using the model shown in Figure 3-2, pathways can be drawn to identify specific influences on the weight-related behaviors of individuals in demographically diverse population groups, within and among the levels shown. Each type of setting shown (top left) and each of the several sectors that can be focal points for intervention (at right) are complex, and these settings and sectors are interrelated. The different levels at which interventions may be undertaken demonstrate how, if taken together, a set of actions across levels might interrelate. Therefore, this figure illustrates the overall complexity of influences on obesity, and shows that preventive actions must be comprehensive and can vary according to the diversity and interrelationships that apply. Homes and families are often listed under "behavioral settings," which would be appropriate. As explained in Chapter 1, however, the committee's approach emphasizes changes in settings and sectors that can accelerate obesity prevention by improving physical activity options and healthful eating, as well as facilitators at both the family or household and individual levels, taking into account their interdependence.

The influence of obesity on the economy, productivity, and population fitness was highlighted in Chapter 2, emphasizing the importance of addressing the epidemic not only for governments but also for businesses and the private sector. The "sectors of influence" on obesity in Figure 3-2 have, therefore, been updated from prior versions to highlight the potential contributions of businesses other than those directly involved in the manufacturing of products related to physical

90

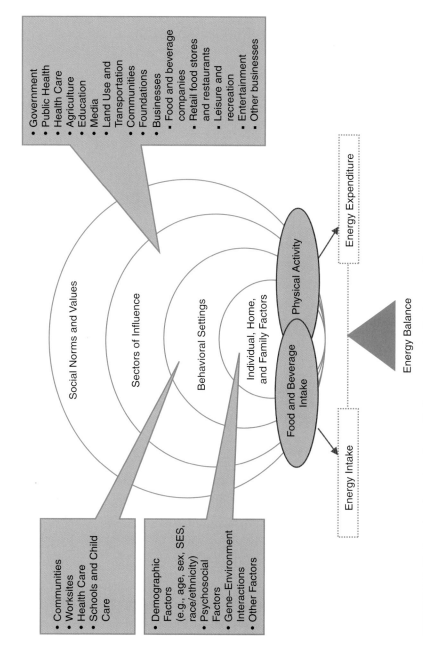

FIGURE 3-2 Various levels and sectors of influence on obesity in populations.
NOTE: SES = socioeconomic status.
SOURCE: Adapted from IOM, 2007.

activity and food. For example, businesses that provide catering or venues where the public eats—such as movie theaters, sporting event venues, and shopping malls—have a role to play in changing the availability of foods and norms about food consumption. Moreover, all employers, both public and private, increasingly are expected to foster work environments—including physical work settings, schedules, and health insurance coverage—that promote weight management and are conducive to good health for both employees and their families (Heinen and Darling, 2009). The *Guide to Community Preventive Services*, which represents the work of the Task Force on Community Preventive Services, recommends worksite programs for obesity control based on strong evidence of their effectiveness (Anderson et al., 2009). Results of a survey by Edelman (2011) indicate that the public expects businesses to contribute to health in a variety of ways in addition to providing health insurance coverage or worksite wellness programs, such as by educating people about the health risks of products or services, creating products and services that are conducive to good health, fostering a dialogue about public priorities related to health, and contributing funds or in-kind services to improve the health of the public. And the Partnership to Build a Healthier America, part of the First Lady's Let's Move campaign, works with food and beverage companies, as well as other companies, to generate meaningful sponsorship commitments that will increase physical activity and improve access to healthy, affordable foods (www.ahealthieramerica.org).

Thus, as emphasized throughout this report, obesity prevention in communities and populations requires social change. The strategies to be employed are similar to those applicable to other situations in which broad actions are needed to affect environments and the rules that apply to them. The Spectrum of Prevention, developed by Cohen and Swift (1999), is a framework for developing multifaceted approaches to address complex health problems and is commonly used in public health and health promotion. It identifies levels of increasing scope and emphasizes that effectiveness in addressing an issue requires integration across those levels: policy and legislative approaches; approaches involving changes in organizational policies, environments, and practices; approaches designed to foster changes in communities and neighborhoods; health communication and social marketing approaches; interventions in health care settings; and finally, multilevel, multisector approaches (IOM, 2010). The relevance of the Spectrum of Prevention as a typology for categorizing strategies relevant to obesity prevention is discussed in detail in the report *Bridging the Evidence Gap in Obesity Prevention: A Framework to Inform Decision Making* (IOM, 2010). Examples from that report are shown in Box 3-4.

As will become evident in Chapter 4, these examples help explain what is meant by population-based obesity prevention and are indicative of the types of actions—individual and combined—that often are recommended for obesity prevention.

A SUCCESSFUL MODEL OF COMPREHENSIVE CHANGE

To date, obesity prevention has not fully employed the complex thinking that is required to address the obesity epidemic. Applying the social change strategies described in this chapter to the community environment in order to encourage increased levels of physical activity, decreased sedentary behaviors, and healthful

Approaches Designed to Foster Changes in Communities and Neighborhoods

Strategies and actions could include advocating for zoning to limit fast-food establishments; facilitating the situating of supermarkets in underserved areas; increasing the availability of farmers' markets; creating and supporting community gardens; supporting safe routes to school; creating and maintaining a walking school bus; increasing the number of bike paths and parks; and enhancing walking infrastructure.

Health Communication and Social Marketing Approaches

Strategies and actions to prevent obesity can be enhanced through communication, marketing, and promotion and new technologies.

Interventions in Health Care Settings

Interventions could include annual screening for obesity, counseling about physical activity and diet, and expanded insurance coverage for behavioral and nutritional counseling.

SOURCE: Based on the "Spectrum of Prevention" in IOM, 2010.

eating is emerging as a practical way to address obesity on a large scale (de Silva-Sanigorski and Economos, 2010). Community-based obesity interventions (targeting policy and environmental changes) require an understanding of how social systems operate, how change occurs within and among systems, and how community changes influence individual behavior and health. Box 3-5 describes a working framework for such a whole-system approach to public health problems.

Shape Up Somerville (SUS): Eat Smart, Play Hard, conducted in Somerville, Massachusetts, illustrates the potential of a whole-system approach. Informed by previous social change models, this initiative was one of the first community-based efforts designed to change the environment to prevent obesity in early elementary school-aged children (Economos et al., 2009). The SUS intervention, as described by de Silva-Sangorski and Economos (2010, p. 59), is:

> focused on creating multilevel environmental change to support behavioral action and its maintenance and to prevent excessive weight gain among early elementary school-aged children through community participation. For example, specific changes within

7. Focus on the **embeddedness of action and policies** for obesity prevention in organizations and systems. Examples of this might include the visibility of obesity as an explicit policy goal or concern for non-health organizations, ongoing strategic commitment to obesity as a local concern, etc.

8. Focus on the **robustness and sustainability** of the system to tackle obesity. Ongoing strategies for resourcing existing and new projects and staff might be an indicator of this feature.

9. **Facilitative leadership.** This is leadership which is not necessarily located at any particular level or organization and is likely to encourage bottom up solutions and activities while providing strong strategic support where needed as well as appropriate resourcing.

10. Well articulated methods for ongoing **monitoring and evaluation** of activities, the results of which feed back into the system and drive change to enhance appropriateness and effectiveness. This relates to notions of the adaptability and learning capabilities of the systems/networks/partnerships established.

SOURCE: Quoted from NICE, 2011, pp. 14-15.

the before-, during-, and after-school environments provided a variety of increased opportunities for physical activity. The availability of less energy-dense foods, with an emphasis on fruits, vegetables, whole grains, and low-fat dairy products, was increased; foods high in fat and sugar were discouraged. Additional changes within the home and the community reinforced opportunities for increased physical activity and improved access to healthier food. To achieve this level of change, many groups and individuals within the community (including children, parents, teachers, school food service providers, city departments, policy makers, health care providers, before- and after-school programs, restaurants, and the media) were engaged in the intervention.

These changes were successful in bringing the community's overall energy equation into balance and were designed to be replicated as a cost-effective community-based action plan (de Silva-Sanigorski and Economos, 2010; Economos and Irish-Hauser, 2007).

Other large-scale, multilevel, community-based childhood obesity prevention initiatives in the United States, including Healthy Eating Active Communities[1] and Healthy Eating Active Living,[2] offer additional lessons for conducting this type of initiative through their resources and publications. These initiatives, begun in 2005-2006 by the California Endowment and Kaiser Permanente, respectively, have funded communities across the state of California (and now spreading across the country) to develop and implement a broad set of interventions focused on improving the physical activity and food environments for children in schools; health care facilities; after-school programs; neighborhoods; marketing and advertising venues; and other places where families live, learn, work, and play.

Similarly, acknowledgment of the responsibility to address obesity in the private and public sectors has been demonstrated globally. As reviewed in 2007, a number of countries and regions have been developing and implementing strategic plans to promote physical activity and healthful eating and to prevent obesity (IOM, 2007). Many of these plans and initiatives continue to evolve, and include the use of multiple types of actions; the development of partnerships, including private and public agreements; and the use of multiple settings, various sectors, and multiple levels of government (WHO, 2007).

An example is EPODE (Together Let's Prevent Childhood Obesity), a multi-stakeholder prevention program that focuses on facilitating the adoption of healthier lifestyles (Borys et al., 2011). Programs developed using the EPODE framework focus on long-term environmental and behavior change without stigmatizing culture, food habits, or overweight and obesity. EPODE began in France in 2003 and has since expanded to cover millions of people in Australia, Belgium, Canada, France, Greece, and Spain.

In 2008, the United Kingdom released a cross-government strategy titled Healthy Weight, Healthy Lives, designed to support people in maintaining a healthy weight. The marketing component of the United Kingdom's government response (called Change4Life[3]), begun in 2009, aims to change behaviors that lead to childhood obesity through a multistakeholder campaign. In 2010, the United

---

[1]Healthy Eating Active Communities. http://www.partnershipph.org/projects/heac (accessed November 14, 2011).

[2]Healthy Eating Active Living. http://www.convergencepartnership.org (accessed November 14, 2011).

[3]Change4Life. http://www.nhs.uk/Change4Life/Pages/change-for-life.aspx (accessed January 3, 2012).

Kingdom released a broader public health strategy entitled Healthy Lives, Healthy People, which sets out the national government's "long-term vision" for the future of public health in England: to provide support to and for local governments as leaders and those responsible for their communities' wellness.

As a final example, in 2008 Switzerland introduced its National Programme on Diet and Physical Activity.[4] This program "defines long-term goals and national priorities and provides a basis for collaboration between the various institutions and organizations working in the field."

PRACTICAL AND POLICY CONSIDERATIONS

This section highlights what the committee views as major practical and policy considerations requiring close attention during the planning of strategies to accelerate obesity prevention. Experience to date provides many examples of issues that can impede progress or lead to unintended adverse consequences. The committee's vision takes into account the need for strategies to be realistic, as well as consistent with fundamental values and principles. At the same time, however, having a diversity of values and priorities among them is itself a principle of U.S. society. Potentially competing values and principles must be reconciled, for example, in considering protections needed for individuals versus the community at large or for the public versus the private sector. Vigilance regarding unintended adverse effects of changes undertaken to address the obesity epidemic also is needed.

Raising awareness of obesity, drawing attention to the associated economic and health care costs, passing new laws or regulations, and implementing community action strategies to mobilize change all require resources, political will, and public support from those whose lives or livelihoods could be affected. Support for changes in living environments or the policies that govern them will vary according to the perception that those changes are needed and sensible, as well as what may be sacrificed if the changes are implemented. The potential for variation in political and public support is illustrated by results of an analysis of variables associated with the passage of state laws designed to reduce obesity prevalence between 2003 and 2005, a period when the number of such laws increased (Cawley and Liu, 2008). The probability of states enacting bills related to physical education, school nutrition, BMI screening, or health education differed according to adult obesity prevalence, the difference between self-reported and ideal weights

---

[4]National Programme on Diet and Physical Activity. http://www.bag.admin.ch/themen/ernaehrung_bewegung/05141/05142/index.html?lang=en (accessed January 3, 2012).

of adults in the state, the percentage of adults with a bachelor's degree or higher, income level, the percentage of the population living below the poverty line, the percentage employed in agricultural occupations, the percentage of blacks in the population, and the political party of the governor. The prevailing economic environment also has an impact. As this report goes to press, the United States continues to wrestle with a major economic crisis that influences the availability of public resources at the national, state, and local levels, as well as private and personal resources (Brown and Lundblad, 2009).

Realities of the Way Americans Live

Perhaps the most prominent and overarching of the practical realities associated with preventing obesity is that Americans are now accustomed to the very societal influences that predispose the average person to gain excess weight. "Obesogenic" environmental forces have been observed not only in the United States but also worldwide, driven by powerful economic and social forces that cannot easily be redirected and for which changes have interconnected and far-reaching effects that must be taken into account (Swinburn et al., 2011; WHO, 2000). Modern, technologically sophisticated lifestyles characterized by dependence on cars; jobs that require limited physical effort; labor-saving devices at home; sedentary entertainment; and the widespread availability of good-tasting, high-calorie foods and beverages are the cultural norm. Americans are steeped in a consumer culture in which many of the rewards of daily life, including food-related pleasures, are increasingly shaped by marketers and in which electronic media are a major source of information, social communication, and recreation for many people (Rideout et al., 2010).

If Americans are in equilibrium with or aspiring to obesity-promoting, modern lifestyles, what—short of a major shock—will it take to motivate and effect changes in the social fabric of the level and scope needed to create routine environments that foster healthy weight? Policy makers and other influential people must be convinced that the adverse health and societal consequences of current lifestyles outweigh the positives. They must then identify and support strategies and actions that will be acceptable with respect to gains and losses. They must resist strong counterpressures from those who see themselves as socially or economically disadvantaged by the changes that are contemplated. Public- and private-sector support and advocacy may be needed for policy adoption. Or, when policies are instituted without the need for public consultation or are not controversial, public- and private-sector support may be critical for implementation and eventual uptake and adoption.

The following example of the types of trade-offs involved is useful in visualizing what might have to happen to effect a major change in the proportion of the population engaging in active transportation such as walking or cycling. Using one's car less is inconvenient but may be acceptable if the cost savings (e.g., low public transportation fares and avoidance of fuel costs and parking fees), convenience (e.g., public transportation routes to necessary or popular destinations), social and aesthetic value (e.g., inviting destinations and pleasant scenery along the way), and safety (e.g., sidewalks along the entire route) of using alternative modes of transportation can be made attractive. Disincentives can also be used to equalize options (e.g., raising parking fees or tolls to discourage bringing cars into urban areas) but would presumably generate much more public opposition than incentive-oriented strategies. Trade-offs also must be balanced to avoid opposition from the automobile industry—including companies that produce and sell cars and the people and communities for whom this industry is a key part of the economy. At the level of social norms and consumer culture, ways to replace the use of cars as a status symbol also may be needed.

Environmental and Policy-Level Intervention Versus Freedom of Choice

Concern that intervening to change environments will inappropriately and unfairly constrain individual freedom of choice is a continuing part of the debate about how to address the obesity epidemic (Kersh, 2009). Such concerns often relate to public policy (i.e., government interventions related to schools and public places), but they may also apply to interventions to change policies or environments at places of employment within private-sector worksites. The importance of protecting individual freedoms has a level of political and public support in the United States that may be unparalleled in other democratic societies. Those who raise concern about the potential loss of individual freedom assert that what people eat (or what their children eat) or whether people walk or use their car or drive their children to school are personal choices, and that government should not intervene to limit these choices. Closely related to this perspective is the argument that obesity results primarily from a failure of personal responsibility to control food intake or, in the case of parents, of the responsibility to feed their children appropriately. This perspective may be waning somewhat given that such "failures"—if signified by overweight and obesity—now affect a majority of adults in the U.S. population and a substantial proportion of the child and adolescent population, but it may still be perpetuated by prevailing biases and negative stereotypes about obese people (Andreyeva et al., 2008; Washington, 2011). Several, related counterarguments to the concern that environmental interventions are inappropriate or unjustified are reviewed below. People differ in the extent to which they are convinced by these counterarguments.

The Context for the Exercise of Free Choice Must Be Improved

Evidence suggests that the current range of choices related to physical activity and food intake is limited and biased toward the unhealthy end of the continuum such that policies are needed to improve the environment for free choice. Commonly cited examples are communities where streets and roads are designed in ways that do not permit pedestrian access, and food outlets or vending machines where all of the choices are relatively unhealthy (Rahman et al., 2011; Sallis and Glanz, 2006). In addition, high-calorie, low-nutrient packaged foods or certain items at fast-food restaurants may be the cheapest ways to obtain calories. Food prices may, therefore, indirectly constrain the range of choices if costs matter. The cost of healthier foods may be higher in terms of price, time needed to shop for healthier foods that are attractive and affordable, time taken away from other pursuits to spend in preparing food, or all of these.

Many Apparent Choices Reflect Habitual or Natural Responses to Environmental Cues

Theory and empirical data from the field of behavioral economics suggest that the majority of physical activity and eating behaviors are routine rather than choices made after deliberation about a set of options (Just and Payne, 2009; Just et al., 2008). In such cases, changing the environmental cues or "default choices" to routinely prompt healthier choices could cause favorable (from a public health perspective) shifts in population behavior (Angell et al., 2009; Frieden et al., 2010).

Individuals' Innate Regulatory Systems Are Overwhelmed

An evolutionary argument is related to the observation that human physiological responses to foods containing fat and sugar still are geared primarily to avoiding hunger and conserving energy, with no innate mechanisms to ensure maintenance of energy balance when such foods are available in high quantities and the demand or opportunity for caloric expenditure is low (WHO, 2000). In this scenario, even conscious efforts to prevent excess weight gain are likely to be ineffective.

Government Has a Responsibility to Protect Health

Ethical principles, as well as numerous precedents, can be cited to support the concept that government has a responsibility to protect the health of the public and therefore the authority to intervene in relevant societal sectors and processes (Economos et al., 2001; IOM, 2005, Appendix A; Kersh and Morone, 2002; Kersh et al., 2011). Precedents include laws that require the use of seat belts in cars or helmets while cycling, restrict the use of certain drugs, make it illegal to drive a vehicle while under the influence of alcohol, or restrict tobacco smoking in public venues, as well as laws supporting water fluoridation or fortification of foods with folic acid. In these cases, governments have determined either that it is essential to ensure that the interventions in question reach the general public without requiring an active choice on the part of each individual (e.g., water and food), or that rules about personal behavior are needed to protect individuals (seat belts or helmets or drugs) or the society at large (driving under the influence, secondhand smoke). Ethical arguments are particularly salient with respect to the government's responsibility to protect children and adolescents. Well-established precedents include child labor laws and policies that restrict the promotion and sale of tobacco and alcohol to children and adolescents (FDA/HHS, 2010; Miller, 2010; Toomey and Wagenaar, 1999).

Public schools, in particular, have an obligation to question and refute poli-cies that do not benefit their students and their communities and a corresponding responsibility to protect students, for whom school attendance is mandated, from harm (Crawford et al., 2011). Children and adolescents spend up to half their waking hours in school, where they may consume as much as one-third to one-half of their daily calories. Therefore, the school food environment is a logical focus for efforts to encourage healthy dietary behaviors. Today, school food ser-vice includes two competing arms—the federally regulated reimbursable National School Lunch and School Breakfast programs and the competitive food and beverage marketplace, which has expanded substantially during recent decades. Competitive foods and beverages are those sold throughout schools in vending machines, school stores, and snack bars and at fundraisers. They are typically of low nutritional quality, such as sweetened beverages, chips and other salty snacks, and sweets such as cookies and pastries (Crawford et al., 2011; Fox et al., 2009; Wechsler et al., 2001). Efforts to encourage children to eat nutritionally sound school meals are undermined by the provision of snacks and beverages that compete with healthier options (Crawford et al., 2011).

Students at schools providing nutritious food offerings still have access to a variety of food choices, along with the option of bringing foods from home. Their freedom of choice is not unjustly breached by limiting the availability of obesogenic foods on campus (Crawford et al., 2011).

Regulation of Food Marketing to Children and Adolescents

Aggressive marketing of high-calorie foods to children and adolescents has been identified as one of the major contributors to childhood obesity (IOM, 2006). The way in which products marketed as oriented to children and adolescents are made available and promoted has been shown to influence children and adolescents' food preferences and selections (IOM, 2006; WHO, 2010). Marketing of non-nutritious foods and beverages on public school grounds (e.g., in classroom materials, on sporting equipment, by signage), a common school fundraising technique in recent decades, undermines attempts to provide nutrition education in the classroom. Frequent exposure to this marketing in schools in low-income areas where children and adolescents are at greater nutritional risk is at odds with fairness and social justice (Crawford et al., 2011).

How to protect children and adolescents from potential adverse effects of such marketing is a major public health policy issue, argued primarily on ethical grounds and, in schools, on economic grounds. Statutory regulation of food marketing to children and adolescents has been proposed, on the grounds that children and adolescents are a vulnerable population in this respect because of their inability to understand the commercial intent of advertising (Hawkes, 2007; Pomeranz, 2010; Swinburn et al., 2008). Attempts to pass laws to this effect have not been successful, however, based on a ruling in 1978 that to restrict advertising would violate the First Amendment of the U.S. Constitution, which guarantees the right to free speech and extends this protection to commercial entities. A prior IOM report on this issue recommends that the food industry voluntarily restrict advertising of unhealthy foods and beverages to children and adolescents (IOM, 2006). A recent evaluation concludes that food and beverage companies have made moderate progress in this respect, with only limited progress being seen in other subsectors of the food industry (Kraak et al., 2011). Public health experts continue to conclude that statutory regulation will be needed to address the problem. They base this conclusion on comparisons of what has been accomplished through voluntary measures and what is perceived as being needed, as well as on increasing changes in advertising practices designed to circumvent the ability of children and adolescents to understand or defend against them (Goren et al., 2010; Harris et al., 2009). Current public- and private-sector efforts to standardize and strengthen ways of classifying foods as appropriate or inappropriate to advertise to children and adolescents could facilitate progress in regulating food marketing to children and adolescents through either voluntary or statutory means.

An important aspect of this challenge is the nature of the food industry—that is, the desirability of having a positive, cooperative relationship with the system that provides our food. Here the difference between the food and tobacco industries is paramount: tobacco products are intrinsically harmful and expendable whereas food is not, although the harm to health from current dietary patterns and excesses is clear. In the framework of Kersh and Morone (2002) regarding the type of climate that is sometimes necessary to generate public action on personal behavior, the tobacco industry can readily be demonized, but doing so is more difficult and less desirable with respect to the food industry. Nevertheless, there are noteworthy similarities in the public policy strategies proposed to change the behavior of the food industry and in the countering strategies used by the industry (Brownell and Warner, 2009), suggesting that strategies to address obesity cannot be naïve.

Effects on Children, Adolescents, and Adults Who Are Obese

Efforts to address the obesity epidemic must consider the potential impact of actions taken on those children, adolescents, and adults who are already obese. Environmental and policy changes that will make it easier to achieve and maintain energy balance should have positive effects across the continuum of body weight. However, the process needed to achieve these changes may inadvertently worsen the day-to-day lives of obese children, adolescents, and adults. The pervasive negative societal attitudes about obese people have been well documented, held by the general public; by employers; by schoolteachers and other professionals, including health professionals; and by children, adolescents, and adults who are obese (Andreyeva et al., 2008; Washington, 2011). Greater awareness of obesity may increase these negative perceptions and the bias and discrimination experienced by obese people. Emphasizing the costs of treating obesity may cause a backlash in which obese people are blamed for rising health care costs, including public expenditures for Medicaid and Medicare. Similarly, emphasizing effects of having a heavier population on infrastructure and other aspects of the economy may increase negative attitudes about obese people. Another potential adverse consequence, of particular importance for children and adolescents, is the inadvertent generation or aggravation of poor body image, low self-esteem, preoccupation with dieting, or inappropriate weight concern, which can impair healthy growth and physical and psychosocial development (Griffiths et al., 2010).

Kersh and Morone (2002) point out the troubling reality that movements toward government action on personal behaviors sometimes take an oversimplified view that begins with public disapproval or demonization of the affected population—e.g., alcoholics, drug users—as weak or irresponsible. Given the prevailing attitudes about obesity and the fact that it is more prevalent in low-income and minority communities, the same effect could occur in the case of the obesity epidemic. Policies and practices to address obesity must take this potential for harm into account and incorporate appropriate safeguards, including the institution of measures to track such outcomes. The case for addressing the obesity epidemic cannot be made at the expense of obese people. Ethical arguments can be and have been made against measures that penalize obese people. For example, when airlines began requiring passengers who were unable to fit safely into one seat to pay full price for a second seat, many major airlines were sued for discrimination. The Canadian Supreme Court formally prohibited airlines from charging obese passengers for additional seats. Despite the opposition, however, some airlines have kept such policies in place.

Careful consideration of the terminology used when discussing the topic and images used to illustrate obesity is warranted to avoid reinforcing negative stereotypes. In addition, making an effective case for universal interventions—that is, environmental and policy-level changes that do not rely on screening and identification of children, adolescents, or adults who are at high risk of obesity or are already obese (IOM, 1995)—will help mitigate potential adverse effects on individuals.

Effects on Racial/Ethnic Minority and Low-Income Populations

The potential for negative stereotyping and social disapproval also applies at the group level. Similar to the considerations for individuals, this means that drawing attention to the high prevalence of obesity in racial/ethnic minority or low-income populations, as in Chapter 1 of this report, must be done not only carefully with respect to terminology and imagery but also accurately with respect to evidence about what is driving the higher obesity rates in these groups. Specifically, a coherent body of evidence implicates relatively greater exposure to the types of environmental contributors that predispose to low levels of physical activity and excess energy intake in higher obesity rates among racial/ethnic minority and low-income populations (Kumanyika et al., 2008). For example, options for safe and affordable leisure-time physical activity are generally less common in racial/ethnic minority and low-income communities (Gordon-Larsen et al., 2006; Powell et al., 2006; Taylor et al., 2006). Likewise, food availability and promotion are less favorable to healthy eating patterns in such communities (e.g., fewer supermarkets selling a greater variety of foods; more fast-food restaurants; and more advertising of fast food and of high-calorie foods and beverages generally) (Grier and Kumanyika, 2008; Kumanyika and Grier, 2006; Taylor et al., 2006; Yancey et al., 2009). Black and Latino children and adolescents are particularly targeted by marketers of sugar-sweetened beverages and fast food, and their vulnerability to such advertising may be increased by their developmental characteristics, limitations on their ability to recognize when advertising is targeting them, and certain techniques used in multicultural marketing (Grier, 2009; Grier and Kumanyika, 2010; Powell et al., 2010; Tharp, 2001). It is unclear whether there are systematic neighborhood differences in the cost of healthy foods in racial/ethnic minority or low-income communities compared with other communities (Grier and Kumanyika, 2008; Krukowski et al., 2010). However, evidence indicates that the lowest-cost foods may be the least healthy (Drewnowski, 2009). Thus, households with limited resources may buy less healthy foods to stretch their dollars. It is worth noting that among immigrant populations, the prevalence of obesity tends to increase with duration of residence in the United States (Oza-Frank and Cunningham, 2010), a fact that also strongly implicates environmental factors in excess weight gain.

Sociocultural influences are part of the environment affecting physical activity and eating habits, and interact with other aspects of the environment (Swinburn et al., 1999). Characteristics of physical activity or food marketing environments and the high prevalence of obesity itself may influence social norms about physical activity and healthy eating, making higher weight, consumption of high-calorie foods and beverages, and sedentary behavior seem normal and appropriate. Body image norms that associate thinness with ill health and larger body sizes with good health and robustness may decrease recognition of clinically significant obesity and undercut motivation for weight control, particularly if large body size is normative in the community (Brown and Konner, 1987; Diaz et al., 2007; Kumanyika, 2008; Liburd et al., 1999). Ethnically targeted marketing, which incorporates cultural preferences, imagery, and traditions and relationship building with the targeted communities (Tharp, 2001), may reinforce cultural attitudes and preferences that favor the consumption of high-fat or high-sugar foods if these are the types of foods marketed. Some cultural preferences are based on foods that may at one time have been difficult to obtain but may now be overabundant in racial/ethnic minority communities (Kumanyika, 2006, 2008). With respect to low-income or food-insecure populations, retail food promotions such as two-for-one deals, 99 cent menus, or large portion sizes, which are for relatively less healthful foods, may hold appeal (Power, 2005). Also, foods that are promoted as normative and desirable for the general population may be attractive to consumers in low-income populations as symbols of belonging or participating in mainstream lifestyles (Power, 2005).

TRACKING PROGRESS IN THE CHANGE PROCESS

Examples of outcomes of interest for tracking progress in the process of change include (1) the quality, scope, reach, and intensity of effects of obesity prevention policies and programs, to answer the questions of what is being done and whether enough of the appropriate types of interventions are occurring to expect success and (2) improvements in intermediate measures of progress toward goals, such as the indicators listed in Boxes 3-1 and 3-2. Assessments should include measures relevant to reaching high-risk populations. Ideally, assessments of progress through interim measures would be traceable to particular intervention approaches and also to obesity outcomes.

The committee that produced *Progress in Preventing Childhood Obesity: How Do We Measure Up?* (IOM, 2007) concluded that the infrastructure for assessing progress was severely underdeveloped and inadequately conceptualized. That report includes specific guidance on needed approaches and provides an evaluation frame-work to facilitate adoption of these approaches. Several advances have since been made in the development of concepts and tools for assessing the success of obesity prevention efforts. These include the aforementioned IOM report on a framework to inform decision making on obesity prevention (IOM, 2010), several ongoing efforts to compile evidence on promising programs (Appendix B in IOM, 2010), recommendations for improving the likelihood that ongoing policies and programs can be well evaluated (Leviton et al., 2010), and the development of a detailed framework and process for assessing the strength of evidence for various policy and environmental change strategies undertaken to prevent childhood obesity (Brennan et al., 2011). With respect to the ability to track progress on interim environmental and policy changes and behavioral trends, the National Collaborative on Childhood Obesity Research (NCCOR [http://www.nccor.org/css]) has developed publicly available, interactive online databases to facilitate the identification of relevant resources—a catalogue of surveillance systems with data related to childhood obesity prevention and a registry of research measures for assessing physical activity and dietary intake (http://www.nccor.org/projects_registry_of_measures.html).

CONCLUSION

Although the obesity epidemic in the United States has been instrumental in bringing worldwide attention to the problem—as noted in Chapter 1 and illustrated by Figures 2-7 and 2-8 in Chapter 2, showing the increases in global as well as U.S. media attention to the problem—the epidemic extends across the globe. Extensive analyses and strategizing on how to approach the epidemic have taken and continue to take place in many countries, particularly in light of the implications of obesity for rising rates of cardiovascular diseases, diabetes, and other noncommunicable diseases globally (OECD, 2010; Swinburn et al., 2011; WHO, 2011). Among the most comprehensive efforts to understand the obesity epidemic, identify effective interventions, and formulate a national action plan was carried out by the Foresight Group in the United Kingdom (Foresight, 2007), which identified a broad range of factors that influence obesity and relationships among key factors in an effort to develop the most effective future responses to obesity for that country.

The consensus among stakeholders engaged in trying to address the obesity problem is that meaningful change on a societal level is needed if individuals' attempts to change their physical activity and eating behaviors are to be effective (Foresight, 2007; White House Task Force on Childhood Obesity, 2010; WHO, 2000). The needed societal changes must be achieved through a public health approach that focuses on policy change and interventions in the environments in which people live, learn, work, and play. Complex realities associated with the obesity epidemic include practical and policy considerations, some of which may impede progress or lead to unintended adverse consequences that must be addressed during the design, implementation, and evaluation of measures to accelerate obesity prevention. These considerations include the nature of modern lifestyles, uncertainty or ambivalence about whether or how governments or other decision makers should use policy strategies to shift population physical activity and eating behaviors, the tensions associated with attempts to regulate food marketing to children and adolescents, and the potential adverse effects of obesity prevention efforts on individuals and population subgroups that are most affected by obesity.

The relevant causal pathways, settings, and sectors for intervention in other high-income countries (e.g., Australia, Canada, Europe, and New Zealand) bear many similarities to those in the United States. Analyses and experiences from these countries—for example, with respect to taxation; regulation of food advertising; and school, health care, or whole-community interventions—or modeling of cost-effectiveness may offer rich opportunities to inform U.S. strategies. The committee recognized the potential value of learning from this broader experience. However, experiences in other countries underscore the importance of tailoring and adapting strategies to policy mechanisms, environmental characteristics, health care systems and other institutional infrastructures, and sociocultural norms and values that apply nationally, regionally, and locally.

REFERENCES

Anderson, L. M., T. A. Quinn, K. Glanz, G. Ramirez, L. C. Kahwati, D. B. Johnson, L. R. Buchanan, W. R. Archer, S. Chattopadhyay, G. P. Kalra, and D. L. Katz. 2009. The effectiveness of worksite nutrition and physical activity interventions for controlling employee overweight and obesity: A systematic review. *American Journal of Preventive Medicine* 37(4):340-357.

Andreyeva, T., R. M. Puhl, and K. D. Brownell. 2008. Changes in perceived weight discrimination among Americans, 1995-1996 through 2004-2006. *Obesity (Silver Spring)* 16(5):1129-1134.

Angell, S. Y., L. D. Silver, G. P. Goldstein, C. M. Johnson, D. R. Deitcher, T. R. Frieden, and M. T. Bassett. 2009. Cholesterol control beyond the clinic: New York City's trans fat restriction. *Annals of Internal Medicine* 151(2):129-134.

Borys, J. M., Y. Le Bodo, S. A. Jebb, J. C. Seidell, C. Summerbell, D. Richard, S. De Henauw, L. A. Moreno, M. Romon, T. L. Visscher, S. Raffin, and B. Swinburn. 2011. EPODE approach for childhood obesity prevention: Methods, progress and international development. *Obesity Reviews*. Epub ahead of print.

Brennan, L., S. Castro, R. C. Brownson, J. Claus, and C. T. Orleans. 2011. Accelerating evidence reviews and broadening evidence standards to identify effective, promising, and emerging policy and environmental strategies for prevention of childhood obesity. *Annual Review of Public Health* 32:199-223.

Brown, G. W., and C. Lundblad. 2009. *The U.S. economic crisis: Root causes and the road to recovery: Return to prosperity requires reversal of excessive consumption, low savings trends.* http://www.journalofaccountancy.com/Issues/2009/Oct/20091781.htm (accessed November 9, 2011).

Brown, P. J., and M. Konner. 1987. An anthropological perspective on obesity. *Annals of the New York Academy of Sciences* 499:29-46.

Brownell, K. D., and K. E. Warner. 2009. The perils of ignoring history: Big tobacco played dirty and millions died. How similar is big food? *Milbank Quarterly* 87(1):259-294.

Cawley, J., and F. Liu. 2008. Correlates of state legislative action to prevent childhood obesity. *Obesity (Silver Spring)* 16(1):162-167.

Cohen, L., and S. Swift. 1999. The spectrum of prevention: Developing a comprehensive approach to injury prevention. *Injury Prevention* 5(3):203-207.

Crawford, P. B., W. Gosliner, and H. Kayman. 2011. The ethical basis for promoting nutritional health in public schools in the United States. *Preventing Chronic Disease* 8(5):A98.

Davison, K. K., C. N. Markey, and L. L. Birch. 2003. A longitudinal examination of patterns in girls' weight concerns and body dissatisfaction from ages 5 to 9 years. *International Journal of Eating Disorders* 33(3):320-332.

de Silva-Sanigorski, A. M., and C. Economos. 2010. Evidence of multi-setting approaches for obesity prevention: Translation to best practice. In *Preventing childhood obesity: Evidence, policy, and practice*, edited by E. Waters, J. C. Seidell, B. A. Swinburn, and R. Uauy. Hoboken, NJ: Wiley-Blackwell. Pp. 57-63.

Diaz, V. A., A. G. Mainous, 3rd, and C. Pope. 2007. Cultural conflicts in the weight loss experience of overweight Latinos. *International Journal of Obesity (London)* 31(2):328-333.

Drewnowski, A. 2009. Obesity, diets, and social inequalities. *Nutrition Reviews* 67(Suppl. 1):S36-S39.

Economos, C. D., and S. Irish-Hauser. 2007. Community interventions: A brief overview and their application to the obesity epidemic. *Journal of Law, Medicine and Ethics* 35(1):131-137.

Economos, C. D., R. C. Brownson, M. A. DeAngelis, P. Novelli, S. B. Foerster, C. T. Foreman, J. Gregson, S. K. Kumanyika, and R. R. Pate. 2001. What lessons have been learned from other attempts to guide social change? *Nutrition Reviews* 59(3 Pt. 2):S40-S56; discussion S57-S65.

Economos, C. D., S. C. Folta, J. Goldberg, D. Hudson, J. Collins, Z. Baker, E. Lawson, and M. Nelson. 2009. A community-based restaurant initiative to increase availability of healthy menu options in Somerville, Massachusetts: Shape Up Somerville. *Preventing Chronic Disease* 6(3):A102.

Edelman. 2011. *Health barometer 2011: Global findings.* http://www.edelman.com/healthbarometer (accessed November 9, 2011).

FDA/HHS (U.S. Food and Drug Administration/U.S. Department of Health and Human Services). 2010. Regulations restricting the sale and distribution of cigarettes and smokeless tobacco to protect children and adolescents. Final rule. *Federal Register* 75(53):13225-13232.

Foresight. 2007. *Tackling obesities: Future choice—Project report, 2nd edition.* London, UK: Government Office for Science.

Fox, M. K., A. Gordon, R. Nogales, and A. Wilson. 2009. Availability and consumption of competitive foods in US public schools. *Journal of the American Dietetic Association* 109(Suppl. 2):S57-S66.

Frieden, T. R., W. Dietz, and J. Collins. 2010. Reducing childhood obesity through policy change: Acting now to prevent obesity. *Health Affairs* 29(3):357-363.

Gordon-Larsen, P., M. C. Nelson, P. Page, and B. M. Popkin. 2006. Inequality in the built environment underlies key health disparities in physical activity and obesity. *Pediatrics* 117(2):417-424.

Goren, A., J. L. Harris, M. B. Schwartz, and K. D. Brownell. 2010. Predicting support for restricting food marketing to youth. *Health Affairs* 29(3):419-424.

Grier, S. 2009. *African American & Hispanic youth vulnerability to target marketing: Implications for understanding the effects of digital marketing.* http://digitalads.org/reports.php (accessed November 11, 2011).

Grier, S. A., and S. K. Kumanyika. 2008. The context for choice: Health implications of targeted food and beverage marketing to African Americans. *American Journal of Public Health* 98(9):1616-1629.

Grier, S. A., and S. Kumanyika. 2010. Targeted marketing and public health. *Annual Review of Public Health* 31:349-369.

Griffiths, L. J., T. J. Parsons, and A. J. Hill. 2010. Self-esteem and quality of life in obese children and adolescents: A systematic review. *International Journal of Pediatric Obesity* 5(4):282-304.

Harris, J. L., J. L. Pomeranz, T. Lobstein, and K. D. Brownell. 2009. A crisis in the marketplace: How food marketing contributes to childhood obesity and what can be done. *Annual Review of Public Health* 30:211-225.

Hawkes, C. 2007. Marketing food to children: Changes in the global regulatory environment 2004-2006. Geneva, Switzerland: WHO.

Heinen, L., and H. Darling. 2009. Addressing obesity in the workplace: The role of employers. *Milbank Quarterly* 87(1):101-122.

Ikeda, J. P., P. B. Crawford, and G. Woodward-Lopez. 2006. BMI screening in schools: Helpful or harmful. *Health Education Research* 21(6):761-769.

IOM (Institute of Medicine). 1995. *Weighing the options: Criteria for evaluating weight-management programs.* Washington, DC: National Academy Press.

IOM. 2005. *Preventing childhood obesity: Health in the balance.* Washington, DC: The National Academies Press.

IOM. 2006. *Food marketing to children and youth: Threat or opportunity?* Washington, DC: The National Academies Press.

IOM. 2007. *Progress in preventing childhood obesity: How do we measure up?* Washington, DC: The National Academies Press.

IOM. 2009. *Weight gain during pregnancy: Reexamining the guidelines.* Washington, DC: The National Academies Press.

IOM. 2010. *Bridging the evidence gap in obesity prevention: A framework to inform decision making.* Washington, DC: The National Academies Press.

Just, D. R., and C. R. Payne. 2009. Obesity: Can behavioral economics help? *Annals of Behavioral Medicine* 38(Suppl. 1):S47-S55.

Just, D. R., B. Wansink, L. Mancino, and J. Guthrie. 2008. *Behavioral economic concepts to encourage healthy eating in school cafeterias: Experiments and lessons from college students, ERR-68.* Washington, DC: USDA.

Kersh, R. 2009. The politics of obesity: A current assessment and look ahead. *Milbank Quarterly* 87(1):295-316.

Kersh, R., and J. Morone. 2002. How the personal becomes political: Prohibitions, public health, and obesity. *Studies in American Political Development* 16(2):162-175.

Kersh, R., D. F. Stroup, and W. C. Taylor. 2011. Childhood obesity: A framework for policy approaches and ethical considerations. *Preventing Chronic Disease* 8(5):A93.

Kraak, V. I., M. Story, E. A. Wartella, and J. Ginter. 2011. Industry progress to market a healthful diet to American children and adolescents. *American Journal of Preventive Medicine* 41(3):322-333; quiz A324.

Krukowski, R. A., D. S. West, J. Harvey-Berino, and T. Elaine Prewitt. 2010. Neighborhood impact on healthy food availability and pricing in food stores. *Journal of Community Health* 35(3):315-320.

Kumanyika, S. K. 2006. Nutrition and chronic disease prevention: Priorities for US minority groups. *Nutrition Reviews* 64(2 Pt. 2):S9-S14.

Kumanyika, S. K. 2008. Environmental influences on childhood obesity: Ethnic and cultural influences in context. *Physiology and Behavior* 94(1):61-70.

Kumanyika, S. K., and S. Grier. 2006. Targeting interventions for ethnic minority and low-income populations. *Future of Children* 16(1):187-207.

Kumanyika, S. K., E. Obarzanek, N. Stettler, R. Bell, A. E. Field, S. P. Fortmann, B. A. Franklin, M. W. Gillman, C. E. Lewis, W. C. Poston, 2nd, J. Stevens, and Y. Hong. 2008. Population-based prevention of obesity: The need for comprehensive promotion of healthful eating, physical activity, and energy balance: A scientific statement from American Heart Association Council on Epidemiology and Prevention, Interdisciplinary Committee for Prevention (formerly the expert panel on population and prevention science). *Circulation* 118(4):428-464.

Leviton, L. C., L. K. Khan, D. Rog, N. Dawkins, and D. Cotton. 2010. Evaluability assessment to improve public health policies, programs, and practices. *Annual Review of Public Health* 31:213-233.

Lewis, C. E., D. R. Jacobs, Jr., H. McCreath, C. I. Kiefe, P. J. Schreiner, D. E. Smith, and O. D. Williams. 2000. Weight gain continues in the 1990s: 10-year trends in weight and overweight from the CARDIA study. Coronary artery risk development in young adults. *American Journal of Epidemiology* 151(12):1172-1181.

Liburd, L. C., L. A. Anderson, T. Edgar, and L. Jack, Jr. 1999. Body size and body shape: Perceptions of black women with diabetes. *Diabetes Educator* 25(3):382-388.

Miller, M. E. 2010. Child labor and protecting young workers around the world. An introduction to this issue. *International Journal of Occupational and Environmental Health* 16(2):103-112.

NICE (National Institute for Health and Clinical Excellence). 2011. *Whole system approaches to obesity prevention: Review of cost-effectiveness evidence.* http://www.nice.org.uk/nicemedia/live/12109/55093/55093.pdf (accessed November 9, 2011).

Norman, J. E., and R. Reynolds. 2011. The consequences of obesity and excess weight gain in pregnancy. *Proceedings of the Nutrition Society* 70(4):450-456.

OECD (Organisation for Economic Co-operation and Development). 2010. *Obesity and the economics of prevention: Fit not fat.* http://www.oecd.org/document/31/0,3746,en_2649_33929_45999775_1_1_1_1,00.html (accessed January 4, 2012).

Oza-Frank, R., and S. A. Cunningham. 2010. The weight of US residence among immigrants: A systematic review. *Obesity Reviews* 11(4):271-280.

Pomeranz, J. L. 2010. Television food marketing to children revisited: The Federal Trade Commission has the constitutional and statutory authority to regulate. *Journal of Law, Medicine and Ethics* 38(1):98-116.

Powell, L. M., S. Slater, F. J. Chaloupka, and D. Harper. 2006. Availability of physical activity-related facilities and neighborhood demographic and socioeconomic characteristics: A national study. *American Journal of Public Health* 96(9):1676-1680.

Powell, L. M., G. Szczypka, and F. J. Chaloupka. 2010. Trends in exposure to television food advertisements among children and adolescents in the United States. *Archives of Pediatrics and Adolescent Medicine* 164(9):794-802.

Power, E. M. 2005. Determinants of healthy eating among low-income Canadians. *Canadian Journal of Public Health. Revue Canadienne de Sante Publique* 96(Suppl. 3):S37-S42.

Rahman, T., R. A. Cushing, and R. J. Jackson. 2011. Contributions of built environment to childhood obesity. *Mount Sinai Journal of Medicine* 78(1):49-57.

Rideout, V. J., U. G. Foehr, and D. F. Roberts. 2010. *Generation M2: Media in the lives of 8- to 18-year-olds.* Menlo Park, CA: Henry J. Kaiser Family Foundation.

Sallis, J. F., and K. Glanz. 2006. The role of built environments in physical activity, eating, and obesity in childhood. *Future of Children* 16(1):89-108.

Seidell, J. C., A. J. Nooyens, and T. L. Visscher. 2005. Cost-effective measures to prevent obesity: Epidemiological basis and appropriate target groups. *Proceedings of the Nutrition Society* 64(1):1-5.

Swinburn, B., G. Egger, and F. Raza. 1999. Dissecting obesogenic environments: The development and application of a framework for identifying and prioritizing environmental interventions for obesity. *Preventive Medicine* 29(6 Pt. 1):563-570.

Swinburn, B., G. Sacks, T. Lobstein, N. Rigby, L. A. Baur, K. D. Brownell, T. Gill, J. Seidell, and S. Kumanyika. 2008. The "Sydney Principles" for reducing the commercial promotion of foods and beverages to children. *Public Health Nutrition* 11(9):881-886.

Swinburn, B. A., G. Sacks, K. D. Hall, K. McPherson, D. T. Finegood, M. L. Moodie, and S. L. Gortmaker. 2011. The global obesity pandemic: Shaped by global drivers and local environments. *The Lancet* 378(9793):804-814.

Taylor, W. C., W. S. C. Poston, L. Jones, and M. K. Kraft. 2006. Environmental justice: Obesity, physical activity, and healthy eating. *Journal of Physical Activity and Health* 3(Suppl. 1):S30-S54.

Tharp, M. 2001. Chapter 3, marketing in a multicultural environment. In *Marketing and consumer identity in multicultural America.* Thousand Oaks, CA: Sage. Pp. 57-90.

Toomey, T. L., and A. C. Wagenaar. 1999. Policy options for prevention: The case of alcohol. *Journal of Public Health Policy* 20(2):192-213.

USDA (U.S. Department of Agriculture)/HHS. 2010. *Dietary Guidelines for Americans, 2010. 7th ed.* Washington, DC: U.S. Government Printing Office.

Washington, R. L. 2011. Childhood obesity: Issues of weight bias. *Preventing Chronic Disease* 8(5):A94.

Wechsler, H., N. D. Brener, S. Kuester, and C. Miller. 2001. Food service and foods and beverages available at school: Results from the school health policies and programs study 2000. *Journal of School Health* 71(7):313-324.

White House Task Force on Childhood Obesity. 2010. *Solving the problem of childhood obesity within a generation: White House Task Force on Childhood Obesity report to the President.* Washington, DC: Executive Office of the President of the United States.

WHO (World Health Organization). 2000. Obesity: Preventing and managing the global epidemic. Report of a WHO consultation. *World Health Organization Technical Report Series* 894:i-xii, 1-253.

WHO. 2007. *Nutrition, physical activity and the prevention of obesity: Policy developments in the WHO European region.* http://www.euro.who.int/__data/assets/pdf_file/0013/111028/E90669.pdf (accessed January 4, 2012).

WHO. 2010. *Set of recommendations on the marketing of foods and non-alcoholic beverages to children.* Geneva, Switzerland: WHO Press.

WHO. 2011. *Global status report on noncommunicable diseases 2010: Description of the global burden of NCDS, their risk factors and determinants*. http://www.who.int/nmh/publications/ncd_report2010/en/ (accessed January 4, 2012).

Williamson, D. F., H. S. Kahn, P. L. Remington, and R. F. Anda. 1990. The 10-year incidence of overweight and major weight gain in US adults. *Archives of Internal Medicine* 150(3):665-672.

Yancey, A. K., B. L. Cole, R. Brown, J. D. Williams, A. Hillier, R. S. Kline, M. Ashe, S. A. Grier, D. Backman, and W. J. McCarthy. 2009. A cross-sectional prevalence study of ethnically targeted and general audience outdoor obesity-related advertising. *Milbank Quarterly* 87(1):155-184.

4

Study Approach

Key Messages

- A systems perspective informed the committee's approach to developing its recommendations and identification of indicators with which to measure progress toward their implementation.

- Guiding principles were developed to inform the committee's decisions, including its critical review of prior obesity-related recommendations and identification of relationships and synergies among them.

- The committee identified five critical areas of focus necessary to accelerate progress in obesity prevention—the physical activity, food and beverage, message, health care and work, and school environments—that are linked as an interrelated system.

- For each critical area, the committee identified goals, recommendations, strategies, and potential actions with the greatest potential reach and impact on preventing obesity as outlined in the committee's guiding principles, based on research evidence and the current level of progress in each area.

- The identification of indicators of progress in implementing the committee's recommendations took into consideration (1) how well an indicator links to the goal of accelerating progress in obesity prevention, (2) its cost, (3) its availability in existing sources or ease of development in cases where sources are lacking, and (4) its ability to measure progress over the next decade.

As discussed in Chapter 1, the committee was tasked with developing a set of recommendations that, if implemented, would be likely to significantly accelerate progress in obesity prevention over the next decade, along with recommendations for tangible, practical indicators with which to measure progress. This chapter first describes the general approach used by the committee to identify critical recommendations for accelerating progress. It then outlines the committee's proposed approach to assessing the progress of these recommendations, including indicators for measuring progress, as well as the need to create a research framework based on the committee's general approach.

Before proceeding, a note on terminology is in order. In reviewing previous obesity-related recommendations as part of its charge, the committee found that a variety of terms were used to frame the advice provided, including "recommendations," "strategies," "actions," and "interventions." In this report, the committee uses the terms "goals," "recommendations," "strategies," and "(potential) actions" to denote levels of increasing specificity (see Box 4-1 for definitions).

BOX 4-1
A Note on Terminology

- **Goals** are the desired outcomes if recommendations are successfully implemented.

- **Recommendations** encompass the broad actions that need to be implemented and the responsible actors.

- **Strategies** are specific means of implementing the recommendations.

- **(Potential) actions** are activities that can help to implement the strategies.

In general, the term "recommendations" is used in the report to denote this full set of terms, whether describing previous work or that of the committee.

THE COMMITTEE'S GENERAL APPROACH

This section describes the approach used by the committee to formulate its recommendations for accelerating progress in obesity prevention, including the systems perspective that informed its deliberations and the development of a set of guiding principles.

A Systems Perspective

As noted in previous chapters, a systems perspective informed every aspect of the committee's approach to its task, including the development of its vision; identification of the need to engage individuals, families, communities, and society to catalyze change; integration of knowledge about the current environment; development of guiding principles; review of prior recommendations; formulation of recommendations, strategies, and actions with the greatest potential to accelerate progress in obesity prevention; and identification of indicators of progress. Systems thinking helped the committee identify areas in which change is needed and how actions taken in these areas can work synergistically to make the greatest impact on obesity prevention. Appendix B provides additional detail on the committee's use of a systems perspective.

Guiding Principles

As described in Chapter 2, obesity has imposed substantial social, health, and economic burdens on the U.S. population. The epidemic is a startling setback to major improvements in child health in the past century. Obesity has many causes; individual energy imbalance is influenced by environmental, cultural, and societal factors (e.g., food policies, the built environment, cultural norms) that ultimately affect personal decisions about physical activity and food intake. Exposure to these influences, both positive and negative, varies by subpopulation, with resulting disparities in the prevalence of obesity.

An urgent need exists to accelerate progress toward obesity prevention because prevention is a more sustainable population-based solution than treatment. Prior recommendations for obesity prevention have been proposed, but their fidelity and degree of implementation and integration have not been thoroughly evaluated.

Informed by a systems perspective as described above; a vision of what society would look like if obesity prevention were achieved (as detailed in Chapter 1); and an understanding of the complex social, political, and economic environment (as detailed in Chapters 2 and 3), the committee developed the following principles to guide its deliberations and decisions:

1. Bold, widespread, and sustained action will be necessary to accelerate progress in obesity prevention.
2. Priority and targeted actions must drive cultural and societal changes to improve environments that influence physical activity and food intake options.
3. Cultural and societal changes are needed to address obesity, and a systems approach must be taken when formulating obesity prevention recommendations so as to address the problem from all possible dimensions.
4. Solutions to the obesity epidemic must come from multiple sources, involve multiple levels and sectors, and take into account the synergy of multiple strategies.
5. Obesity prevention recommendations should be based on the best available scientific evidence as outlined in the Locate Evidence, Evaluate Evidence, Assemble Evidence, Inform Decisions (L.E.A.D.) framework (IOM, 2010).
6. The cost, feasibility, and practicality of implementing prior and further recommendations must be considered.
7. Unintended consequences of obesity prevention efforts must be considered.
8. Obesity prevention recommendations should incorporate ongoing evaluation of progress toward achieving benchmarks and of the need for any course corrections.
9. Recommendations to accelerate progress in obesity prevention must include an assessment of the potential for high impact, the reach and scope of potential effects, the timeliness of effects, the ability to reduce disparities and promote equity, and clearly measureable outcomes.

Approach to the Development of Recommendations

From the outset, a key aspect of this study was the tension between the reality that complementary interventions in multiple areas are needed and the fact that evidence and decisions about specific interventions often are generated without consideration of the larger systemic context. Therefore, the committee evaluated all potential recommendations for their potential impact on obesity based both on their theoretical or documented effects on physical activity or eating and on their potential links to other recommendations. The committee's step-by-step approach to the development of recommendations, which was informed throughout by the guiding principles outlined above, is depicted in Figure 4-1, described below, and discussed in greater detail in Appendix B.

Identification, Grouping, Organization, Review, and Filtering of Prior Recommendations and Identification of Gaps

As a first step, the committee was charged with reviewing previous obesity-related recommendations. To this end, the committee identified approximately 800 recommendations to review, as shown on the left of Figure 4-1. It then grouped and organized these recommendations and developed a process for reviewing and filtering them. The committee identified prior recommendations with the greatest reach and potential impact on obesity prevention, and prioritized them using the best available scientific evidence according to the L.E.A.D. framework, a framework that was developed to inform decisions on obesity prevention, integrating research evidence into a broader policy context (IOM, 2010). In this process, the committee took into consideration the progress made in implementing the recommendations, their ability to be evaluated or measured to assess progress or impact, the timeliness of their effects, any unintended consequences, their potential to reduce disparities in the risk of obesity, and the feasibility and practicality of their implementation. Throughout the process, gaps were identified and considered in formulating the committee's final set of recommendations. The process of locating, evaluating, and assembling the evidence is further detailed in Appendix B.

Identification of Linkages Among Filtered Recommendations

As recommended by the L.E.A.D. framework, the committee's approach included identifying relationships among recommendations and implementing strategies with the most promise to accelerate progress in obesity prevention and determining whether they could work together to make a larger impact. This process was informed by guidance from an expert in systems modeling and centered

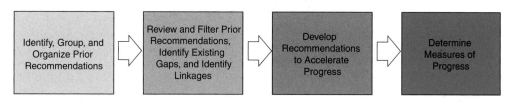

FIGURE 4-1 Overview of committee's approach to identifying recommendations to accelerate progress in obesity prevention.

around whether the recommendations and strategies of interest required, would enhance, or would be enhanced by any of the others under consideration. A qualitative tool—a systems map—was developed as an aid to visualizing and better understanding the interconnectedness of the recommendations and strategies and other factors that could improve or act as barriers to their implementation.

The results of this effort included the identification of five critical areas of focus for this study (see Figure 4-2)

- physical activity environments,
- food and beverage environments,
- message environments,
- health care and work environments, and
- school environments.

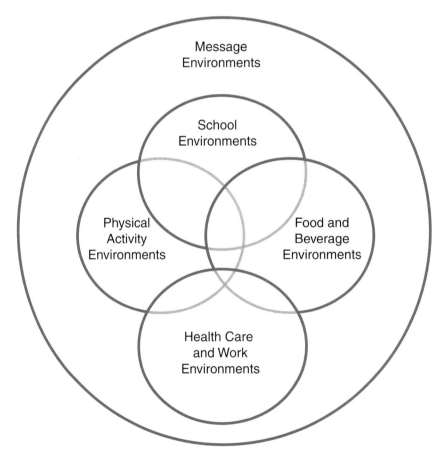

FIGURE 4-2 A simplified systems map illustrating the interconnectedness of the five areas of focus of the Committee on Accelerating Progress in Obesity Prevention.

These five areas constitute those in which major reforms are necessary to accelerate progress in obesity prevention: access to and opportunities for physical activity; widespread reductions in the availability of unhealthy food and beverage options and increases in access to healthier food and beverage options at affordable, competitive prices; an overhaul of messages that surround Americans (through marketing and education) with respect to physical activity and food consumption; expansion of the obesity prevention support structure provided by health care providers, insurers, and employers in every health care and workplace setting; and schools being made a major national focal point for obesity prevention. Appendix B provides the committee's detailed systems map, along with discussion of its development and interpretation; Chapters 5-9 each contain a simplified systems map (similar to Figure 4-2) highlighting the area addressed in that chapter. While a Venn diagram such as that in Figure 4-2 cannot illustrate the many and diverse interactions and feedback loops revealed by a systems map (as presented in Appendix B), it does reflect the critical areas of concern and their interrelationships.

Development of Recommendations

The final step was to formulate a recommendation in each of the five areas outlined above and to articulate the goal associated with each of these recommendations. The committee identified three to five strategies for each recommendation that, if acted upon, would have the greatest potential reach and impact on preventing obesity, based on research evidence and the current level of progress in each area, with guidance from the L.E.A.D. framework. For each strategy, the committee then devised a set of actions that would be likely to make a positive contribution to the implementation of that strategy based on research evidence or, where evidence is lacking or limited, have a logical connection with the strategy's implementation. The committee's stepwise approach to the development of recommendations, goals, strategies, and potential actions is illustrated in Figure 4-3. Chapters 5 through 9, respectively, present the committee's recommendations and goals in the five focus areas, the associated strategies and actions, the supporting research evidence, and the current level of progress in each area.

As described earlier in this chapter, the committee determined that accelerating obesity prevention will require synergy among various strategies and actions that, although important in themselves, would yield even greater benefit through complementary effects and mutual positive feedback. Box 4-2 provides an example to illustrate how action in a particular area might enhance or be enhanced by action

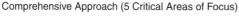

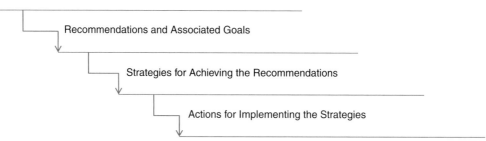

Comprehensive Approach (5 Critical Areas of Focus)

Recommendations and Associated Goals

Strategies for Achieving the Recommendations

Actions for Implementing the Strategies

FIGURE 4-3 The committee's stepwise development of goals, recommendations, strategies, and potential actions.

in other areas, previewing some of the strategies recommended in the critical area of school environments and linkages identified in the systems map (see Chapter 9 and Appendix B).

Finally, the committee considered the important role of two issues—leadership and prioritization—in the implementation of its recommendations and the acceleration of progress in obesity prevention over the next decade (see Chapter 10).

ASSESSMENT OF PROGRESS

Recommending potential indicators that can act as markers of progress in obesity prevention was one aspect of the committee's charge. Moreover, the committee believes that, to accelerate progress in obesity prevention, it is critical to identify and track progress in achieving each of the recommended strategies included in this report, as well as the overarching goal of reducing the prevalence and incidence of obesity and overweight. The committee's charge clearly stated that indicators of progress should be capable of being evaluated readily through the use of existing databases and/or measures or surveys that could be developed and implemented quickly in cases where existing sources failed to exist.

For purposes of this report, the committee defined an *indicator of progress* as "an objective measure that can be used to assess the effect of, or association with, a given strategy in accelerating progress toward obesity prevention." In identifying potential indicators of progress, the committee considered the following key factors

- the extent to which existing and/or potential indicators were linked with the overarching goal of accelerating progress in obesity prevention and/or with the individual strategies tied to each recommendation,

BOX 4-2
Example of Linkages Among the Committee's Recommendations

Consider a school district that would like to implement actions to improve its students' physical activity and food environments. Chapter 9 describes the committee's three strategies for implementing its recommendation related to school environments—making schools a focal point for obesity prevention: (1) require quality physical education and opportunities for physical activity in schools; (2) ensure strong nutritional standards for all foods and beverages sold or provided through schools; and (3) ensure food literacy, including skill development, in schools. Individually, the implementation of these evidence-based strategies will be important to prevent obesity, but they can most likely make a larger impact on accelerating obesity prevention by working together. Furthermore, it will be important for school districts to understand how these changes will influence, reinforce, or even be affected by other strategies that are implemented (or not implemented) outside of school. If schools invest in sports fields and open spaces as opportunities for students to participate in physical activity during the school day, not only will the activity level of the students be increased, but also will that of their families and others in the community if these spaces are available to them. That is, investing in and allowing joint use of the physical environment at the school will reinforce opportunities for activity for students after school and may encourage their families and other community members to make physical activity routine. Additionally, these school-based strategies support strategies in a variety of other areas. For example, physical education and physical activity in schools will contribute to making physical activity an integral and routine part of life (another critical recommendation). Also, food literacy in schools can help reduce overconsumption of sugar-sweetened beverages (a recommended strategy for food and beverage environments). This example illustrates how the committee's full set of recommendations and strategies support each other as a system for preventing obesity, increasing overall effectiveness from multiple directions and among multiple actors.

The systems map in Appendix B provides additional linkages among and across the committee's critical recommendations and related strategies.

- cost,
- the availability of an existing indicator or the ease of an indicator's development, and
- the ability to measure progress in the given strategy over the next decade.

A multilevel framework for developing the indicators of progress was developed. This framework (Figure 4-4) was designed to ensure that relevant and measurable indicators would be identified at multiple levels.

Referring to Figure 4-4, four levels of indicators of progress are used in this report. *Overarching indicators* focus on tracking progress in reducing the incidence and prevalence of obesity and overweight. These indicators are assumed to be the data that most clearly measure progress toward obesity prevention.

Primary indicators focus on measuring progress in factors most closely related to energy balance, the physiologic precursor to obesity. These indicators are those

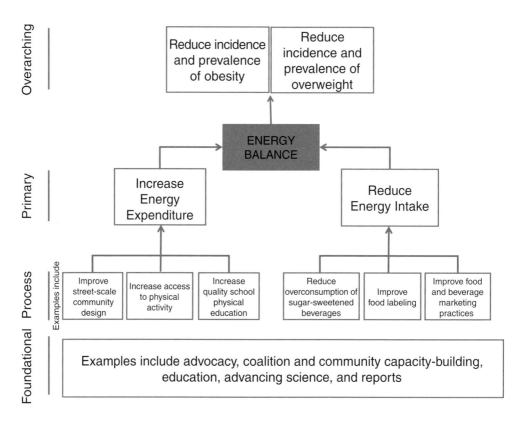

FIGURE 4-4 Framework for developing indicators of progress in accelerating obesity prevention.

most closely related to higher energy expenditure (increased physical activity) and lower energy intake (lower caloric consumption)—the two components of energy balance. If achieved, they should affect the overarching indicators of accelerating progress in obesity prevention.

Process indicators are more distal and relate to policies and environmental strategies designed to result in increasing the likelihood of energy balance. Examples include increasing the proportion of states and municipalities that adopt policies promoting enhancements to the physical and built environment that support increased physical activity.

Finally, *foundational indicators* relate to actions even further upstream that influence the broader dynamics involved in accelerating progress in obesity prevention (e.g., adoption of federal legislative and regulatory policies to increase domestic production of fruits and vegetables). Foundational indicators also relate to actions designed to specifically address health disparities for population subgroups disproportionately affected by obesity, physical inactivity, or excess caloric intake (e.g., reduced consumption of sugar-sweetened beverages among populations with higher rates of consumption of such beverages, including non-Hispanic blacks, Mexican Americans, and lower-income individuals).

The committee carefully reviewed each recommended strategy against existing data sources to identify indicators of progress at each level of the above framework. Additionally, the committee held a public workshop in March 2011 to obtain input on potential indicators and to identify areas in which systems for tracking progress on a given indicator are clearly needed. Because of the committee's emphasis on accelerating progress in obesity prevention nationwide, the focus was on identifying national data sources as the primary sources for proposed indicators that currently exist. As indicated in the committee's charge, however, indicators do not yet exist for many of the strategies recommended in this report. Therefore, it was necessary to identify new indicators that must rely heavily on commercial data or require the development of new data sources. The proposed indicators (both existing and new) are identified after each recommended strategy (throughout Chapters 5 through 9) and for the system of recommendations (near the conclusion of Chapter 10). Additionally, because many of the proposed indicators do not yet exist, the committee has identified this as an area in which additional work is clearly needed moving forward (see Chapter 10).

Finally, in conjunction with the identification of indicators of progress, the committee believes an important opportunity exists to create a research framework that would further the committee's systems approach. At the conclusion of Chapter 10, the committee offers a brief discussion of quantitative systems-science methodologies that could be used to further test and refine the set of recommendations in this report and in turn facilitate future decisions that may be necessary to address this dynamic, complex problem.

SUMMARY

In accordance with its charge, the committee drew on approximately 800 prior obesity prevention recommendations to identify critical areas for intervention that are fundamental to accelerating progress against the obesity epidemic. This process involved reviewing the evidence that supports these interventions, evaluating potential interventions according to a set of guiding principles, determining what indicators could be used to assess progress related to these interventions, and using a systems perspective to understand the potential for these actions to influence each other and drive change. The committee identified five critical environments for intervention: physical activity environments, food and beverage environments, message environments, health care and workplace environments, and school environments. These areas serve as the basis for the committee's five recommendations and respective goals, along with specific strategies and potential actions for implementation, as detailed in Chapters 5 through 9. When reading these next five chapters, it is important to remember that each recommendation, strategy, and potential action has positive potential to accelerate obesity prevention. However, the committee also emphasizes that its recommendations should be viewed together as a system, taking into account the potential for combined impacts (or synergies) and recognizing likely positive and negative interactions and feedback loops.

REFERENCE

IOM (Institute of Medicine). 2010. *Bridging the evidence gap in obesity prevention: A framework to inform decision making.* Washington, DC: The National Academies Press.

5

Physical Activity Environments

Physical Activity Environments: Goal, Recommendation, Strategies, and Actions for Implementation

Goal: Make physical activity an integral and routine part of life.

Recommendation 1: Communities, transportation officials, community planners, health professionals, and governments should make promotion of physical activity a priority by substantially increasing access to places and opportunities for such activity.[1]

Strategy 1-1: Enhance the physical and built environment. Communities, organizations, community planners, and public health professionals should encourage physical activity by enhancing the physical and built environment, rethinking community design, and ensuring access to places for such activity.

Potential actions include

- communities, urban planners, architects, developers, and public health professionals developing and implementing sustainable strategies for improving the physical environment of communities that are as large as several square miles or more or as small as a few blocks in size in ways that encourage and support physical activity; and

---

[1] Note that physical education and opportunities for physical activity in schools are covered in Recommendation 5, on school environments.

- communities and organizations developing and maintaining sustainable strategies to create and/or enhance access to places and programs where people can be physically active in a safe and enjoyable way.

Strategy 1-2: Provide and support community programs designed to increase physical activity. Communities and organizations should encourage physical activity by providing and supporting programs designed to increase such activity.

Potential actions include

- developing and implementing ongoing physical activity promotion campaigns that involve high-visibility, multiple delivery channels and multiple sectors of influence;

- developing and implementing physical activity strategies that fit into people's daily routines—strategies that are most effective when tailored to specific interests and preferences; and

- developing and implementing strategies that build, strengthen, and maintain social networks to provide supportive relationships for behavior change with respect to physical activity.

Strategy 1-3: Adopt physical activity requirements for licensed child care providers. State and local child care and early childhood education regulators should establish requirements for each program to improve its current physical activity standards.

Potential actions include

- requiring each licensed child care site to provide opportunities for physical activity, including free play and outdoor play, at a rate of 15 minutes per hour of care; as a minimum, immediate first step, each site providing at least 30 minutes of physical activity per day for half-day programs and 1 hour for full-day programs.

Strategy 1-4: Provide support for the science and practice of physical activity.

Federal, state, and local government agencies should make physical activity a national health priority through support for the translation of scientific evidence into best-practice applications.

For **federal-level government agencies,** potential actions include

- the Department of Health and Human Services establishing processes for the regular and routine communication of scientific advances in understanding the health benefits of physical activity, particularly with respect to obesity prevention (these processes could include, but are not limited to, regularly scheduled updates of the Physical Activity Guidelines for Americans and reports of the U.S. Surgeon General); and

- all federal government agencies with relevant interests developing priority strategies to promote and support the National Physical Activity Plan, a trans-sector strategy for increasing physical activity among Americans.

For **state and local health departments,** potential actions include

- developing plans and strategies for making promotion of physical activity a health priority at the state and local levels.

Physical activity is defined as any movement requiring "skeletal muscles that results in energy expenditure" (Caspersen et al., 1985, p. 126); exercise refers to a specific type of physical activity that is planned, repetitive, and purposeful in increasing physical activity (Caspersen et al., 1985). National guidelines for recommended levels of physical activity for the general health of both adults and children are for adults to engage in 150 minutes of moderate-intensity or 75 minutes of vigorous physical activity each week and for children to engage in at least 60 minutes of a combination of aerobic, muscle-strengthening, and bone-strengthening physical activity per day (see also Box 3-3 in Chapter 3). (It should be noted that, although 60 minutes or more of physical activity per day is recommended for children and adolescents, some studies suggest that a longer time period per day is more likely to be optimal [Andersen et al., 2006; HHS, 2008].)

Both physical activity and exercise are relevant to obesity prevention because both contribute to energy balance. Energy balance—defined as a total energy expenditure that is roughly equal to energy intake—is a steady state in which weight gain is minimized or prevented. Caloric excess occurs when total energy intake is greater than total energy expended. Total energy expenditure reflects the expenditure from physiologic functioning (metabolism) in a person of a given body size, as well as energy expended through routine activities of daily living, activities undertaken specifically for work and recreation, and exercise undertaken for health reasons. It is the routine or voluntary component of physical activity that is the focus of physical activity (or exercise) guidelines. Expending calories through activity raises the level of caloric intake associated with maintaining energy balance, i.e., before calories are "excess."

RECOMMENDATION 1

Communities, transportation officials, community planners, health professionals, and governments should make promotion of physical activity a priority by substantially increasing access to places and opportunities for such activity.

As described in the previous chapter, a simplified systems map illustrates the interrelationships among the five areas that structure the committee's recommendations. Figure 5-1 highlights physical activity environments, one of these five areas. Although the focus of this report is on accelerating obesity prevention, physical activity has far more health-enhancing benefits. Strong evidence indicates that participation in physical activity at or above the minimal equivalent of 150 minutes/week at moderate intensity for adults reduces the risk of coronary artery disease, stroke, type 2 diabetes mellitus, cancers of the colon and breast, hypertension, and an adverse lipid/lipoprotein profile (Physical Activity Guidelines Advisory Committee, 2008). Strong evidence also indicates that this amount of physical activity reduces the risk of depression and cognitive dysfunction specifically in older adults (Physical Activity Guidelines Advisory Committee, 2008). Moreover, there is moderate and emerging evidence for a variety of other beneficial health outcomes of physical activity in adults.

For children and adolescents, evidence indicates that 60 minutes of physical activity (including aerobic and bone- and muscle-strengthening activity) every day

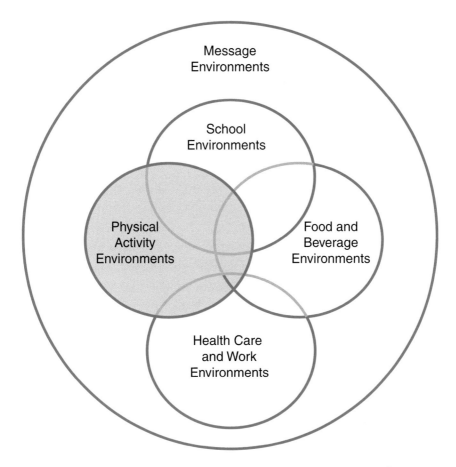

FIGURE 5-1 Five areas of focus of the Committee on Accelerating Progress in Obesity Prevention.
NOTE: The area addressed in this chapter is highlighted.

leads to important health benefits, including positive impacts on physical fitness, body fatness, cardiovascular and metabolic risks, bone health, and depression and anxiety (Physical Activity Guidelines Advisory Committee, 2008). In children, effects on body mass index (BMI) have been seen with 30 to 60 minutes of physical activity three to five times per week (HHS, 2008).

Physical activity promotion should therefore be a health priority. Currently, however, Americans are not meeting the physical activity recommendations summarized above. Results of the 2009 Behavioral Risk Factor Surveillance System survey indicate that approximately half of all U.S. adults engage in enough physical activity to meet the recommended time and intensity for substantial health benefits (CDC, 2009). Furthermore, the 2009 Youth Risk Behavior Surveillance System found that just more than 18 percent of adolescents (grades 9 through 12) nationwide are engaged in the recommended amount of physical activity, and almost one-quarter of adolescents are generally inactive (i.e., did not participate in the recommended 60 minutes of physical activity on any day during the week preceding the survey) (Eaton et al., 2010).

Any strategy that increases energy expenditure (when combined with restriction of energy intake) should be considered as a potential contributor to obesity prevention. Priority should therefore be given to evidence-based strategies for promoting physical activity at both the community and individual levels. Such evidence-based strategies exist (Heath et al., 2006; Kahn et al., 2002). However, studies specifically examining the role of energy expenditure in the prevention of obesity are limited; rather, the literature generally has focused on combinations of energy expenditure and energy restriction for weight loss. Indeed, age, gender, genetics, physical fitness, and other factors all appear to contribute to slightly different levels of energy expenditure in different people. Thus, creating a single-recommendation or target for physical activity to prevent obesity (without also considering energy intake) is nearly impossible. Some people are able to control their weight while being physically inactive, while others must constantly be physically active and restrict caloric intake to maintain a stable weight.

According to the 2008 Physical Activity Guidelines for Americans, "people who are at a healthy body weight but slowly gaining weight can either gradually increase the level of physical activity (toward the equivalent of 300 minutes a week of moderate-intensity aerobic activity), or reduce caloric intake, or both, until their weight is stable. By regularly checking body weight, people can find the amount of physical activity..." and the type of that activity that are individually effective in preventing unhealthy weight gain (HHS, 2008, p. 26). The guidelines further state that "it is important to remember that all activities—both routine and physical activity—'count' toward energy balance. Active choices, such as taking the stairs rather than the elevator or adding short episodes of walking to the day, are examples of activities that can be helpful in weight control" (HHS, 2008, p. 26). Associated with increases in physical activity, decreases in inactivity (or time spent at or near resting metabolism) should be minimized.

The amount of physical activity required to accelerate progress in obesity prevention requires understanding several concepts, including the volume, duration, intensity, and frequency of physical activity and volume of sedentary time:

- Total volume of physical activity is directly related to energy expenditure: the higher the total volume of physical activity, the higher the energy expenditure.
- The volume of physical activity in an individual in a defined time period is a function of duration (or length of time per physical activity event), absolute intensity, and frequency (or physical activity events per time period). Thus, the amount of activity is one expression of activity dose. Changes in duration, intensity, and frequency of physical activity will result in changes (increases or decreases) in energy expenditure. Energy expenditure is frequently used as a marker of activity dose.
- The intensity of the activity being performed is important. Intensity of physical activity is expressed as either relative or absolute. Relative intensity of physical activity is a measure of energy expenditure or work intensity based on the capacity of a person's physiologic systems to exercise. For weight control, vigorous-intensity activity (done at or above 6 times resting metabolism) is far more time-efficient than moderate-intensity activity (between 3 and 5.9 times resting metabolism) (Physical Activity Guidelines Advisory Committee, 2008). For prevention of weight gain and, by extension, prevention of obesity, absolute intensity of physical activity appears to be more important than relative intensity. Absolute intensity is the energy or work required to perform a given activity independent of the physiologic capacity of the individual. For aerobic activity, absolute intensity can be expressed as the rate of energy expenditure (e.g., kilocalories per minute, multiples of resting energy expenditure [metabolic equivalent of the task, or MET]) or, for some activities, simply as the speed of the activity (e.g., walking at 3 miles per hour, jogging at 6 miles per hour). For resistance exercise, absolute intensity is expressed as total weight lifted or force exerted (e.g., pounds, kilograms) (Physical Activity Guidelines Advisory Committee, 2008).
- Changes in energy expenditure can be assessed by increases in the total volume of physical activity or by increases (or decreases) in the total volume of sedentary time. Sedentary time is defined as total time in a defined period that an individual may spend engaged in activities with an energy demand at or near that which is required at rest.

Although increased attention has been paid in recent years to understanding the role of sedentary behavior in health and specifically in weight control, very little information is currently available on the relationship between reduced sedentary behavior (time spent at or near resting metabolic rate) and obesity prevention. A key part of obesity prevention is increased energy expenditure, and reducing sedentary behavior would appear to be a logical strategy for accomplishing this. It is unclear, however, whether a reduction in one type of sedentary behavior results in an actual increase in energy expenditure or a "transfer" of one sedentary behavior to another (e.g., reductions in television time may increase time spent reading or working at a computer). Studies of weight loss suggest that reductions in sedentary behavior (primarily television and video game time) may impact BMI (Robinson, 1999). However, evidence from recent randomized controlled trials suggests that the impact may paradoxically be due to changes in energy intake rather than expenditure (Epstein et al., 2008). More work is needed to understand the effectiveness of reducing sedentary behavior and its role in promoting energy expenditure for obesity prevention.

It is important to emphasize that the physical activity patterns of Americans cannot be changed solely by focusing on individual behaviors. Major technological innovations have substantially reduced the physical requirements of daily life. The dominance of the automobile as the most practical and convenient mode of personal travel and the steady decentralization of metropolitan-area population and employment (including schools, neighborhoods, shopping, and transit stops) to low-density, widely dispersed suburban locations have played a role in reducing physical activity (TRB and IOM, 2005). Barriers to walking, cycling, and other forms of physical activity for individuals and families are likely to differ among communities. And school-aged and more preschool-aged children in families with working parents are spending a significant amount of time in school and school-related activities and in child care for extended numbers of hours every day. Together, these environmental and lifestyle changes have influenced how much physical activity Americans engage in every day and where—recreationally, at home, at work, and everywhere in between.

To change American's physical activity patterns, the committee recommends that promotion of physical activity be a health priority in all sectors and organizations where children, adolescents, and adults live, work, play, worship, and attend school. Increasing the prevalence of children, adolescents, and adults who meet the 2008 Physical Activity Guidelines for Americans (HHS, 2008), coupled with appropriate caloric intake, should accelerate progress toward obesity prevention. The Task Force on Community Preventive Services (Heath et al., 2006; Kahn et al., 2002) has offered evidence-based recommendations for strategies to increase physical activity. These recommendations can be defined operationally as focusing on (1) environmental and policy strategies to enhance opportunities for physical activity, (2) strategies to promote school-based physical education and physical activity, and (3) individual behavior change strategies. The committee recommends these and other, related evidence-based strategies and implementing actions as the primary means of increasing physical activity in individuals and populations. These strategies and actions are detailed in the remainder of this chapter, with the exception of those related to physical education and opportunities for physical activity in schools, which are covered in Chapter 9, on school environments. Indicators for measuring progress toward the implementation of each strategy, organized according to the scheme presented in Chapter 4 (primary, process, foundational) are presented in a box following the discussion of that strategy.

STRATEGIES AND ACTIONS FOR IMPLEMENTATION

Strategy 1-1: Enhance the Physical and Built Environment

Communities, organizations, community planners, and public health professionals should encourage physical activity by enhancing the physical and built environment, rethinking community design, and ensuring access to places for such activity.

Potential actions include

- communities, urban planners, architects, developers, and public health professionals developing and implementing sustainable strategies for improving the physical environment of communities that are as large as several square miles or more or as small as a few blocks in size in ways that encourage and support physical activity; and
- communities and organizations developing and maintaining sustainable strategies to create and/or enhance access to places and programs where people can be physically active in a safe and enjoyable way.

Context

This strategy focuses on the environmental determinants of physical activity. The built environment is shaped by transportation and land use planning and policies, and can promote (or inhibit) physical activity during recreational/leisure time, work, household activities, and travel. It therefore provides an opportunity to address the decline in physical activity that has contributed to the obesity epidemic.

Over the past half-century, Americans have become more reliant on the automobile, and patterns of land use have been decentralized (TRB and IOM, 2005). These and other trends in travel behavior and where people live (urban, suburban, rural), changes in occupations, and zoning restrictions for mixed-use land development (e.g., for parking, multifamily houses, commercial use) have been influenced by institutional and regulatory policies and arrangements that have created today's built environment. Additionally, some of these policies and arrangements may over time have reinforced economic and racial separation (TRB and IOM, 2005). These and other broad societal trends have been thought to reduce opportunities for daily purposeful physical activity, giving way to the need to emphasize leisure-time physical activity or recreational physical activity and exercise.

Three intersecting characteristics that influence physical activity are part of the built environment: transportation infrastructure, land use patterns, and urban design (Frank and Engelke, 2001; Frank et al., 2003). Transportation infrastructure comprises the built elements designed to connect facilities and services, including roads and interstate highways, trails, sidewalks, and bicycle paths. Land use patterns (how land is used) are commonly characterized as residential; commercial; office; industrial; and nonresidential, such as parks or open space. Finally, urban design (the shape, form, function, and appeal of public spaces) includes the appearance and arrangement of physical elements within public spaces.

With reference to physical activity, the built environment consists of three geospatial scales. The smallest scale is the building or site, such as places of employment or schools. Next is the street scale, conceptualized as one or more city blocks around a certain point. Finally, the community or regional level of the built environment can include an entire municipal or metropolitan area or district that can measure several square miles.

Evidence

The Task Force on Community Preventive Services (Heath et al., 2006) recommends the use of evidence-based environmental and policy strategies to increase physical activity. Environmental and policy strategies to promote physical activity are designed to create or enhance opportunities, support, and cues to help people be more physically active. They may involve changes to the physical and built environment, changes in organizational norms and policies, or legislation. These strategies often are combined with informational outreach activities to enhance their effectiveness. Creating or enhancing access to places for physical activity—such as through community-scale and street-scale urban design and land use policies and practices—is one such evidence-based strategy found to be effective in increasing physical activity (Heath et al., 2006). Additionally, a recent review (Ding et al., 2011) suggests scientific support for environmental walkability, traffic speed/volume, access/proximity to recreation facilities, land use mix, and residential density as key environmental correlates of physical activity, specifically for children and adolescents. If coupled with restriction of energy intake, successful implementation of these strategies should accelerate progress toward obesity prevention.

Implementation

Enhancing the physical and built environment for physical activity involves changes in land use policies and practices designed to make entire communities and neighborhoods more amenable to physical activity, whether that activity is transportation related or exercise done purposefully in recreational or discretionary time. These changes can be applied to urban areas of several square miles or larger or to smaller, street-scale areas the size of a few square blocks. Implementation of many such changes is not a short-term strategy and will not likely result in immediate changes in physical activity patterns. Policy changes that seek to enhance the physical and built environment may take years to realize the goal of increasing physical activity participation.

Examples of communitywide strategies include improved connectivity of transportation arteries; landscaping and lighting to enhance the aesthetics and perceived safety of the community; tax incentives for developers to build sidewalks and trails in new developments; zoning changes to require pedestrian access; a communitywide program to encourage bicycling; coordinated policies to promote bicycle commuting; and community design planning and zoning that serve to increase the proximity of residential areas to such destinations as workplaces, schools, and areas for leisure and recreation to make them reachable safely by walking or bicycling. Examples of street-scale strategies include enhancements to increase safety and aesthetics for pedestrians and cyclists, such as marked street-crossing areas or pedestrian bridges over multilane highways; traffic-calming strategies, such as traffic circles, stop lights, and signs or speed bumps; bicycle lanes; and lighting, landscaping, and repair of street-level eyesores such as broken windows and graffiti.

Studies that have examined the utility of increased access to opportunities for physical activity have focused on strategies that make it easier for people to be physically active by changing the physical environment. Converting a former railroad bed to a hike and bike trail, reducing the cost of fitness center membership for employees in a company (economic access), and unlocking the school playground basketball court so it can be used on weekends are all simple strategies for increasing access. Such efforts should be accompanied by appropriate (and targeted) information that will communicate the existence of the resource to users.

Indicators for Assessing Progress in Obesity Prevention for Strategy 1-1

Primary Indicator

- Increase in the proportion of children, adolescents, and adults meeting the 2008 Physical Activity Guidelines for Americans.
  Sources for measuring indicator: BRFSS, NHANES, NHIS, YRBSS

Process Indicators

- Increase in the proportion of states and municipalities that adopt policies and supports for policies designed to promote enhancements to the physical and built environment that are supportive of increased physical activity.
  Source needed for measurement of indicator.

- Increase in the proportion of municipalities that enhance their physical and built environment infrastructure in ways that support physical activity consistent with the Task Force on Community Preventive Services Recommendations.
  Source needed for measurement of indicator.

- Increase in the proportion of municipalities with community-scale or street/neighborhood-scale enhancements that promote physical activity consistent with the *Guide to Community Preventive Services Task Force Recommendations.*
  Source needed for measurement of indicator.

- Increase in the proportion of municipalities that adopt and implement policies designed to promote access to places to be physically active.
  Source needed for measurement of indicator.

Foundational Indicators

- Increase in leadership in multiple sectors to increase awareness of the importance of the physical and built environment in promoting physical activity. *Source needed for measurement of indicator.*

- Increase in awareness of neighborhood and community disparities in characteristics of the physical and built environment that support physical activity. *Source needed for measurement of indicator.*

NOTES: BRFSS = Behavioral Risk Factor Surveillance System; NHANES = National Health and Nutrition Examination Survey; NHIS = National Health Interview Survey; YRBSS = Youth Risk Behavior Surveillance System.

Strategy 1-2: Provide and Support Community Programs Designed to Increase Physical Activity

Communities and organizations should encourage physical activity by providing and supporting programs designed to increase such activity.

Potential actions include

- developing and implementing ongoing physical activity promotion campaigns that involve high-visibility, multiple delivery channels and multiple sectors of influence;
- developing and implementing physical activity strategies that fit into people's daily routines—strategies that are most effective when tailored to specific interests and preferences; and
- developing and implementing strategies that build, strengthen, and maintain social networks to provide supportive relationships for behavior change with respect to physical activity.

Context

Routine physical activity will not just happen. It is important to support this behavior change by improving knowledge of the benefits of physical activity, increasing awareness of opportunities for physical activity in a community, and helping people participate in the activities that are available (Kahn et al., 2002). Additionally, careful consideration of the needs of specific populations in developing physical activity programs will increase the effectiveness and success of these interventions (Ransdell et al., 2009).

Evidence

This strategy focuses on the individual determinants of physical activity. The Task Force on Community Preventive Services (Kahn et al., 2002) recommends the use of evidence-based informational and behavioral and social strategies to increase physical activity. Examples include communitywide campaigns and behavioral and social support strategies. Such strategies have been shown to be effective in organizations (such as worksites) and communities for increasing physical activity in target populations.

Implementation

Communitywide campaigns Communitywide campaign strategies involve broad, cross-sectoral (e.g., transportation, education, parks and recreation, business, other community-based sectors), highly visible approaches to promoting physical activity. Such efforts can be combined with dietary change campaigns or focused solely on physical activity promotion. Information outreach to support such efforts should use multiple media (e.g., television, radio, Internet) to raise awareness of the program, disseminate various physical activity-related health messages, and reinforce behavior change. Targeted mailings and communications with key influences on people's attitudes and behavior, such as places of worship and community centers, can support the information campaign. Communitywide informational campaigns encompass many sectors. They frequently include highly visible, broadly targeted strategies and are part of broader health promotion strategies, such as heart disease prevention or cancer screening.

The scientific literature suffers from a lack of standardization in this area. Precise, unbiased and randomized evaluations of, and comparisons across, communitywide campaigns are difficult, and more proximal evidence may suggest an ambiguity in the effectiveness of such campaigns (Baker et al., 2011).

There is, however, reasonable evidence to support this type of strategy (Kahn et al., 2002), particularly if it is tailored to the target population. For example, the 10,000 Steps Rockingham program (Brown et al., 2006) was designed to increase physical activity in the entire adult population of Rockingham, Australia. The program made use of substantial social marketing strategies to increase awareness through information outreach, combined with other strategies, including use of pedometers. Results showed a nearly 5 percent increase in the number of women in the population who were classified as physically active relative to a comparison community. Although similar results were not found among men, these results suggest that such approaches can be effective.

Behavioral and social support strategies Behavioral and social support strategies for promoting physical activity involve either imparting behavior change and management skills or structuring the social environment so that it is conducive to such activity. Behavioral and social approaches may be designed to increase participation in physical activity as part of leisure, occupation, transportation, and/or at-home activities.

Individually adapted behavior change programs are tailored to the needs and preferences of individuals or groups. Such programs are designed to teach behavioral skills needed to make successful behavior adaptations to increase participation in physical activity. Social support strategies focus on building, strengthening, and maintaining social networks that provide supportive relationships for behavior change related to physical activity (e.g., setting up a buddy system, making contracts between people to complete specified levels of physical activity, establishing walking or other groups to provide friendship and support) (Task Force on Community Preventive Services, 2002). Social approaches are one way to make it easier to use those skills.

Largely unexplored, but with potential to increase the social support and behavioral strategies around individually adapted behavior change, are innovations in digital communications that allow for real-time prompting and tailoring of messaging relative to proximal circumstances. Such approaches, while transforming communication strategies in society at large, have only just begun to be integrated into health promotion strategies (Gibbons et al., 2011; Gold et al., 2011). Currently, there is no evidence of their effectiveness in physical activity promotion.

Strategy 1-3: Adopt Physical Activity Requirements for Licensed Child Care Providers

State and local child care and early childhood education regulators should establish requirements for each program to improve its current physical activity standards.

Potential actions include

• requiring each licensed child care site to provide opportunities for physical activity, including free play, and outdoor play, at a rate of 15 minutes per hour of care; as a minimum, immediate first step, each site providing at least 30 minutes of physical activity per day for half-day programs, and 1 hour for full-day programs.

Context

The first years of life are important to health and well-being throughout the life span. Data from the Centers for Disease Control and Prevention suggest that young children are not immune to the obesity epidemic. About 10 percent of infants and toddlers have high weight for length, and slightly more than 20 percent of children aged 2-5 are already overweight or obese (Ogden et al., 2010). Considerable evidence illustrates the importance of early-life strategies for the prevention of childhood overweight and obesity. Children do not "grow out of" obesity; rather, childhood obesity tends to persist into later life and can increase the risk for obesity-related disease in adulthood (IOM, 2011; Pocock et al., 2010).

The 2011 Institute of Medicine (IOM) report *Early Childhood Obesity Prevention Policies* notes that very little research has been conducted on the relationship between physical activity and health in infants, and that limited research has been undertaken on the relationship between physical activity and body weight in toddlers and preschoolers. Nonetheless, the prevalence of overweight and obesity clearly has increased in children within these age groups over the past 30 years (Ogden et al., 2010), and expert panels frequently have recommended that increased physical activity be targeted as one strategy for reducing the prevalence of obesity among these children (IOM, 2005; Strong et al., 2005).

The Early Childhood Program Participation Survey of the National Household Education Surveys Program found that approximately 80 percent of preschool-aged children with employed mothers were enrolled in some form of child care for an average of almost 40 hours a week (ECPP-NHES, 2006). Center-based care arrangements (e.g., child care centers, preschools, Head Start programs) were used by the majority of working parents; approximately 10 percent of working parents' children were enrolled in family child care homes. With such a high proportion of preschool children in child care arrangements, it is important to consider the role of child care providers in ensuring that children are receiving adequate amounts of physical activity while in their care (Larson et al., 2011).

Evidence

The committee that developed the recent IOM report on obesity in early childhood (IOM, 2011) was charged with conducting a comprehensive examination of the literature on factors related to overweight and obesity in infants, toddlers, and preschoolers (aged birth to 5 years), with a focus on nutrition, physical activity, and sedentary behavior; identifying gaps in knowledge; and making recommendations for policies to prevent early childhood obesity, taking into account the differences between children aged birth to 2 years and 2 to 5 years. Because many children in this age group spend much of their time in child care settings, that committee also examined the role of child care providers in ensuring that infants and young children are receiving adequate time and opportunities for physical activity.

Studies have found that infants should be provided time each day to move freely and explore their surroundings, with adequate supervision and a secure perimeter; although evidence in this area is limited, physical activity in infancy may help control excessive weight gain and maximize infants' developmental potential (IOM, 2011). In addition, studies suggest that structured physical activity sessions implemented in child care settings can be effective in increasing physical activity levels among preschool-aged children (Eliakim et al., 2007; Trost et al., 2008; Williams et al., 2009). The issue of whether prolonged bouts of sedentary behavior may have negative health consequences has been studied in adults (Hamilton et al., 2007; Hu et al., 2003) but not yet in young children. Nonetheless, the 2011 IOM report concludes that, based on the available data, it appears to be appropriate for young children to avoid long periods of inactivity in order to increase their opportunities for energy expenditure.

Implementation

After fully considering the available evidence, the committee that developed the 2011 IOM report formulated goals for increasing physical activity in young children. The report recommends asking child care regulatory agencies to "require child care providers and early childhood educators to provide infants, toddlers, and preschool children with opportunities to be physically active throughout the day," and to "require child care providers and early childhood educators to allow infants, toddlers, and preschoolers to move freely by limiting the use of equipment that restricts infants' movement and by implementing appropriate strategies to ensure that the amount of time toddlers and preschoolers spend sitting or standing still is limited." The report also provides potential actions for achieving these goals. The report recommends further that, because physical activity in child care settings provides children with important opportunities to expend energy, child care facilities ensure that toddlers and preschoolers are active for at least one-quarter of the time they spend in the facility, a documented median of activity for children of this age (IOM, 2011).

Strategy 1-4: Provide Support for the Science and Practice of Physical Activity

Federal, state, and local government agencies should make physical activity a national health priority through support for the translation of scientific evidence into best-practice applications.

For **federal-level government agencies,** potential actions include

• the Department of Health and Human Services establishing processes for the regular and routine communication of scientific advances in understanding the health benefits of physical activity, particularly with respect to obesity prevention (these processes could include, but are not limited to, regularly scheduled updates of the Physical Activity Guidelines for Americans and reports of the U.S. Surgeon General); and
• all federal government agencies with relevant interests developing priority strategies to promote and support the National Physical Activity Plan, a trans-sector strategy for increasing physical activity among Americans.

For **state and local health departments,** potential actions include

- developing plans and strategies for making promotion of physical activity a health priority at the state and local levels.

Context

Evidence-based strategies that increase caloric expenditure, when balanced with appropriate caloric intake, are likely to accelerate progress toward obesity prevention. The substantive increases in physical activity necessary to accelerate progress on obesity prevention will be difficult to achieve unless government agencies make this a scientific and public health priority. This strategy focuses on making physical activity a priority at the national, state, and local levels by advancing the science and practice of physical activity promotion. Progress has begun on this recommendation, but sustained, concerted, and multilevel efforts must be strengthened and continued.

Implementation

The establishment of science-based guidelines and recommendations is a cornerstone of public health leadership. Because increases in physical activity are necessary to accelerate progress toward obesity prevention, advancing science with respect to understanding of the health effects of physical activity and effective strategies for physical activity promotion is critical. The first and only U.S. Surgeon General's Report on *Physical Activity and Health* was published in 1996 (HHS, 1996), and the first and only comprehensive Physical Activity Guidelines for Americans were published by the Department of Health and Human Services in 2008 (HHS, 2008). These efforts served as point summaries for the state of the science regarding physical activity and health. Although the science base is continually expanding, however, there are currently no processes in place for regularly scheduled updates of these reports.

The U.S. Physical Activity Plan was published in 2009 (Coordinating Committee and Working Groups for the Physical Activity Plan, 2010). It represents the first comprehensive approach to organizing policies, programs, and initiatives that will increase participation in physical activity among the American population. Recommendations in the plan are organized around eight societal sectors: business and industry; education; health care; mass media; parks, recreation, fitness, and sports; public health; transportation; land use and community design; and volunteer and nonprofit. The long-term viability of the efforts associated with the U.S. Physical Activity Plan is critical to creating a culture in the United States in which physical activity becomes and remains a health priority.

Texas and West Virginia recently developed plans to help make physical activity a state and local health priority (Duke, 2010; West Virginia Physical Activity Plan, 2010). These efforts are focused on translating evidence and national-level recommendations on strategies to promote physical activity for state and local organizations. Such efforts must be supported and maintained if physical activity is to become a national health priority.

Indicators for Assessing Progress in Obesity Prevention for Strategy 1-4

Process Indicator

- Increase in the prevalence of state and local public health planning efforts specifically designed to promote physical activity.
  Source needed for measurement of indicator.

Foundational Indicators

- Processes in place for scheduled updates to the Physical Activity Guidelines for Americans.
  Source needed for measurement of indicator.

- Evidence from federal agencies (e.g., HHS, DOT, DOE) and national nonprofits (e.g., YMCA, BGCA, NRPA) that the U.S. Physical Activity Plan is guiding decision making and program prioritization.
  Source needed for measurement of indicator.

NOTE: BGCA = Boys and Girls Club of America; DOE = U.S. Department of Education; DOT = U.S. Department of Transportation; HHS = U.S. Department of Health and Human Services; NRPA = National Parks and Recreation Association; YMCA = Young Men's Christian Association.

INTEGRATION OF STRATEGIES FOR ACCELERATING PROGRESS IN OBESITY PREVENTION

Increases in energy expenditure through increases in physical activity at the individual and population levels are central to maintaining energy balance and weight stability and therefore to obesity prevention. Evidence-based strategies for promoting physical activity exist, and implementation of these strategies, as well as strategies to help all children, adolescents, and adults avoid inactivity, should be a health priority for all sectors of society and all organizations.

Each individual strategy to increase physical activity proposed in this chapter has been shown to be effective in increasing physical activity. Taken together as part of an overall systems approach (Figure 5-1), these strategies, when coupled with appropriate energy intake, have the potential to substantially accelerate progress toward obesity prevention by helping all people meet the minimal physical activity guidelines set forth in the 2008 Physical Activity Guidelines for Americans (HHS, 2008).

REFERENCES

Andersen, L. B., M. Harro, L. B. Sardinha, K. Froberg, U. Ekelund, S. Brage, and S. A. Anderssen. 2006. Physical activity and clustered cardiovascular risk in children: A cross-sectional study (the European Youth Heart Study). *Lancet* 368(9532):299-304.

Baker, P. R., D. P. Francis, J. Soares, A. L. Weightman, and C. Foster. 2011. Community wide interventions for increasing physical activity. *Cochrane Database System Reviews* (4):CD008366.

Brown, W. J., K. Mummery, E. Eakin, and G. Schofield. 2006. 10,000 steps Rockingham: Evaluation of a whole community approach to improving population levels of physical activity. *Journal of Physical Activity and Health* 3(1):1-14.

Caspersen, C. J., K. E. Powell, and G. M. Christenson. 1985. Physical activity, exercise, and physical fitness: Definitions and distinctions for health-related research. *Public Health Reports* 100(2):126-131.

CDC (Centers for Disease Control and Prevention). 2009. *Physical activity—2009. Adults with 30+ minutes of moderate physical activity five or more days per week, or vigorous physical activity for 20+ minutes three or more days per week.* http://apps.nccd.cdc.gov/BRFSS/list.asp?cat=PA&yr=2009&qkey=4418&state=All (accessed October 31, 2011).

Coordinating Committee and Working Groups for the Physical Activity Plan. 2010. *US national physical activity plan.* http://www.physicalactivityplan.org/ (accessed January 26, 2012).

Ding, D., J. F. Sallis, J. Kerr, S. Lee, and D. E. Rosenberg. 2011. Neighborhood environment and physical activity among youth a review. *American Journal of Preventive Medicine* 41(4):442-455.

Duke, H. P. 2010. *Active Texas 2020. Taking action to promote physical activity.* Washington, DC: Directors for Health Promotion and Education.

Eaton, D. K., L. Kann, S. Kinchen, S. Shanklin, J. Ross, J. Hawkins, W. A. Harris, R. Lowry, T. McManus, D. Chyen, C. Lim, L. Whittle, N. D. Brener, and H. Wechsler. 2010. Youth risk behavior surveillance—United States, 2009. *Morbidity and Mortality Weekly Report Surveillance Summaries* 59(5):1-142.

ECPP-NHES (Early Childhood Program Participation Survey of the National Household Education Surveys Program). 2006. *Table 44. Number of children under 6 years old and not yet enrolled in kindergarten, percentage in center-based programs, average weekly hours in nonparental care, and percentage in various types of primary care arrangements, by selected child and family characteristics: 2005.* http://nces.ed.gov/programs/digest/d09/tables/dt09_044.asp (accessed October 28, 2011).

Eliakim, A., D. Nemet, Y. Balakirski, and Y. Epstein. 2007. The effects of nutritional-physical activity school-based intervention on fatness and fitness in preschool children. *Journal of Pediatric Endocrinology and Metabolism* 20(6):711-718.

Epstein, L. H., J. N. Roemmich, J. L. Robinson, R. A. Paluch, D. D. Winiewicz, J. H. Fuerch, and T. N. Robinson. 2008. A randomized trial of the effects of reducing television viewing and computer use on body mass index in young children. *Archives of Pediatrics and Adolescent Medicine* 162(3):239-245.

Frank, L., and P. O. Engelke. 2001. The built environment and human activity patterns: Exploring the impacts of urban form on public health. *Journal of Planning Literature* 16:202-218.

Frank, L. D., P. Engelke, and T. L. Schmid. 2003. *Health and community design: The impact of the built environment on physical activity.* Washington, DC: Island Press.

Gibbons, M. C., L. Fleisher, R. E. Slamon, S. Bass, V. Kandadai, and J. R. Beck. 2011. Exploring the potential of Web 2.0 to address health disparities. *Journal of Health Communication* 16(Suppl. 1):77-89.

Gold, J., A. E. Pedrana, R. Sacks-Davis, M. E. Hellard, S. Chang, S. Howard, L. Keogh, J. S. Hocking, and M. A. Stoove. 2011. A systematic examination of the use of online social networking sites for sexual health promotion. *BMC Public Health* 11:583.

Hamilton, M. T., D. G. Hamilton, and T. W. Zderic. 2007. Role of low energy expenditure and sitting in obesity, metabolic syndrome, type 2 diabetes, and cardiovascular disease. *Diabetes* 56(11):2655-2667.

Heath, G. W., R. C. Brownson, J. Kruger, R. Miles, K. E. Powell, L. T. Ramsey, and Task Force on Community Preventive Services. 2006. The effectiveness of urban design and land use and transport policies and practices to increase physical activity: A systematic review. *Journal of Physical Activity & Health* 3(Suppl. 1):S55-S76.

HHS (U.S. Department of Health and Human Services). 1996. *Physical activity and health: A report of the US Surgeon General.* Washington, DC: HHS.

HHS. 2008. *Physical activity guidelines for Americans.* Washington, DC: HHS.

Hu, F. B., T. Y. Li, G. A. Colditz, W. C. Willett, and J. E. Manson. 2003. Television watching and other sedentary behaviors in relation to risk of obesity and type 2 diabetes mellitus in women. *Journal of the American Medical Association* 289(14):1785-1791.

IOM (Institute of Medicine). 2005. *Preventing childhood obesity: Health in the balance*, edited by J. P. Koplan, C. T. Liverman, and V. A. Kraak. Washington, DC: The National Academies Press.

IOM. 2011. *Early childhood obesity prevention policies.* Washington, DC: The National Academies Press.

Kahn, E. B., L. T. Ramsey, R. C. Brownson, G. W. Heath, E. H. Howze, K. E. Powell, E. J. Stone, M. W. Rajab, and P. Corso. 2002. The effectiveness of interventions to increase physical activity. A systematic review. *American Journal of Preventive Medicine* 22(Suppl. 4):73-107.

Larson, N., D. S. Ward, S. B. Neelon, and M. Story. 2011. What role can child-care settings play in obesity prevention? A review of the evidence and call for research efforts. *Journal of the American Dietetic Association* 111(9):1343-1362.

Ogden, C. L., M. D. Carroll, L. R. Curtin, M. M. Lamb, and K. M. Flegal. 2010. Prevalence of high body mass index in US children and adolescents, 2007-2008. *Journal of the American Medical Association* 303(3):242-249.

Physical Activity Guidelines Advisory Committee. 2008. *Physical Activity Guidelines Advisory Committee report.* Washington, DC: HHS.

Pocock, M., D. Trivedi, W. Wills, F. Bunn, and J. Magnusson. 2010. Parental perceptions regarding healthy behaviours for preventing overweight and obesity in young children: A systematic review of qualitative studies. *Obesity Reviews* 11(5):338-353.

Ransdell, L., M. Dinger, J. Huberty, and K. Miller. 2009. *Developing effective physical activity programs.* Champaign, IL: Human Kinetics.

Robinson, T. N. 1999. Reducing children's television viewing to prevent obesity: A randomized controlled trial. *Journal of the American Medical Association* 282(16):1561-1567.

Strong, W. B., R. M. Malina, C. J. Blimkie, S. R. Daniels, R. K. Dishman, B. Gutin, A. C. Hergenroeder, A. Must, P. A. Nixon, J. M. Pivarnik, T. Rowland, S. Trost, and F. Trudeau. 2005. Evidence based physical activity for school-age youth. *Journal of Pediatrics* 146(6):732-737.

Task Force on Community Preventive Services. 2002. Recommendations to increase physical activity in communities. *American Journal of Preventive Medicine* 22(Suppl. 4):67-72.

TRB (Transportation Research Board) and IOM. 2005. *Does the build environment influence physical activity? Examining the evidence.* Washington, DC: National Academy of Sciences.

Trost, S. G., B. Fees, and D. Dzewaltowski. 2008. Feasibility and efficacy of a "move and learn" physical activity curriculum in preschool children. *Journal of Physical Activity & Health* 5(1):88-103.

West Virginia Physical Activity Plan. 2010. *Active WV 2015. Can we do it?* http://www.wvphysicalactivity.org/?pid=0 (accessed October 28, 2011).

Williams, C. L., B. J. Carter, D. L. Kibbe, and D. Dennison. 2009. Increasing physical activity in preschool: A pilot study to evaluate animal trackers. *Journal of Nutrition Education and Behavior* 41(1):47-52.

6

Food and Beverage Environments

Food and Beverage Environments:
Goal, Recommendation, Strategies, and Actions for
Implementation

Goal: Create food and beverage environments that ensure that healthy food and beverage options are the routine, easy choice.

Recommendation 2: Governments and decision makers in the business community/private sector[1] should make a concerted effort to reduce unhealthy food and beverage options[2] and substantially increase healthier food and beverage options at affordable, competitive prices.

[1] The business community/private sector includes private employers and privately owned and/or operated locations frequented by the public, such as movie theaters, shopping centers, sporting and entertainment venues, bowling alleys, and other recreational/entertainment facilities.
[2] Although there is no consensus on the definition of "unhealthy" foods/beverages, the term refers in this report to foods and beverages that are calorie-dense and low in naturally occurring nutrients. Such foods and beverages contribute little fiber and few essential nutrients and phytochemicals, but contain added fats, sweeteners, sodium, and other ingredients. Unhealthy foods and beverages displace the consumption of foods recommended in the Dietary Guidelines for Americans and may lead to the development of obesity.

Strategy 2-1: Adopt policies and implement practices to reduce over-consumption of sugar-sweetened beverages. Decision makers in the business community/private sector, in nongovernmental organizations, and at all levels of government should adopt comprehensive strategies to reduce over-consumption of sugar-sweetened beverages.[3]

For **schools and other locations where children and adolescents are cared for**, potential actions include

- prohibiting access to sugar-sweetened beverages;

- providing a variety of beverage options that are competitively priced and are recommended by and included in the Dietary Guidelines for Americans; and

- making clean, potable water available.

For the **business community/private sector, nongovernmental organizations, and governments**, potential actions include

- making clean, potable water readily available in public places, worksites, and recreation areas;

- making a variety of beverage options that are competitively priced readily available in public places, worksites, and recreation areas;

- implementing fiscal policies aimed at reducing overconsumption of sugar-sweetened beverages through (1) pricing and other incentives to make healthier beverage options recommended by the Dietary Guidelines for Americans more affordable and, for governments, (2) substantial and specific excise taxes on sugar-sweetened beverages (e.g., cents per ounce of liquid, cents per teaspoon of added sugar), with the revenues being dedicated to obesity prevention programs;

---

[3]Sugar-sweetened beverages are defined to include all beverages containing added caloric sweeteners, including, but not limited to, sugar- or otherwise calorically sweetened regular sodas, less than 100 percent fruit drinks, energy drinks, sports drinks, and ready-to-drink teas and coffees.

- supporting the work of community groups and coalitions to educate the public about the risks associated with overconsumption of sugar-sweetened beverages; and

- developing social marketing campaigns aimed at reducing overconsumption of sugar-sweetened beverages.

For the **food and beverage industry**, potential actions include

- developing and promoting a variety of beverage options for consumers, including a range of healthy beverage options, beverages with reduced sugar content, and smaller portion sizes (e.g., 8-ounce containers).

For **health care providers**, such as physicians, dentists, registered dietitians, and nurses, potential actions include

- performing routine screening regarding overconsumption of sugar-sweetened beverages and counseling on the health risks associated with consumption of these beverages.

Strategy 2-2: Increase the availability of lower-calorie and healthier food and beverage options for children in restaurants. Chain and quick-service restaurants should substantially reduce the number of calories served to children and substantially expand the number of affordable and competitively priced healthier options available for parents to choose from in their facilities.

Potential actions include

- developing a joint effort (modeled after the Healthy Weight Commitment initiative) to set a specific goal for substantially reducing the total annual calories served to children in these facilities; and

- ensuring that at least half of all children's meals are consistent with the food and calorie guidelines of the Dietary Guidelines for Americans for moderately active 4- to 8-year-olds and are competitively priced.

Strategy 2-3: Utilize strong nutritional standards for all foods and beverages sold or provided through the government, and ensure that these healthy options are available in all places frequented by the public. Government agencies (federal, state, local, and school district) should ensure that all foods and beverages sold or provided through the government are aligned with the age-specific recommendations in the current Dietary Guidelines for Americans. The business community and the private sector operating venues frequented by the public should ensure that a variety of foods and beverages, including those recommended by the Dietary Guidelines for Americans, are sold or served at all times.

For **government agencies**, potential actions include

- the federal government expanding the healthy vending/concession guidelines to include all government-owned and/or -operated buildings, worksites, facilities,[4] and other locations where foods and beverages are sold/served; and

- all state and local government-owned and -operated buildings, worksites, facilities, and other locations where foods and beverages are sold/served (including through vending machines and concession stands) adopting and implementing a healthy food and beverage vending/concession policy.

For the **business community/private sector**, potential actions include

- the business community and private-sector entities that operate places frequented by the public ensuring that a variety of food and beverage options are competitively priced and available for purchase and consumption in

---

[4]"Government-owned and -operated buildings, worksites, and facilities" is defined broadly to include not only places of work but, also, locations such as government-owned and/or -operated child care centers, hospitals, and other health care/assisted living facilities, military bases, correctional facilities, and educational institutions.

these places,[5] including foods and beverages that are aligned with the recommendations of the Dietary Guidelines for Americans.

Strategy 2-4: Introduce, modify, and utilize health-promoting food and beverage retailing and distribution policies. States and localities should utilize financial incentives such as flexible financing or tax credits, streamlined permitting processes, and zoning strategies, as well as cross-sectoral collaborations (e.g., among industry, philanthropic organizations, government, and the community) to enhance the quality of local food environments, particularly in low-income communities. These efforts should include encouraging or attracting retailers and distributors of healthy food (e.g., supermarkets) to locate in underserved areas and limiting the concentration of unhealthy food venues (e.g., fast-food restaurants, convenience stores). Incentives should be linked to public health goals in ways that give priority to stores that also commit to health-promoting retail strategies (e.g., through placement, promotion, and pricing).

Potential actions include

- states creating cross-agency teams to analyze and streamline regulatory processes and create tax incentives for retailing of healthy foods in underserved neighborhoods;

- states and localities creating cross-sectoral collaborations among the food and beverage industry, philanthropy, the finance and banking sector, the real estate sector, and the community to develop private funding to facilitate the development of healthy food retailing in underserved areas; and

- localities utilizing incentive tools to attract retailing of healthy foods (e.g., supermarkets and grocery stores) to underserved neighborhoods, such as through flexible financing or tax credits, streamlined permitting processes, zoning strategies, grant and loan programs, small business/economic development programs, and other economic incentives.

---

[5]"Places frequented by the public" includes, but is not limited to, privately owned and/or operated locations frequented by the public such as movie theaters, shopping centers, sporting and entertainment venues, bowling alleys, and other recreational/entertainment facilities.

Strategy 2-5: Broaden the examination and development of U.S. agriculture policy and research to include implications for the American diet. Congress, the Administration, and federal agencies should examine the implications of U.S. agriculture policy for obesity, and should ensure that such policy includes understanding and implementing, as appropriate, an optimal mix of crops and farming methods for meeting the Dietary Guidelines for Americans.

Potential actions include

- the President appointing a Task Force on Agriculture Policy and Obesity Prevention to evaluate the evidence on the relationship between agriculture policies and the American diet, and to develop recommendations for policy options and future policy-related research, specifically on the impact of farm subsidies and the management of commodities on food prices, access, affordability, and consumption;

- Congress and the Administration establishing a process by which federal food, agriculture, and health officials would review and report on the possible implications of U.S. agriculture policy for obesity prevention to ensure that this issue will be fully taken into account when policy makers consider the Farm Bill;

- Congress and the U.S. Department of Agriculture (USDA) developing policy options for promoting increased domestic production of foods recommended for a healthy diet that are generally underconsumed, including fruits and vegetables and dairy products, by reviewing incentives and disincentives that exist in current policy;

- as part of its agricultural research agenda, USDA exploring the optimal mix of crops and farming methods for meeting the current Dietary Guidelines for Americans, including an examination of the possible impact of smaller-scale agriculture, of regional agricultural product distribution chains, and of various agricultural models from small to large scale, as well as other efforts to ensure a sustainable, sufficient, and affordable supply of fresh fruits and vegetables; and

- Congress and the Administration ensuring that there is adequate public funding for agricultural research and extension so that the research agenda can include a greater focus on supporting the production of foods Americans need to consume in greater quantities according to the Dietary Guidelines for Americans.

The 2010 Dietary Guidelines for Americans provide science-based recommendations that Americans aim to maintain energy balance so as to achieve and sustain a healthy weight; emphasize nutrient-dense foods and beverages in their diets; and reduce their intake of excess calories, such as those attributable to added sugars and solid fats (as described in Appendix B) (HHS/USDA, 2010). To achieve these dietary goals, the guidelines identify specific foods to increase and others to reduce (Box 6-1).

Among the consumer behaviors that the Dietary Guidelines suggest to help Americans achieve these goals are to (HHS/USDA, 2010)

- consume foods and drinks to meet, not exceed, calorie needs;
- limit calorie intake from solid fats and added sugars;
- increase intake of fruits, vegetables, and whole grains;
- increase intake of fat-free or low-fat milk and milk products and replace higher-fat milk and milk products with lower-fat options;
- choose water, fat-free milk, 100 percent fruit juice, or unsweetened tea or coffee as drinks instead of sugar-sweetened beverages;
- choose a variety of foods from protein sources;
- consume fewer foods and beverages high in solid fats, added sugars (including sugar-sweetened beverages), and sodium;
- reduce intake of refined grains;
- reduce portion sizes; and
- cook and eat more meals at home rather than eating out and, when eating out, consider choosing healthier options.

Nutrients that the Dietary Guidelines direct Americans to reduce, such as trans and saturated fatty acids, sodium, and added sugars, are often added to foods during processing. Processing also may result in an increase in caloric density and the removal of beneficial nutrients, such as fiber (Ludwig, 2011). While processing of many foods in this way is intended in part to increase their palatability, some have suggested that it has unintended consequences, in that some of the biological mechanisms that help us monitor and control the consumption of calories are bypassed. The result is said to be an "addictive consumption" of food that leads to dependence, with physiological symptoms upon withdrawal (Blumenthal and Gold, 2010; Garber and Lustig, 2011; Gearhardt et al., 2011; Ifland et al., 2009; Lenoir et al., 2007). While this line of reasoning is speculative, it is likely that

Foods and Nutrients to Increase

- Increase vegetable and fruit intake.

- Eat a variety of vegetables, especially dark-green and red and orange vegetables and beans and peas.

- Consume at least half of all grains as whole grains. Increase whole-grain intake by replacing refined grains with whole grains.

- Increase intake of fat-free or low-fat milk and milk products, such as milk, yogurt, cheese, or fortified soy beverages.

- Choose a variety of protein foods, which include seafood, lean meat and poultry, eggs, beans and peas, soy products, and unsalted nuts and seeds.

- Increase the amount and variety of seafood consumed by choosing seafood in place of some meat and poultry.

- Replace protein foods that are higher in solid fats* with choices that are lower in solid fats and calories and/or are sources of oils.

- Use oils to replace solid fats* where possible.

- Choose foods that provide more potassium, dietary fiber, calcium, and vitamin D, which are nutrients of concern in American diets. These foods include vegetables, fruits, whole grains, and milk and milk products.

---

*Fats with a high content of saturated and/or trans fatty acids, which are usually solid at room temperature. Common examples of solid fats include butter, beef fat, lard, shortening, coconut oil, palm oil, and milk fat, which is solid at room temperature but is suspended in fluid milk by homogenization (HHS/UDSA, 2010).

Foods to Reduce

- Reduce daily sodium intake to less than 2,300 milligrams (mg) and further reduce intake to 1,500 mg among persons who are 51 and older and those of any age who are black or have hypertension, diabetes, or chronic kidney disease. The 1,500 mg recommendation applies to about half of the U.S. population, including children and the majority of adults.

- Consume less than 10 percent of calories from saturated fatty acids by replacing them with monounsaturated and polyunsaturated fatty acids.

- Consume less than 300 mg per day of dietary cholesterol.

- Keep trans fatty acid consumption as low as possible by limiting foods that contain synthetic sources of trans fats, such as partially hydrogenated oils, and by limiting other solid fats.

- Reduce the intake of calories from solid fats and added sugars.

- Limit the consumption of foods that contain refined grains, especially refined grain foods that contain solid fats, added sugars, and sodium.

- If alcohol is consumed, it should be consumed in moderation—up to one drink per day for women and two drinks per day for men—and only by adults of legal drinking age.

SOURCE: HHS/USDA, 2010.

reductions in the degree of processing would result in diets more likely to meet the Dietary Guidelines.

At present, solid fats and added sugars represent approximately 35 percent of calories consumed by Americans—children, adolescents, adults, and older adults, and both males and females—and contribute significantly to excess calorie intake without contributing significantly to overall nutrient adequacy. In an eating pattern within calorie limits, calories from solid fats and added sugars are more likely to contribute to weight gain than calories from other food sources. Furthermore, as solid fats and added sugars increase in the diet, it becomes difficult for individuals to meet nutrient needs while staying within calorie limits. Most Americans can accommodate only 5-15 percent of calories from solid fats and added sugars in an eating pattern that meets nutrient needs within calorie limits (USDA/HHS, 2010).

The amount of calories consumed should vary based on a person's age, sex, and physical activity level (see Chapter 5 for recommendations related to physical activity). Table 6-1 summarizes estimated daily calorie needs by age, sex, and activity level. Most Americans consume too many calories on a daily basis given their age, sex, and activity level, and the calories they consume are often high in added sugars and solid fats rather than the items recommended by the Dietary Guidelines (Figure 6-1).

RECOMMENDATION 2

Governments and decision makers in the business community/private sector[6] should make a concerted effort to reduce unhealthy food and beverage options[7] and substantially increase healthier food and beverage options at affordable, competitive prices.

Food and beverage environments are one of the five critical areas for accelerating progress in obesity prevention identified by the committee (Figure 6-2). Increasing access to healthy food and beverage options and decreasing consumption of solid fats and added sugars are important steps toward achieving energy

---

[6]The business community/private sector includes private employers and privately owned and/or operated locations frequented by the public, such as movie theaters, shopping centers, sporting and entertainment venues, bowling alleys, and other recreational/entertainment facilities.

[7]Although there is no consensus on the definition of "unhealthy" foods/beverages, the term refers in this report to foods and beverages that are calorie-dense and low in naturally occurring nutrients. Such foods and beverages contribute little fiber and few essential nutrients and phytochemicals, but contain added fats, sweeteners, sodium, and other ingredients. Unhealthy foods and beverages displace the consumption of foods recommended in the Dietary Guidelines for Americans and may lead to the development of obesity.

TABLE 6-1 Estimated Calorie Needs per Day by Age, Sex, and Physical Activity Level[a]

Sex	Age (years)	Physical Activity Level[b]		
		Sedentary	Moderately Active	Active
Child (female and male)	2-3	1,000-1,200[c]	1,000-1,400[c]	1,000-1,400[c]
Female[d]	4-8	1,200-1,400	1,400-1,600	1,400-1,800
	9-13	1,400-1,600	1,600-2,000	1,800-2,200
	14-18	1,800	2,000	2,400
	19-30	1,800-2,000	2,000-2,200	2,400
	31-50	1,800	2,000	2,200
	51+	1,600	1,800	2,000-2,200
Male	4-8	1,200-1,400	1,400-1,600	1,600-2,000
	9-13	1,600-2,000	1,800-2,200	2,000-2,600
	14-18	2,000-2,400	2,400-2,800	2,800-3,200
	19-30	2,400-2,600	2,600-2,800	3,000
	31-50	2,200-2,400	2,400-2,600	2,800-3,000
	51+	2,000-2,200	2,200-2,400	2,400-2,800

NOTE: Estimates are rounded to the nearest 200 calories. An individual's calorie needs may be higher or lower than these average estimates.
[a]Based on estimated energy requirement (EER) equations, using reference heights (average) and reference weights (healthy) for each age/gender group. For children and adolescents, reference height and weight vary. For adults, the reference man is 5 feet, 10 inches tall and weighs 154 pounds. The reference woman is 5 feet, 4 inches tall and weighs 126 pounds. EER equations are from IOM (2002).
[b]Sedentary means a lifestyle that includes only the light physical activity associated with typical day-to-day life. Moderately active means a lifestyle that includes physical activity equivalent to walking about 1.5 to 3 miles per day at 3 to 4 miles per hour, in addition to the light physical activity associated with typical day-to-day life. Active means a lifestyle that includes physical activity equivalent to walking more than 3 miles per day at 3 to 4 miles per hour, in addition to the light physical activity associated with typical day-to-day life.
[c]The calorie ranges shown are to accommodate needs of different ages within the group. For children and adolescents, more calories are needed at older ages. For adults, fewer calories are needed at older ages.
[d]Estimates for females do not include women who are pregnant or breastfeeding.
SOURCE: HHS/USDA, 2010.

balance when implemented together with adequate levels of physical activity (Chapter 5). The eating patterns of Americans cannot be changed in isolation. Major changes in the nation's food system and food and eating environments have occurred in recent decades, driven by technological advances; U.S. food and agriculture policies; population growth; and economic, social, and lifestyle changes (Story et al., 2008). Food now is readily available and accessible in many settings throughout the day. The current U.S. food supply contains a large amount

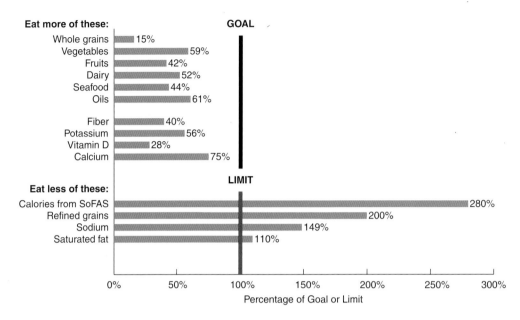

Eat more of these:

Whole grains 15%
Vegetables 59%
Fruits 42%
Dairy 52%
Seafood 44%
Oils 61%

Fiber 40%
Potassium 56%
Vitamin D 28%
Calcium 75%

GOAL

Eat less of these:

LIMIT

Calories from SoFAS 280%
Refined grains 200%
Sodium 149%
Saturated fat 110%

0%   50%   100%   150%   200%   250%   300%
Percentage of Goal or Limit

FIGURE 6-1 Comparison of typical American diets with Dietary Guidelines for Americans.
NOTE: SoFAS = solid fats and added sugars.
SOURCE: HHS/USDA, 2010.

of energy-dense foods, many of which consist of refined grains and foods high in fats and/or sugars and low in nutrients. Many of these foods are often available in increasingly large portion sizes at relatively low prices (Story et al., 2008). Americans also are eating out more often and consuming more calories away from home than ever before (Keystone Forum, 2006), and families are eating fewer meals together (Neumark-Sztainer et al., 2003). In addition, the school food environment is radically different than it was a few decades ago, with many schools now offering and promoting high-calorie, low-nutrition foods throughout the school day (Fox et al., 2009). Food marketing aimed at children using multiple channels, such as digital media, has increased dramatically as well (RWJF, 2011). Finally, an exodus of grocery stores and an influx of fast-food restaurants in lower-income urban areas have contributed to income and racial/ethnic disparities in access to healthier foods (IOM, 2005). Together, these environmental changes have influenced what, where, and how much Americans eat and have played a large role in the current obesity epidemic (IOM, 2009).

To change American's eating patterns, a sustained, systematic and comprehensive approach is required that empowers consumers to make healthy choices;

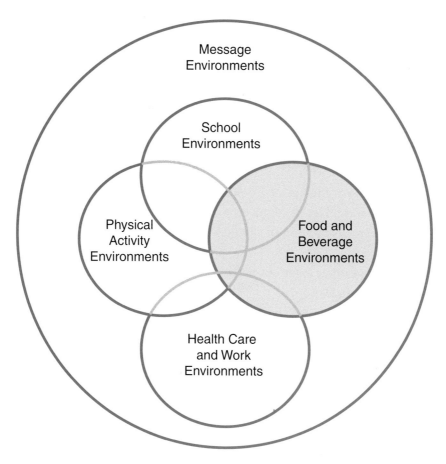

FIGURE 6-2 Five areas of focus of the Committee on Accelerating Progress in Obesity Prevention.
NOTE: The area addressed in this chapter is highlighted.

that gives them a variety of affordable, healthy options from which to choose; that promotes consistent messages about the importance of healthy eating in concert with daily physical activity; that makes healthy food options readily available and accessible; and that cuts across all sectors of society—from government, to schools, to restaurants and privately run places of public access, to health care settings, to farming. Absent a multifaceted approach, the nation will be no better off in 2022 than it is in 2012. The time for change is now. The committee recommends making the healthy option the routine, readily available, and affordable option and provides five strategies and potential actions for implementing this recommendation. These strategies and actions are detailed in the remainder of this chapter. Indicators for measuring progress toward the implementation of each strategy, organized according to the scheme presented in Chapter 4 (primary, process, foundational) are presented in a box following the discussion of each strategy.

STRATEGIES AND ACTIONS FOR IMPLEMENTATION

Strategy 2-1: Adopt Policies and Implement Practices to Reduce Overconsumption of Sugar-Sweetened Beverages

Decision makers in the business community/private sector, in nongovernmental organizations, and at all levels of government should adopt comprehensive strategies to reduce overconsumption of sugar-sweetened beverages.[8]

For **schools and other locations where children and adolescents are cared for,** potential actions include

- prohibiting access to sugar-sweetened beverages;
- providing a variety of beverage options that are competitively priced and are recommended by and included in the Dietary Guidelines for Americans; and
- making clean, potable water available.

For the **business community/private sector, nongovernmental organizations, and governments,** potential actions include

- making clean, potable water readily available in public places, worksites, and recreation areas;
- making a variety of beverage options that are competitively priced readily available in public places, worksites, and recreation areas;
- implementing fiscal policies aimed at reducing overconsumption of sugar-sweetened beverages through (1) pricing and other incentives to make healthier beverage options recommended by the Dietary Guidelines for Americans more affordable and, for governments, (2) substantial and specific excise taxes on sugar-sweetened beverages (e.g., cents per ounce of

---

[8]Sugar-sweetened beverages are defined to include all beverages containing added caloric sweeteners, including, but not limited to, sugar- or otherwise calorically sweetened regular sodas, less than 100 percent fruit drinks, energy drinks, sports drinks, and ready-to-drink teas and coffees.

Accelerating Progress in Obesity Prevention

liquid, cents per teaspoon of added sugar), with the revenues being dedicated to obesity prevention programs;

- supporting the work of community groups and coalitions to educate the public about the risks associated with overconsumption of sugar-sweetened beverages; and
- developing social marketing campaigns aimed at reducing overconsumption of sugar-sweetened beverages.

For the **food and beverage industry**, potential actions include

- developing and promoting a variety of beverage options for consumers, including a range of healthy beverage options, beverages with reduced sugar content, and smaller portion sizes (e.g., 8-ounce containers).

For **health care providers** such as physicians, dentists, registered dietitians, and nurses, potential actions include

- performing routine screening regarding overconsumption of sugar-sweetened beverages and counseling on the health risks associated with consumption of these beverages.

Context

Consumption of sugar-sweetened beverages is the single largest contributor of calories and added sugars to the American diet (HHS/USDA, 2010; NCI, 2010b; Welsh et al., 2011). Such beverages also displace healthier, more nutrient-dense beverages such as milk, 100 percent fruit juice, and water (Woodward-Lopez et al., 2010).

According to National Health and Nutrition Examination Survey (NHANES) 2005-2006 dietary intake data, sugar-sweetened beverages represent the largest share of calories in the diets of all individuals aged 2 and above[9]—more calories than are contributed by any other food category, including grain-based desserts, yeast breads, and chicken and chicken mixed dishes. Using the same NHANES data, Reedy and Krebs-Smith (2010) show that for children and adolescents aged

---

[9]This figure is calculated by summing all persons' mean intake of energy (in kilocalories) from two categories—soda/energy/sports drinks (114 kcal) and fruit drinks (36 kcal)—to obtain 150 kcal, which is a higher proportion of total calories than that represented by any other food group. This is likely a conservative estimate, because it does not include calories from other sugar-sweetened beverages, such as sweetened, ready-to-drink teas and coffee drinks (NCI, 2010b).

2-18, sugar-sweetened beverages were the largest contributor—22 percent—to empty calorie intake (that is, calories from solid fat and added sugars).

On a given day, one-half of the U.S. population aged 2 and older consumes sugared drinks (excluding ready-to-drink sugar-sweetened teas and coffees) (Ogden et al., 2011). According to NHANES data for 2005-2008, 25 percent of Americans drink more than one sugared drink daily (200 kcal/day), 20 percent consume one to four such drinks a day (200-566 kcal/day), and 5 percent drink more than four such drinks daily (567 kcal/day) (Ogden et al., 2011).

Consumption of sugar-sweetened beverages is not limited to particular segments of the U.S. population, although certain groups are more likely to consume them than others. According to Ogden and colleagues (2011), males are more likely than females to consume sugared drinks, with males aged 2-19 most likely to do so (70 percent) on a given day and females aged 20 and older least likely to do so (40 percent). At the same time, sugared drinks represent a greater percentage of daily caloric intake for certain racial/ethnic groups (Ogden et al., 2011). Sugared drink consumption represents 8.5 percent of total daily kilocalories for non-Hispanic black children and adolescents aged 2-19 as compared with 7.7 percent and 7.4 percent of total daily kilocalories for non-Hispanic whites and Mexican American children and adolescents, respectively (Ogden et al., 2011). For Americans aged 20 and over, the racial/ethnic disparity in sugared drink consumption is even greater—8.6 percent of total daily kilocalories consumed by non-Hispanic blacks were from sugared drinks as compared with 5.3 and 8.2 percent for non-Hispanic whites and Mexican Americans aged 20 and over, respectively (Ogden et al., 2011). Consumption of sugared drinks also is lower among higher-income than lower-income persons, with such differences being particularly noticeable among adults aged 20 and over (Ogden et al., 2011).

Of particular concern are the added sugars attributable to excess consumption of sugar-sweetened beverages overall. According to NHANES 2005-2006 dietary intake data, sugar-sweetened beverages are the largest contributor to added sugars in the diets of all individuals aged 2 and above.[10] While added sugar intake has declined for Americans aged 2 and older, largely because of reduced consumption of regular sodas, added sugar intakes continue to exceed dietary recommendations, and rates of consumption of energy drinks as a source of added sugars have increased significantly over the past decade (Welsh et al., 2011). If people are to

---

[10]This figure is calculated by summing all persons' mean intake of added sugars (in teaspoons) from two categories—soda/energy/sports drinks (35.7 tsp) and fruit drinks (10.5 tsp)—which yields a higher proportion of added sugars than that represented by any other food group (NCI, 2010a).

meet the Dietary Guidelines for Americans' recommended food pattern/caloric intake for their age, sex, and activity level, they must minimize their intakes of all solid fats and added sugars. While the maximum recommended limits for solid fats and added sugars vary by age, sex, and level of physical activity, these limits are intended to reflect intakes of both solid fats and added sugars. Yet in most cases, more than half of the recommended calories from solid fats and added sugars being consumed are from sugared drinks; in many cases, more than two-thirds of the recommended calories from solid fats and added sugars are attributable to sugared drink consumption (Figure 6-3). In other words, Americans' current rates of sugared drink consumption leave very little room in their diet for any additional solid fats and added sugars, and in some cases (e.g., males aged 6-8 and 12-13), they exceed the daily recommendations for solid fats and added sugars with their sugared drink consumption alone. As the Keystone Forum[11] (2006) notes in its recommendations for preventing weight gain and obesity, several dietary factors contribute to the development of obesity (a detail that the Forum participants recognized), "and one of those factors is excess caloric intake. A decrease in caloric beverage consumption is just one of many necessary strategies in the effort to reduce obesity."

Evidence

Despite the complexity of the etiology of obesity and the difficulty of quantifying relative contributions to the obesity epidemic, researchers have found strong associations between intake of sugar-sweetened beverages and weight gain. Although the exact mechanisms of how sugar-sweetened beverages contribute to obesity are not fully known, their link to obesity is stronger than that observed for any other food or beverage, as described in the 2010 Dietary Guidelines for Americans advisory report (DGAC, 2010). Woodward-Lopez and colleagues (2010) found that sugar-sweetened beverages account for at least 20 percent of the increases in weight in the United States from 1977 to 2007. Others have concluded that liquid calories supplied approximately half of the 150- to 300-calorie increase in daily energy intake observed over the past 30 years (Johnson et al., 2009), concomitant with no apparent change in physical activity (Briefel and Johnson, 2004; Nielsen et al., 2002). Additional evidence supporting the reduction of sugar-sweetened beverages in order to promote energy balance is predicated on evidence suggesting that liquid calories from sweet, energy-dense beverages are poorly compensated for by reduced

---

[11] The Keystone Forum of the Keystone Center is a nonprofit public policy and dispute resolution organization that brought together participants from industry, government, civic organizations, and academia.

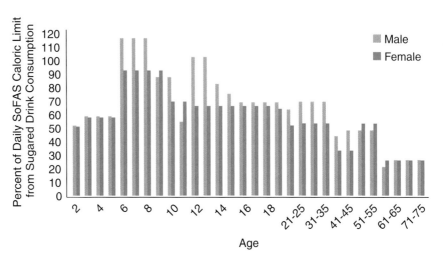

FIGURE 6-3 Percentage of daily caloric limit of solid fats and added sugars from sugared drink consumption for given ages, assuming moderate activity level.

NOTES: Moderate physical activity is defined as a lifestyle that includes physical activity equivalent to walking about 1.5-3 miles per day at 3-4 miles per hour, in addition to the light physical activity associated with typical day-to-day life (HHS/USDA, 2010, p. 78). The definition of sugared drinks is based on that used in Ogden et al. (2011) and Reedy and Krebs-Smith (2010). Sugared drinks include fruit drinks, sodas, energy drinks, sports drinks, and sweetened bottled waters. Sugared drinks in this analysis do not include sweetened teas or flavored milks, nor do they include 100 percent fruit juices or diet drinks. The percentage of daily limit of solid fats and added sugars attributable to sugared drinks was computed by dividing the average daily caloric intake of sugar drinks from Ogden et al. (2011) by the maximum calories from solid fats and added sugars for the given age/sex, assuming a moderate physical activity level, from the Dietary Guidelines for Americans (HHS/USDA, 2010). Note that some of the age categories do not directly correspond to the age categories reported in Ogden et al. (2011). In these cases, the calories were assigned based on the earlier year in the age range (e.g., 19-20 reflects the calories for 12- to 19-year-olds, whereas 21-25 reflects the calories for 20- to 39-year-olds from Ogden et al. [2011]).

SoFAS = solid fats and added sugars.

SOURCE: Computed based on Dietary Guidelines for Americans, Appendix 7 (HHS/USDA, 2010; Ogden et al., 2011).

dietary intake from other sources (Bellisle and Rolland-Cachera, 2001; DiMeglio and Mattes, 2000; Mattes, 1996; Popkin and Duffey, 2010).

The 2010 Dietary Guidelines Advisory Committee (DGAC) concluded that for adults, "limited evidence shows that intake of SSBs [sugar-sweetened beverages] is linked to higher energy intake . . . a moderate body of epidemiologic evidence suggests that greater consumption of SSBs is associated with increased body weight in adults, and a moderate body of evidence suggests that under isocaloric controlled conditions, added sugars, including sugar-sweetened beverages, are no more likely to cause weight gain than any other source of energy" (DGAC, 2010, p. 301). The 2010 DGAC found a more robust link between sugar-sweetened beverages and childhood adiposity, concluding that "strong evidence supports the conclusion that greater intake of SSBs is associated with increased adiposity in children." The DGAC recommended a "greatly reduced" intake of sugar-sweetened beverages to prevent excess weight among children, noting that consumption should also be discouraged because of the need to replace empty calories with nutrient-rich energy for optimal growth and development (DGAC, 2010, p. 12).

The contributions of the consumption of sugar-sweetened beverages to childhood obesity also will likely lead to greater future prevalence of adult obesity. The established habitual nature of consumption of these beverages suggests that their consumption is likely to persist into adulthood, further increasing the risk for obesity (Popkin and Duffey, 2010).

Because 100 percent fruit juice is suggested as an alternative to sugar-sweetened beverages and there may be concern that its calorie content will promote obesity, the committee cites the DGAC report, which states: "limited and inconsistent evidence suggests that for most children, intake of 100 percent fruit juice is not associated with increased adiposity when consumed in amounts that are appropriate for age and energy needs of the child." The report also notes, however, that intake of 100 percent fruit juice has been prospectively associated with increased adiposity in children who are overweight or obese (DGAC, 2010). Furthermore, the report explains that although 100 percent fruit juice provides nutrients and can be part of a healthy diet when consumed in moderation,[12] it lacks dietary fiber and can contribute extra calories when consumed in excess; thus, the majority of fruit servings should come from whole fruits.

Implementation

Recognizing the trends described above, a number of prior Institute of Medicine (IOM) committees have recommended strategies aimed at reducing consumption of and exposure to sugar-sweetened beverages, as well as encouraging consumption of healthier beverages. *Nutrition Standards for Foods in Schools: Leading the Way Toward Healthier Youth* (IOM, 2007a) recommends that beverages provide no more than 35 percent of calories from total sugars per packaged portion, with the

---

[12]The American Academy of Pediatrics (AAP) recommends not introducing 100 percent fruit juice into the diet before 6 months of age, and recommends daily upper limits of 4-6 ounces for children aged 1-6 and 8-12 ounces for older children, up to age 18 (AAP Committee on Nutrition, 2001).

exception of 100 percent fruit juices and 100 percent vegetable juices without added sugars and unflavored nonfat and lowfat milk. The same report also recommends that sports drinks be available in schools only for student-athletes participating in vigorous-intensity sports for at least 1 hour. Likewise, the IOM (2009) has recommended that local governments ensure that publicly run entities promote healthy beverages. It has also recommended that restaurants promote healthier options, such as by serving nonfat milk instead of soda in children's meals (IOM, 2006b, 2009); that food, beverage, restaurant, retail, and marketing industry trade associations improve the availability and selection of healthful beverages accessible at eye level and reach in grocery stores and retail environments (IOM, 2006b); that the media promote healthful beverages (IOM, 2006b); that industry shift product portfolios and advertising and marketing emphasis toward beverages substantially lower in total calories and added sugars and higher in nutrient content (IOM, 2006b); and that caregivers of young children (birth to 4 years) build skills to foster the selection of healthful beverages (IOM, 2006b).

Likewise, a number of medical, public health, scientific, policy-making, non-profit, and consensus-building bodies have specifically identified reduced consumption of sugar-sweetened beverages and/or excess caloric intake associated with such consumption as key issues requiring a societal response that involves not only governments but also, just as important, schools, industry, food service providers, and medical care providers. The Dietary Guidelines for Americans (HHS/USDA, 2010), the American Academy of Pediatrics in association with the American Heart Association (Gidding et al., 2006), and the American Medical Association (AMA, 2007) all recommend reducing intake of sugar-sweetened beverages because they are the leading contributor to excess sugar consumption in the American diet. And the Centers for Disease Control and Prevention (CDC) (2010) has identified seven recommended strategies for reducing consumption of sugar-sweetened beverages that are aligned with actions outlined above by the committee. The following discussion briefly summarizes the evidence, positions, and, where available, implementation experiences related to the overall strategy of reducing consumption of sugar-sweetened beverages.

Access to sugar-sweetened beverages in public places and schools The U.S. Surgeon General (2010), the Department of Health and Human Services (National Prevention Council, 2011), the National Governors Association (Mulheron and Vonasek, 2009), the National Association of Local Boards of Health (2010), CDC (Khan et al., 2009), the Alliance for a Healthier Generation (2006), the American

Dental Association (2005), and the American Academy of Pediatric Dentistry (AAPD, 2010) all recommend a range of strategies for reducing consumption of sugar-sweetened beverages. These strategies include eliminating or restricting access to sugar-sweetened beverages, including those sold through vending machines and in schools, child care/early learning centers, and other government facilities and public places and increasing access to healthier options, such as bottled water and non- or low-fat milk. Likewise, given the wide availability of sugar-sweetened beverages in workplaces, schools, recreation facilities, entertainment venues, and other places frequented by the public, a number of organizations have recognized the need to ensure that Americans have sufficient alternatives to such beverages available, and have identified specific strategies to that end. The Keystone Forum (2006, p. 11) specifically called upon food service providers to "develop, make available, and promote beverage options that help consumers to reduce caloric intake," including through smaller portion sizes and a range of low-calorie[13] and zero-calorie beverage choices, increased selections of low-fat and nonfat milk beverages, and pricing strategies that make smaller sizes and lower-calorie options more appealing. Although the beverage industry has sold sugar-sweetened beverages with smaller portion sizes (e.g., 7.5 ounce cans) for some time, they are not priced favorably (CSPI, 2010), nor are they marketed to encourage consumers to choose them in lieu of the larger options (e.g., 12 ounce cans, 20 ounce bottles).

Given the relationship between consumption of sugar-sweetened beverages and child and adolescent overweight and obesity, most policy interventions to date have focused on the elementary and, to a lesser extent, secondary school environments. In 2006, the Alliance for a Healthier Generation (an alliance between the William J. Clinton Foundation and the American Heart Association) brokered an agreement with three major beverage firms to limit access to sugar-sweetened beverages in schools. The resulting School Beverage Guidelines limit portion sizes of and set standards for the calorie and nutrient content of beverages sold in schools; the restrictions are tighter in elementary and middle schools than in high schools. An industry report following implementation of the guidelines indicated an 88 percent reduction in beverage calories shipped to schools by the middle of the 2009-2010 school year (ABA, 2010). Independent researchers reported that based on a nationally representative mail-back survey, high-calorie beverages and beverages not allowed by national guidelines were still available in

---

[13]Because its charge was to focus specifically on strategies for accelerating progress in obesity prevention, the committee did not deliberate on the effects of low-calorie, artificially sweetened beverages on population health and did not take a position on this issue.

elementary schools during the 2008-2009 school year. They noted that beverages in schools may be obtained from school stores or vending machines that are outside of formal contracts with beverage suppliers (Turner and Chaloupka, 2010). Additionally, concern has been expressed about the less restrictive guidelines for high schools, where intake of sugar-sweetened beverages occurs more frequently than in other schools; about the lack of nonindustry evaluation funding; and about the fact that the guidelines fail to address other beverages, such as calorie-dense sports drinks, diet drinks (for which brand marketing continues to be offered), and new drink categories such as energy drinks (Sharma et al., 2010).

Levy and colleagues (2011) reviewed the literature on school nutrition policies directed at consumption of sugar-sweetened beverages by children and adolescents, finding that policies limiting the availability of such beverages and improving food offerings in school lunches generally have been associated with reduced consumption of these beverages. In middle schools, restricting access can reduce the percentage of students consuming sugar-sweetened beverages by 25 percent and the energy they consume by 30 percent. In high schools, 30 percent reductions in energy intake were observed among student buyers of sugar-sweetened beverages when access policies were in place.

Briefel and colleagues (2009a,b), Levy and colleagues (2011), and Taber and colleagues (2011) conclude that restrictions on in-school access to sugar-sweetened beverages reduce in-school consumption, and that reduced intake of such beverages in schools is unlikely to be offset by increased consumption outside of schools. Recent experience in Boston public schools confirms that students do not compensate for reduced access to sugar-sweetened beverages by buying those beverages outside of school (Cradock et al., 2011) (see Box 6-2).

Access to water Recognizing that if governments, employers, schools, public places, and other locations encouraged reduced consumption of sugar-sweetened beverages, consumers would need alternative options readily available, the IOM (2007a, 2009), the National Association of County and City Health Officials (NACCHO, 2010), the Department of Health and Human Services (HHS/USDA, 2010), and CDC (Khan et al., 2009) all recommend increasing the availability of safe, free drinking water and healthier beverages such as non-fat/low-fat milk and 100 percent juices in schools and other places where beverages are sold and served. Increasing water intake may help limit excess weight gain among children, adolescents, and adults (Daniels and Popkin, 2010; Dennis et al., 2010; Stookey et al., 2007, 2008). Replacing sugar-sweetened beverages with water is associated with reductions in total energy intake for children and adolescents (Wang et al., 2009), and installing water fountains in public places and facilities can increase water intake and prevent and reduce overweight and obesity (Muckelbauer et al., 2009). The *Healthy, Hunger-Free Kids Act of 2010*[14] requires schools participating in federally funded child nutrition programs to make water available during meal periods at no cost to students, and mandates that child care facilities provide free water throughout the day. After a survey revealed that 40 percent of responding California school districts reported lack of access to free drinking water in cafeterias for students, a state law was implemented requiring schools to make free, fresh drinking water available during meals (California Food Policy Advocates, 2011).

Pricing strategies and fiscal policies At least three IOM committees have considered fiscal policies (taxes and incentives) to discourage consumption of unhealthy foods and beverages such as sugar-sweetened beverages or encourage consumption of healthier alternatives. Two committees (IOM, 2005, 2006b) concluded that evidence was insufficient to draw a definite conclusion or develop a strong recommendation either for or against imposing a tax on less healthful foods. In 2009, however, the IOM recommended that local governments "implement fiscal policies and local ordinances to discourage the consumption of calorie-dense, nutrient poor foods and beverages (e.g., taxes, incentives, land use and zoning regulations)" (IOM, 2009, p. 62). That committee highlighted "implement[ing] a tax strategy to discourage consumption of foods and beverages of minimal nutritional value, such as sugar-sweetened beverages" as an action with considerable promise, noting the growing interest in and broad reach of such a strategy (IOM, 2009, p. 63). One of the earlier IOM committees recommended that governments consider incentives, including tax incentives, to encourage and reward food, beverage, and restaurant companies that develop, provide, and promote healthier beverages for children and adolescents in the settings in which they typically consume beverages (IOM, 2006b). Likewise, the 2009 IOM report recommends creating incentive programs to enable small food store owners in underserved areas to carry healthier, affordable food items. That report also recommends offering incentives or subsidies to government programs and localities that provide healthy foods at competitive prices and limit calorie-dense, nutrient-poor foods.

Non-IOM reports also have recommended fiscal policies to discourage consumption of less healthy foods and beverages and encourage consumption of

---

[14]Public Law 111-296, 111th Cong., 2d sess. (December 13, 2010), 124, 3183.

Case Study of the Impact of Boston Public Schools'
Policy on Consumption of Sugar-Sweetened Beverages

Boston Public Schools instituted a policy in 2004 restricting the sale of sugar-sweetened beverages (soft drinks, non-100 percent fruit and vegetable juices, and sports drinks) anywhere in school buildings or campuses. Concurrent activities included the introduction of nutrition-related curricula in elementary and middle schools, presentation of the policy to school administrators, and negotiation of new vending contracts to provide more healthful beverage options. Two years later, more than 2,000 students were surveyed to determine whether consumption of sugar-sweetened beverages declined after the policy was implemented (Cradock et al., 2011). The student body is diverse (37 percent black, 39 percent Hispanic, 13 percent white, and 9 percent Asian), and almost three-quarters of the students are eligible for free or reduced-price meals. On average, students reported consuming 1.71 servings of sugar-sweetened beverages in 2004 and 1.38 servings in 2006; servings of soda (−0.16), other sugar-sweetened beverages (−0.14), and total sugar-sweetened beverages (−0.30) declined during that period. The percentage of students reporting no consumption of these beverages rose from 4.5 percent in 2004 to 9.8 percent in 2006. During the same time (2004-2006), national data from the National Health and Nutrition Examination Survey showed no significant changes in adolescent consumption of sugar-sweetened beverages, ruling out the possibility that consumption decreased in general during this time. The study authors concluded that students did not compensate for reduced school access to sugar-sweetened beverages by buying

healthier alternatives. The California Legislature Task Force on Diabetes and Obesity (Greenwood et al., 2009) has recommended creating tax incentive programs to encourage employers to adopt workplace policies that make healthy eating easier for employees, as well as offering incentives to mobile carts within one-half mile of school campuses to offer healthy and restrict unhealthy foods. The Robert Wood Johnson Foundation Action Strategies Toolkit for state and local leaders (RWJF, 2009) encourages state and local policy makers, through financial or other incentives, to motivate restaurants to provide price reductions for healthier foods, and convenience stores and bodegas to provide affordable healthy those beverages elsewhere, and that restricting their sale in schools may be a promising strategy for reducing unnecessary energy intake among adolescents.

This case study illustrates policies restricting access to sugar-sweetened beverages in schools coinciding with reductions in consumption of these beverages. Given that these beverages are a leading sources of calories in the diets of Americans aged 2-18,* this case study is illustrative of the potential impact of this implementation action for Strategy 2-1. The investigators did not examine sales or beverage substitution behaviors because these outcomes were beyond the scope of the study, which focused exclusively on sugar-sweetened beverage consumption patterns.

SOURCE: Cradock et al., 2011.

---

*This figure is calculated by summing 2- to 18-year-olds' mean intake of energy (in kilocalories) from two categories—soda/energy/sports drinks (118 kcal) and fruit drinks (55 kcal)—to obtain 173 kcal, which is a higher proportion of total calories than that represented by any other food group for this age subgroup. Available http://riskfactor.cancer.gov/diet/foodsources/energy/table1b.html (accessed December 19, 2011).

options. CDC (Khan et al., 2009) has recommended that communities provide incentives for food retailers to locate in underserved areas and offer healthy food and beverage choices. CDC also has issued a series of strategies for reducing consumption of sugar-sweetened beverages. Finally, the White House Task Force on Childhood Obesity (2010) has recommended an analysis of the effect of state and local taxes on less healthy, energy-dense foods.

While available research on existing small sales taxes (ranging from 1.0 to 7.25 percent) (Bridging the Gap Program, 2011) finds little or no impact on consumption, body mass index (BMI), or obesity rates (Finkelstein et al., 2010; Kim and Kawachi, 2006; Powell and Chriqui, 2011; Powell et al., 2009; Sturm et al., 2010), many believe that more sizable, nontrivial pricing interventions could have measurable effects on weight outcomes, particularly for children and adolescents, populations of low socioeconomic status, and those most at risk for overweight (Finkelstein et al., 2010; Powell and Chaloupka, 2009; Powell et al., 2009; Sturm et al., 2010). Although a number of state and local governments recently have attempted to enact sizable taxes on sugar-sweetened beverages (on the order of 1 cent per liquid ounce) (Rudd Center for Food Policy and Obesity, 2011), none have succeeded in doing so to date. The rationale for these proposals is grounded largely in the considerable body of evidence for the impact of food pricing on weight outcomes and in an emerging literature that examines the impact of taxes or price increases (amounting to a 10-20 percent price increase) on consumption of sugar-sweetened beverages and weight outcomes. Note that estimates of the impact of a tax on sugar-sweetened beverages will likely vary because of the length of the causal pathway between prices of these beverages and weight outcomes and the complexity of the variables involved in this pathway.

The effectiveness of a tax on sugar-sweetened beverages depends in part on the degree to which consumers change their food and beverage purchasing and consumption behavior in response to higher sugar-sweetened beverages prices (price elasticity). In a review that includes studies based on large survey data sets, Andreyeva and colleagues (2010) show that food consumption or expenditure is generally price sensitive. Smith and colleagues (2010) estimate that a 10 percent price increase for sweetened beverages would reduce grocery store purchases of these items by 12.6 percent, and also note that when taxes are large, estimated elasticities may underestimate actual consumer reactions. Another study (Wendt and Todd, 2011) reports that inflation-adjusted prices for carbonated drinks have fallen over the past 30 years and that responses to changes in price vary, particularly across income levels and BMI range. In the past, 10 percent higher prices for carbonated beverages were associated with a decrease in the average child's BMI. The effect was significant for boys but not for girls. The effect also was greater for children in households with income below 200 percent of the federal poverty level, a finding that is not surprising because economic theory suggests that lower-income households are more price-responsive than their higher-income counterparts. The effect was larger for children with lower BMI, perhaps because these children are less likely to substitute caloric drinks (such as juice) (see the discussion below) or because their preferences for carbonated beverages are less entrenched, so their price sensitivity for these beverages is higher. Notwithstanding

Accelerating Progress in Obesity Prevention

available estimates, Smith and colleagues (2010) conclude that the literature lacks the demand elasticity estimates needed to fully examine the effect of a tax on sugar-sweetened beverages in practice.

A number of studies have predicted the effect of sizable taxes and/or price increases on consumption of sugar-sweetened beverages. According to one recent estimate, a 10 percent price increase for soft drinks would reduce their consumption by 8-10 percent (Andreyeva et al., 2010). Another analysis indicates that a penny-per-ounce tax would reduce per capita consumption of sugar-sweetened beverages by 24 percent and could reduce per capita calorie intake from such beverages by about 50 calories/day (approximately 5 pounds/year), assuming no substitution of other caloric beverages or foods (Andreyeva et al., 2011). Some of these same studies suggest that a 20 percent increase in the price of sugar-sweetened beverages or a penny-per-ounce tax could significantly reduce per capita calorie intake, translating to a reduction in body weight ranging from approximately 1.5 to 5.0 pounds a year, assuming no substitution of other caloric beverages (Andreyeva et al., 2011; Dharmasena and Capps, 2011; Smith et al., 2010). Chaloupka and colleagues (2011b) modeled a penny-per-ounce tax on sugar-sweetened beverages in the state of Illinois, showing that the frequency of consumption of such beverages (≥2 times/day) would fall sharply as a result of the tax. They estimated an overall 23.5 percent drop in consumption of sugar-sweetened beverages and an average weight reduction of 1.7 pounds annually based on the assumption that half of the calorie deficit from reduced consumption of such beverages would be offset by increases in energy intake from other sources. Wang and colleagues (2012) estimated that a penny-per-ounce sugar-sweetened beverages tax would reduce sugar-sweetened beverages consumption by 15 percent among adults aged 25-64, after factoring in the assumption that 40 percent of the calorie deficit from reduced sugar-sweetened beverages consumption would be compensated for by consumption of other caloric beverages (such as milk and juice) in equal measure. They also projected the sugar-sweetened beverages tax's impact on downstream health benefits and medical costs savings over a 10-year period (2010-2020), finding that it could reduce new cases of type 2 diabetes by 2.6 percent and the prevalence of obesity by 1.5 percent. Over 10 years these reductions would result in 95,000 fewer coronary heart events, 8,000 fewer strokes, and 26,000 fewer premature deaths, avoiding more than $17 million in medical costs while generating approximately $13 billion in tax revenue.

The extent to which calories from nontaxed foods and caloric beverages are substituted for calories in taxed items is a key consideration when translating tax-induced reductions in caloric intake into decreased body weight and obesity (Chaloupka et al., 2011b). The literature in this area is mixed. Fletcher and colleagues (2011b) maintain that substitution of other high-calorie drinks for soft drinks may blunt the effect of soft drink taxes on obesity; they cite the lack of evidence supporting the argument that if taxes are large enough, consumption of sugar-sweetened beverages will fall substantially. However, others have estimated only modest increases in calories from other caloric beverages and continue to observe a net caloric deficit when examining a hypothetical 20 percent price increase in sugar-sweetened beverages (Dharmasena and Capps, 2011; Smith et al., 2010). While those researching this topic agree almost universally that more research is needed, Fletcher and colleagues (2011a) point out that convincing evidence may not be available until a large tax is instituted in a state or locality. Despite the apparent lack of research examining substitution effects, analyses that examine weight outcomes are implicitly capturing the substitution that occurs, and a negative impact of taxing sugar-sweetened beverages on BMI and/or obesity prevalence indicates that full compensation from substitution of other calorie sources does not occur.

The committee considered the potential allegation that taxes on sugar-sweetened beverages are regressive, that is, that they would disproportionately affect low-income and minority consumers, who spend a larger proportion of their income on food than those with higher incomes and whites. Brownell and colleagues (2009) observe that taxes on such beverages may be most beneficial to the former populations because they are disproportionately affected by obesity, may consume more soft drinks than other populations, and may be more price-sensitive—all supporting the argument that they may stand to benefit substantially from reduced consumption of sugar-sweetened beverages, especially if they are the focus of the obesity prevention programs funded by the taxes on these beverages. Furthermore, sugar-sweetened beverages are not an essential dietary component, and as explained above, hinder Americans from achieving dietary intakes aligned with the Dietary Guidelines for Americans. Finally, water, a no-cost alternative to sugar-sweetened beverages, is readily available (Brownell et al., 2009).

Even though predicted reductions in body weight resulting from a substantial tax on sugar-sweetened beverages may be relatively small or still must be tested in practice, the committee believes that fiscal policies such as incentivizing the purchase of healthier beverages or taxing sugar-sweetened beverages are one action that can be taken to reduce consumption of these beverages. The current evidence does not indicate that fiscal policies alone can solve the obesity problem. Rather, it suggests that fiscal policies would act synergistically with other actions to reduce consumption of sugar-sweetened beverages, thereby advancing the achievement of a comprehensive obesity prevention strategy, particularly if the revenues from taxes on such beverages were directed toward obesity prevention programs, as recommended by the public health community (Brownell and Ludwig, 2011; Chaloupka et al., 2011a; Powell and Chriqui, 2011). The public also is more supportive of taxes on sugar-sweetened beverages if revenues will support activities to reduce obesity. A December 2008 poll found that 52 percent of New Yorkers supported a "soft drink tax," and support increased to 72 percent when respondents were told the revenues would be earmarked to prevent obesity and to avoid service cuts in schools, health care, mass transit, or law enforcement (Citizens' Committee for Children of New York, Inc., 2008). Likewise, a 2011 poll of 500 Massachusetts voters found that 69 percent would support a sales tax on soda if the revenues funded local schools or anti-obesity programs targeting children, but the sample was split nearly 50-50 if they were not told how the revenues would be used. The Rudd Center has compiled additional results from eight other polls demonstrating public support for a tax on sugar-sweetened beverages, particularly when the revenues would be earmarked for obesity prevention (Rudd Center for Food Policy and Obesity, 2010).

Social marketing campaigns Social marketing has been used to impact a variety of health and risk behaviors among children, adolescents, and adults. Because many health-based social marketing campaigns are insufficiently funded and not sustained over significant periods of time, assessing their effectiveness accurately is difficult (Randolph and Viswanath, 2004; Wakefield et al., 2010). However, evidence from carefully designed studies indicates that media campaigns can have a positive impact on health behaviors if they are carefully crafted, well tested, fully funded, highly targeted (in terms of audience and behavior), and sustained over a long period of time (Wakefield et al., 2010). Social marketing campaigns are discussed in greater detail in Chapter 7, under Strategy 3-1.

Social marketing campaigns aimed at reducing consumption of sugar-sweetened beverages are emerging rapidly and are encouraged by health professional organizations. For example, the American Academy of Pediatric Dentistry "encourages collaboration with other dental and medical organizations, governmental agencies, education officials, parent and consumer groups, and corporations to increase public awareness of the negative effects of frequent and/or inappropriate intake of sweetened drinks (carbonated and noncarbonated) and low nutrient dense snack foods on infant, child, and adolescent oral health, nutrition, and general health" (AAPD, 2010, p. 56).

In 2011, a campaign titled "Life's Sweeter with Fewer Sugary Drinks" debuted with the goal of decreasing average consumption of such drinks (regular soda, fruit drinks with less than 100 percent juice, sweetened teas, lemonade, energy drinks, and sports drinks) to approximately three cans per person per week by 2020 (CSPI, 2011). The campaign brings together health experts, civic organizations, youth groups, and others to meet this goal. It also encourages employers, hospitals, and government agencies to adopt policies designed to decrease soda consumption. The campaign has been embraced by the American Diabetes Association, the American Heart Association, the Center for Science in the Public Interest, and more than 100 local and national health organizations. At the same time, local and state governments from across the country—including Boston, New York City, Philadelphia, Seattle and King County, and the Rhode Island Department of Health, to name a few—have been developing and implementing social marketing campaigns aimed at reducing consumption of sugar-sweetened beverages.

Role of health care providers All health care providers should adopt standards of practice for prevention, screening, and counseling regarding overweight and obesity to help their patients achieve and maintain a healthy weight (see Chapter 8, Strategy 4-1). Given the linkage between consumption of sugar-sweetened beverages and obesity, particularly among children and adolescents, and the fact that these beverages are the leading source of added sugars in the American diet, health care providers such as physicians, dentists, registered dietitians, and nurses have a unique opportunity to screen and/or counsel patients on the risks associated with overconsumption of these beverages. The American Academy of Pediatrics (2011) calls for pediatricians to educate children, adolescents, and their parents about the linkage among consumption of sports drinks, excess caloric intake, and obesity and overweight, as well as dental erosion; to promote water as the principal source of hydration for children and adolescents; and to limit consumption of sports drinks to circumstances in which rapid replenishment of carbohydrates and/or electrolytes is necessary, such as during periods of prolonged, vigorous physical activity. Additionally, given the risk of dental caries associated with excessive sugar consumption, the AAP Section on Pediatric Dentistry and Oral Health (2008) recommends that pediatricians counsel parents and caregivers on the importance of reducing children's exposure to added sugars in foods and beverages, including limiting sugared drinks, avoiding carbonated beverages and juice drinks containing less than 100 percent juice, and encouraging children to drink only water and milk between meals.

In summary, sugar-sweetened beverages make a substantial contribution to the energy intake of Americans and are linked to increased weight gain/body weight, particularly in children. Moreover, availability of and exposure to such beverages are widespread in all sectors of society. Therefore, the committee believes an integrated, comprehensive approach will be needed to cause Americans to reduce consumption of these beverages as part of an effort to ensure a balanced diet that includes a variety of foods and beverages recommended in the Dietary Guidelines for Americans.

Indicators for Assessing Progress in Obesity Prevention for Strategy 2-1

Primary Indicator

- Reduction in energy intake from consumption of sugar-sweetened beverages.
  Source for measuring indicator: NHANES

Process Indicators

- Reduction in consumption of sugar-sweetened beverages such that they account for a smaller proportion of solid fats and added sugars in the daily diet.
  Source for measuring indicator: NHANES

- Adoption by states and school districts of policies that prohibit the sale of sugar-sweetened beverages in schools and require that schools offer a variety of no- or low-calorie beverage options that are favorably priced.
  Sources for measuring indicator: CDC's School Health Policies and Practices Survey and CLASS (NCI)

- Adoption by states and school districts of policies that require schools to provide access to free, clean, potable water throughout the school setting.
  Source for measuring indicator: CDC's School Health Policies and Practices Survey

Foundational Indicators

- USDA's prohibition of the sale of sugar-sweetened beverages in schools as part of the competitive food and beverage regulations to be developed for the Healthy, Hunger-Free Kids Act of 2010.
Source for measuring indicator: USDA

- Reduction in energy intake from consumption of sugar-sweetened beverages among populations with higher rates of consumption of such beverages, including non-Hispanic blacks, Mexican Americans, and lower-income individuals.
Source for measuring indicator: NHANES

NOTE: CDC = Centers for Disease Control and Prevention; CLASS = Classification of Laws Associated with School Students; NCI = National Cancer Institute; NHANES = National Health and Nutrition Examination Survey; USDA = U.S. Department of Agriculture.

Strategy 2-2: Increase the Availability of Lower-Calorie and Healthier Food and Beverage Options for Children in Restaurants

Chain and quick-service restaurants should substantially reduce the number of calories served to children and substantially expand the number of affordable and competitively priced healthier options available for parents to choose from in their facilities.

Potential actions include

- developing a joint effort (modeled after the Healthy Weight Commitment initiative) to set a specific goal for substantially reducing the total annual calories served to children in these facilities; and
- ensuring that at least half of all children's meals are consistent with the food and calorie guidelines of the Dietary Guidelines for Americans for moderately active 4- to 8-year-olds and are competitively priced.

Accelerating Progress in Obesity Prevention

Context

On any given day, it is estimated that 30-40 percent of children and adolescents (aged 4-19) eat fast food (Bowman et al., 2004; Kant and Graubard, 2004; Paeratakul et al., 2003). Approximately one-third of calories consumed by all Americans (aged 2 and older) are consumed outside the home (ERS, 2004). Most quick-service and chain restaurants offer children's meals. Limited research has addressed the nutritional profile of these meals. Relative to established expert guidelines (i.e., the Dietary Guidelines for Americans [HHS/USDA, 2010], Healthier School Challenge [FNS, 2011a], the Dietary Reference Intakes [IOM, 2006a], IOM school meal guidelines [IOM, 2007a]), however, two studies found that a majority of children's meals at chain and fast-food restaurants exceed the recommended calories, are considered high in saturated fat and sodium, and offer limited healthful choices (Harris et al., 2010; Wootan et al., 2008). In 2007 only 3 percent of meals marketed to children at 10 popular quick-service restaurants met the current National School Lunch Guidelines (O'Donnell et al., 2008). The caloric content of meals studied ranged from 180 to 880 kcal (O'Donnell et al., 2008).

To date, much of the attention related to reducing childhood obesity has focused on marketing of foods and beverages to children and adolescents, especially items to be consumed in the home, such as cereals and snack foods. Voluntary initiatives (CFBAI, 2011; Healthy Weight Commitment Foundation, 2011) have sought to address such marketing through nutrition standards and have resulted in some product reformulation and the introduction of some healthier foods (Kraak et al., 2011). As of this writing, however, the membership of Children's Food and Beverage Advertising Initiative (CFBAI) includes just two restaurants, and the Healthy Weight Commitment includes just one. Thus, this avenue offers substantial potential for accelerating progress in obesity prevention. Expectations are that by the end of 2015, food manufacturing companies will reduce annual calories by 1.5 trillion and sustain that level (Gable, 2011). An individual evaluation of the Healthy Weight Commitment began in 2010 to study calorie sources and eating pattern shifts (UNC Carolina Population Center, 2011). Such evaluation efforts present many opportunities and challenges, but clearly show that work is under way to measure progress.

In recent years, several fast-food and chain outlets have started developing healthier options for children's meals. In 2006, for example, Disney began offering a healthier children's meal as the default option at its theme parks (The Walt Disney Company, 2011). In 2011 the National Restaurant Association announced an initiative in which 19 chains, including Burger King, agreed to provide at least one children's meal option with no more than 600 calories (NRA, 2011). Also in 2011, McDonald's announced that low-fat milk will be the default drink option with Happy Meals, apples will be included in every Happy Meal, and the portion of french fries offered with Happy Meals will be reduced, resulting in a 20 percent calorie reduction compared with the traditional Happy Meal (the company did not release the specific number of calories) (McDonald's, 2011).

Although these developments sound encouraging, a recent analysis of the availability of healthy items on fast-food menus (as of January 2010) revealed that much more progress is needed (Harris et al., 2010). Just 12 of the 3,039 possible children's meal combinations that were studied met nutrition criteria for preschoolers, while 15 met the criteria for older children and adolescents (Harris et al., 2010). Although almost all of the top quick-service chains offer at least one healthy side dish and nutritious beverages, very few of the main dish options qualify as nutritious (Harris et al., 2010). In sum, industry has begun to respond to the need to provide healthier options for parents, but given the magnitude of the health challenge posed by childhood obesity, much more needs to be done, and on a far more urgent basis. Industry must truly step up and take, as the IOM has recommended, a "transforming" leadership role (IOM, 2006b).

Evidence

The IOM and other observers have long recommended that fast-food and chain restaurants play a larger role in addressing obesity, particularly childhood obesity. One IOM report recommends that full-service and fast-food restaurants expand healthier food options (IOM, 2005), and another calls on restaurant trade associations to assume "transforming leadership roles" on behalf of healthful diets for children and adolescents (IOM, 2006b). Similarly, the White House Task Force on Childhood Obesity has recommended that the restaurant industry "develop or reformulate more healthful foods for children and young people" (White House Task Force on Childhood Obesity, 2010, p. 60). And the Healthy Eating, Active Living Convergence Partnership has recommended encouraging restaurants to provide healthy foods and beverages by "reformulating existing menu items, adding healthier menu items (e.g., fruits, vegetables, and whole grains), offering affordable and reasonably sized portions, [and] providing healthier combinations for meals," and specifically suggested "making healthier items the standard for children's meals" (Lee et al., 2008, p. 7).

Children and adolescents who eat more meals from restaurants (sit-down and fast-food) have higher caloric intakes and poorer diet quality (i.e., more fat and sugar-sweetened beverages and less fruit, vegetables, and milk) (Befort et al., 2006; Boutelle et al., 2004; Bowman et al., 2004; French et al., 2001b; Lin et al., 1999; Paeratakul et al., 2003; Schmidt et al., 2005; Wiecha et al., 2006; Zoumas-Morse et al., 2001). Some studies have had mixed results regarding the association between frequency of eating out and higher BMI or body fatness; however, two longitudinal studies found that greater intake of fast food in adolescence is associated with an increase in body weight or BMI in young adulthood (Niemeier et al., 2006; Thompson et al., 2004). It has been reported that specific populations of children and adolescents consume higher amounts of fast food (males, non-Hispanic blacks, older adolescents, those with higher household incomes, and those who reside in the South) and that children, adolescents, and young adults consume more fast food than adults (Bowman et al., 2004; Paeratakul et al., 2003).

Implementation

Given the substantial number of calories consumed by children and adolescents away from home and particularly at quick-service and full-service restaurant chains, the committee believes this recommendation has the potential to accelerate progress in obesity prevention by effecting substantial reduction in the calories and fat consumed by children and adolescents. This recommendation may have the added benefit of reducing disparities in obesity rates for those young people who consume more food away from home—those who are male, non-Hispanic black, of higher household income, and older (i.e., adolescents).

Some companies have begun to make healthier options the default selection unless the customer requests otherwise, and other companies are beginning to offer healthier (lower-calorie) children's meals. After Disney began offering a healthier children's meal as the default option at its theme parks in 2006, more than 50 percent of customers stayed with the healthier choice (The Walt Disney Company, 2011). When McDonald's began offering apple dippers on request as a substitute for french fries in Happy Meals, the chain reported that less than 11 percent of customers requested the apples instead of the fries (McDonald's, 2011). In summer 2011, McDonald's announced it would be including apples, a smaller portion of french fries, and 20 percent fewer calories overall in the "most popular" Happy Meals. In 2011, the National Restaurant Association announced that 19 large restaurant chains had agreed to provide at least one children's meal option with no more than 600 calories (NRA, 2011).

These and other new restaurant industry efforts will need further evaluation to determine the impact of these new offerings on purchase requests and consumption patterns. The vast majority of children's menu items in quick-service and chain outlets currently fail to meet the Dietary Guidelines for Americans (Harris et al., 2010); if they did so, a meaningful reduction in calories would result. The success of some outlets (for example, Disney) in making healthier children's meals the default option indicates that many children and parents will make the healthier choice. At the same time, it must be noted that a majority of the food purchased for older children and adolescents in quick-service restaurants does not come from the available items on children's menus (Harris et al., 2010). Instead, ordering from such menus for older children has declined, while purchases of items from value menus have increased. In particular, parents of elementary-age children are more likely to order items for their children from the regular menu than from the children's menu (Harris et al., 2010). Therefore, it will be important to monitor the overall amount of calories consumed by children and adolescents in quick-service and chain restaurants to ensure that the unintended effect of shifting children's choices to higher-calorie, less-nutritious menu items does not occur. A multiyear effort will be required in which industry leaders make a joint commitment to reformulating menus and substantially reducing calories in child and adolescent meal offerings.

In sum, a significant number of calories consumed by children and adolescents come from fast-food and chain restaurants. Offering healthier selections and lower-calorie options should result in a more opportunities for children and adolescents (and parents) to select these items, thus improving the quality of diets, reducing caloric intake, and likely reducing BMI or weight.

Indicators for Assessing Progress in Obesity Prevention for Strategy 2-2

Process Indicators

- Reduction in caloric intake by children and adolescents in chain and quick-service restaurants.
  Source for measuring indicator: NPD Group (a consumer market research firm)

- Increase in the proportion of children's meals offered by chain and quick-service restaurants that meet the Dietary Guidelines for Americans.
  Source for measuring indicator: Update to study or similar to 2010 "Fast Food FACTS: Evaluating Fast Food Nutrition and Marketing to Youth" (Yale Rudd Center for Food Policy and Obesity)

- Increase in the proportion of restaurant outlets that offer a healthier option as the default menu choice.
  Source needed for measurement of indicator.

- Increase in the proportion of purchased children's meals that are labeled as "healthy."
  Source for measuring indicator: NPD Group (a consumer market research firm)

- Maintenance of or reduction in the percentage of adult meals, value meals, or à la carte items consumed by children and adolescents in chain or quick-service restaurants.
  Source for measuring indicator: NPD Group (a consumer market research firm)

Foundational Indicators

- Increase in the proportion of chain and quick-service restaurants that join the Children's Food and Beverage Advertising Initiative.
  Source for measuring indicator: CFBAI

- Increase in the percentage of chain and quick-service restaurants that join the Healthy Weight Commitment.
  Source for measuring indicator: HWC

- Increase in the proportion of chain and quick-service restaurants that commit to offering at least 50 percent of all children's meals meeting the Dietary Guidelines for Americans.
  Sources for measuring indicator: NRA and the associated press.

NOTE: CFBAI = Children's Food and Beverage Advertising Initiative; HWC = Healthy Weight Commitment; NRA = National Restaurant Association.

Strategy 2-3: Utilize Strong Nutritional Standards for all Foods and Beverages Sold or Provided Through the Government, and Ensure That These Healthy Options Are Available in All Places Frequented by the Public

Government agencies (federal, state, local, and school district) should ensure that all foods and beverages sold or provided through the government are aligned with the age-specific recommendations in the current Dietary Guidelines for Americans. The business community and the private sector operating venues frequented by the public should ensure that a variety of foods and beverages, including those recommended by the Dietary Guidelines for Americans, are sold or served at all times.

For **government agencies,** potential actions include

- the federal government expanding the healthy vending/concession guidelines to include all government-owned and/or -operated buildings, worksites, facilities,[15] and other locations where foods and beverages are sold/served; and
- all state and local government-owned and -operated buildings, worksites, facilities, and other locations where foods and beverages are sold/served (including through vending machines and concession stands) adopting and implementing a healthy food and beverage vending/concession policy.

For the **business community/private sector,** potential actions include

- the business community and private-sector entities that operate places frequented by the public ensuring that a variety of food and beverage options are competitively priced and available for purchase and consumption in these places,[16] including food and beverages that are aligned with the recommendations of the Dietary Guidelines for Americans.

---

[15] "Government-owned and -operated buildings, worksites, and facilities" is defined broadly to include not only places of work but also locations such as government-owned and/or -operated child care centers, hospitals, and other health care/assisted living facilities, military bases, correctional facilities, and educational institutions.

[16] "Places frequented by the public" includes, but is not limited to, privately owned and/or operated locations frequented by the public such as movie theaters, shopping centers, sporting and entertainment venues, bowling alleys, and other recreational/entertainment facilities.

Context

In 2010, 47.9 percent of all food spending, or more than $594 million, was for food consumed away from home (which includes food purchased by families and individuals for other-than-home consumption, expense-account meals, food furnished to employees, food furnished to inmates and patients, and food and cash donated to schools and institutions) (ERS, 2011a,b). Thus, attention must be paid to those places Americans frequent on a regular basis where they have ready access to food to ensure that they have a range of food options, including those that are healthy and affordably priced.

The food environment and points of access to that environment are vast. Outside of the home, Americans have access to food on a daily basis through government-run and/or -operated buildings and facilities, at work, at school and in child care settings, in recreational and entertainment settings, and in other locations (e.g., institutional facilities, military bases). Yet many of these locations are often overlooked as critical in affecting Americans' access to healthy, affordable foods that are recommended by the Dietary Guidelines for Americans.

Evidence

To maintain energy balance and focus on nutrient-dense foods and beverages, Americans must have access to a wide range of foods and beverages and not be inundated predominantly with those options that the Dietary Guidelines recommend limiting. Given that foods consumed outside of the home represented approximately 34 percent of the energy intake of children and adolescents by 2006 (Poti and Popkin, 2011) and 47.9 percent of all food spending (ERS, 2011b), it is critical to focus on such foods, including those consumed in government-owned and -operated buildings, worksites, and facilities, as well as places owned and operated by private enterprise but frequented by the public.

There is a positive relationship between eating behaviors and access to healthy foods (Larson et al., 2009). Studies have found that individuals with access to a greater amount of healthy foods consume more fresh produce and other healthful items (Treuhaft and Karpyn, 2010). Increasing consumption of the foods and beverages recommended by the Dietary Guidelines will depend heavily upon their availability and affordability. In fact, a 2011 IOM workshop on hunger and obesity explained that the keys to maximizing the purchase of healthier food options are increased availability, reduced price, and promotion of healthier choices (IOM, 2011). The evidence is clear that decreasing the prices of healthy food items relative to less-healthy items is effective in promoting purchases of the healthier items

(Epstein et al., 2006, 2007; French, 2003; French et al., 1997, 2001a; Michels et al., 2008; Ni Mhurchu et al., 2010), and that higher beverage prices lead to reduced consumption (Powell and Chaloupka, 2009; Smith et al., 2010).

Implementation

Federal, state, and local government Federal, state, and local government agencies are providers of food and should not be overlooked as part of the food environment. Various government programs procure food for their own restaurant/food service operations or provide assistance to allow others to do so (IOM, 2010). These programs range from food purchases for public worksites, health care facilities, senior centers, and military bases to foods sold in vending machines in city parks and other public places. More than 19 million individuals are employed at the federal, state, and local levels of government (U.S. Census Bureau, 2007), and this figure does not include members of the public who frequent or reside in government-owned or operated buildings, worksites, or facilities. Further, more than 1,400,000 people are on active duty in the U.S. military worldwide (Defense Manpower Media Center, 2011); the most recent estimate indicates that the military purchases more than $800 million in food to feed these personnel (GAO, 2000). According to the U.S. Census Bureau, between 2005 and 2009 more than 2 million people resided in adult correctional facilities, more than 1.8 million in nursing facilities/skilled nursing facilities, and more than 2 million in college/university housing (U.S. Census Bureau, 2011). Additionally, a number of federal programs use government funds for the purchase of food (GAO, 2000). The ability of these settings to institute public food standards may vary given their purpose, operating constraints, and reach (see Table 6-2).

Early child care and school settings also are key points of food access. More than 8 million children aged 3-5 were enrolled in early child care programs in 2009, and more than 55 million children and adolescents were projected to be enrolled in public and private secondary schools in 2010 (NCES, 2010, 2011). (See the discussion of school food standards in Chapter 9.)

Research has shown that changes in the workplace and child care settings (in addition to changes in the school setting addressed in Recommendation 5 [Chapter 9]) are effective in increasing the consumption of healthy options or in limiting access to unhealthy options. Strong evidence shows that worksite obesity prevention and control programs can reduce weight in employees and create habits that could be modeled at home. Some of these effective programs include interventions that improve access to healthy foods by changing cafeteria and

TABLE 6-2 Federal Agencies and Programs That Directly Purchase Foods or Use or Set Standards for Food Purchases

Agency	Program
U.S. Department of Agriculture	National School Lunch Program School Breakfast Program Supplemental Nutrition Assistance Program (SNAP) Summer Food Service Program Child and Adult Care Food Program Commodity Supplemental Food Program Food Distribution Program on Indian Reservations Nutrition Program for the Elderly The Emergency Food Assistance Program Food Assistance for Disaster Relief Fresh Fruit and Vegetable Program Special Supplemental Nutrition Program for Women, Infants, and Children (WIC) Nutrition Services Incentive Program
Department of Defense	Regular feeding of troops Fresh Fruit and Vegetable Program Defense Supply Center Philadelphia's Subsistence Directorate (link between the Armed Forces and the food industry; provides subsistence for military personnel and federal agencies worldwide)
Department of Justice (Bureau of Prisons)	Subsistence program purchases food for prisons
Department of Veterans Affairs	Food purchases for Veterans Affairs facilities
Department of Labor	Job Corps Center (provides training and employment for severely disadvantaged youths, generally in a residential setting)

SOURCES: Defense Logistics Agency, 2011; FNS, 2011b; GAO, 2000.

vending machine options as part of a multicomponent program (Anderson et al., 2009). (See also the discussion of Strategy 4-3 in Chapter 8.) Likewise, research suggests that in child care settings, the nutritional quality of meals and snacks can be poor, and activity levels may be inadequate (see the discussion of Strategy 1-4 in Chapter 5) (Ball et al., 2008; Padget and Briley, 2005; Story et al., 2006). Furthermore, children model the behavior of adults (Pearson et al., 2009). Thus, ensuring that publicly run worksites and child care centers are offering foods and beverages that are aligned with the Dietary Guidelines for Americans is essential to making the healthy choice the default choice (IOM, 2009; Ritchie et al., 2012).

Governments nationwide are in fact adopting and implementing nutrition standards to ensure the availability of a wide variety of foods and beverages, including those recommended by the Dietary Guidelines for Americans, in government-run or -regulated facilities and programs and applying those standards to food and beverage procurement and contracting (see Box 6-3). Such standards were recommended by a prior IOM committee and other experts (IOM, 2009, 2011). They build on the work done in schools nationwide to create healthy eating environments through state, district, and federal policies (the latter with the implementation of the *Healthy, Hunger-Free Kids Act of 2010*[17]) that restrict fats, sugars, calories, and other items that the Dietary Guidelines recommend limiting (CDC, 2011; Chriqui et al., 2010; Trust for America's Health and RWJF, 2011).

By instituting nutrition standards for all foods purchased with government dollars, local and state authorities can reduce the calories consumed by their residents across a variety of environments, model healthier eating, and potentially drive reformulation as companies respond to new product specifications. Furthermore, local and state governments can have considerable influence over a number of diverse food purchase and distribution locations. The introduction of nutrition standards is an area of increasing activity that offers an opportunity to influence diet at the population level. Beyond federal programs, state and local governments often are relatively large purchasers of food. They purchase or contract with restaurant/food service operators to supply the foods sold in employee cafeterias, schools and child care centers, public hospitals, senior centers, parks, and numerous other facilities (IOM, 2010).

Business community Foods are readily available in public places such as movie theaters, sports venues, and theme parks, to name a few, and attendance at these public places is not trivial. In 2010, more than 1.3 billion movie tickets were sold in the United States and Canada; 68 percent of all Americans and Canadians— or 222.7 million people—attended at least one movie in 2010 (Motion Picture Association of America, 2010). Furthermore, 339 million people attended theme parks during 2009, and 132 million attended professional sporting events such as Major League Baseball, National Football League, and National Basketball

---

[17]Public Law 111-296 (December 13, 2010).

BOX 6-3
Government Nutrition Standards

A number of states, counties, and cities have adopted nutrition standards for the meals and snacks they serve or provide to clients, employees, and the public. The introduction of nutrition standards for snacks and drinks sold in vending machines located on government-owned or -operated property, most commonly schools and hospital systems, is another area of recent local government engagement. When nutrition standards for foods sold in machines are incorporated into vending machine contracts, government further supports normalizing the consumption of healthier foods (IOM, 2010).

Federal Worksites

The Department of Health and Human Services and the General Services Administration developed Health and Sustainability Guidelines for Federal Concessions and Vending Operations (CDC, 2011). The goal of these guidelines is to assist contractors in increasing the availability of healthy food and beverage options and maintaining sustainable practices at federal worksites.

New York City

In 2009, New York City adopted standards for meals/snacks purchased and served by city agencies to agency clients that include schools, senior centers, homeless shelters, child care centers, after-school programs, correctional facilities, public hospitals and parks, and other agency facilities and programs and for beverage vending machines (New York City Department of Health and Mental Hygiene, 2011). The beverage vending machine standards affect all machines on city property. Twelve city agencies purchase or serve food that is covered by the meal/snack standards. These standards and those for beverage vending machines are being adopted voluntary by some private hospitals, workplaces, and community organizations (personal communication, T. Farley, New York City Department of Health and Mental Hygiene, May 25, 2011).

continued

Based on agency reports, the New York City Department of Health and Mental Hygiene estimates that the standards affect more than 260 million meals and snacks served each year by city agencies (New York City Department of Health and Mental Hygiene, 2011). Five (of the nine) city agencies that serve meals provide three meals a day to their clients, while the other four agencies serve one or two meals a day (personal communication, T. Farley, New York City Department of Health and Mental Hygiene, May 25, 2011). Some of the clients are seen every day (in day care and after school), while others are transient populations (the hospitalized, the homeless).

Since the adoption of the standards for meals/snacks in 2009, the New York City agency procurement practices and purchasing patterns have changed. The standards have been included in contracts with food suppliers and caterers. The result has been discontinuation of the purchase of some items (e.g., sugary drink mixes or items that require deep frying), the purchase of healthier alternative products (e.g., fruit packed in juice, not syrup), and the reformulation of some products to meet the standards (e.g., reducing the sodium in canned vegetables and reducing the sodium and fat in beef patties) (personal communication, T. Farley, New York City Department of Health and Mental Hygiene, May 25, 2011). Overall, implementation of the standards has resulted in the availability of more healthy options among the foods purchased and served by New York City agencies.

Massachusetts

In 2009, the Governor of Massachusetts issued an executive order mandating that all food purchased and sold by state agencies on state property conform to certain nutrition standards established by the public health department (Executive Order 509, 2009). Vending machines and other independent concessions are exempted. This order is aimed at food served to clients by state agencies and their vendors. These clients are dependent on the state for a package of services that

Association games—all venues where food is sold for immediate consumption and all hosting a captive audience or consumer base seeking a wide range of food and beverage options, including those recommended by the Dietary Guidelines for includes the provision of food and beverages. The executive order applies to 9 of the state's 58 agencies, responsible for approximately 110,980 meals each day (personal communication, Cynthia Taft Bayerl, Massachusetts Department of Public Health, August 24, 2011).

As of August 2011, the language of the executive order had been incorporated into a request for proposals for bakery products and catering to serve the nine affected agencies. As a result, the availability of healthy food choices has improved for these agencies. The larger agencies have larger food budgets, which allow them to balance the reduction in unhealthy food options (e.g., high-calorie foods and snacks) with the increased cost of healthy food options (e.g., whole-grain rather than white bread). The smaller agencies report the most difficulty in offering healthier foods. These agencies lack the buying power of the larger state agencies. Given their limited number of clients and storage space, these sites purchase smaller amounts of food at the local supermarket.

Public-service venues, vendings, and concessions are exempt from the executive order. However, they are encouraged to follow the state's *Healthy Meeting and Event Guide* (Massachusetts Department of Public Health, 2007).

Delaware State Parks

In June 2010, Delaware State Parks adopted a "Munch Better" initiative that will provide healthy foods for sale and in vending machines. For the first year, the goal is for at least 75 percent of the food and beverage products sold by parks to be either a "Go" or a "Slow" food (i.e., no more than 25 percent will be a "Whoa" food). This initiative was developed through a partnership among the Division of Parks and Recreation, the Nemours Health and Prevention Services (which developed the food and beverage guidelines), and the Delaware Health and Social Services' Division of Public Health (which will monitor progress) (Delaware State Parks, 2011).

Americans (Motion Picture Association of America, 2010). Indeed, the business community has been improving the foods and beverages offered for sale at entertainment and sporting events (see Box 6-4 for examples).

Examples of Improved Food and Beverage Offerings at Entertainment and Sporting Events

Improvements in food and beverage offerings are not limited to government settings. Positive steps in this regard also are occurring in the business community through improvements in the foods and beverages offered for sale in public venues such as entertainment and sporting events. Two illustrative examples follow.

Movie Theaters

In March 2010, the chairman and CEO of Sony Pictures Entertainment, Michael Lynton, asked the nation's theater owners to offer healthier snacks at their concession stands alongside the traditional candy, popcorn, and soda (James, 2010). In April 2011, AMC Theaters introduced AMC Smart MovieSnacks at all of its U.S. theaters for $7.00, compared with the roughly $10 cost of popcorn and a soda (AMC Entertainment, 2011; Carollo, 2011). The snack packs contain "the best of nutritious snack choices, yet still allow guests to indulge, albeit smartly, when snacking at the movies" (AMC Entertainment, 2011). They include

- Chiquita Fruit Chips consisting of 100 percent real fruit;

- Dasani purified water;

- Odwalla Bar Chocolate Chip Trail Mix with chocolate chips, rolled oats, peanuts, raisins, coconut, sunflower seeds, and Vitamins A, C, and E plus folic acid and calcium; and

- PopCorners—chip-like corn snacks that are air popped with real corn and all natural ingredients.

In sum, the committee believes that implementation of this strategy, in concert with the other strategies recommended in this chapter and in the report as a whole, represents an important step toward reducing the obesogenic environment in which Americans live, work, and play. Implementation of this strategy by

The new snack bundle has about 450 calories and 10 grams of fat (Carollo, 2011).

AMC's initiative to improve access to more nutritious snacks at the movies included working with the Alliance for a Healthier Generation and testing hundreds of products with guest panelists. AMC modeled its Smart MovieSnacks on the Alliance's school competitive food and beverage guidelines (AMC Entertainment, 2011).

Baseball Stadiums

At Dodger Stadium in Los Angeles, Kaiser Permanente has partnered with the stadium's restaurant group to offer healthier options at "Healthy Plate" carts in three locations around the stadium. Menu items include "Curried Chicken Lettuce Wraps served with radish, cucumber, cottage cheese and cherry tomatoes; Spicy Shrimp Cocktail, a refreshing gazpacho-like dish; Fresh Fruit Salad using only fruits that are in season; Greek Salad made with basil, feta cheese, tomatoes and red onions with low-fat balsamic vinaigrette; assorted sushi including California rolls, spicy tuna rolls and cucumber rolls; and a turkey sandwich served on whole wheat with avocado. Gluten-free beer and snacks will also be available at the Kaiser Permanente Healthy Plate Carts" (Dodgers, 2010). With the original recipe, the curried chicken salad ($8.75) weighs in at 313 calories and 15 grams of fat per serving, but the ballpark serving will be a couple of ounces bigger and include a scoop of cottage cheese. The farmers' market Greek salad ($8.75) has 130 calories and 11 grams of fat per serving, and the fruit and yogurt parfait ($5.25) with granola topping has 222 calories and 2 grams of fat (both per original recipes) (Stein, 2009).

governments and the business community would go a long way toward providing Americans with access to foods and beverages recommended by the Dietary Guidelines for Americans in places where they spend their work and leisure time.

Indicators for Assessing Progress in Obesity Prevention for Strategy 2-3

Primary Indicators

- Increase in the proportion of energy intake attributable to consumption of foods and beverages recommended by the Dietary Guidelines for Americans. *Source for measuring indicator:* NHANES

- Reduction in energy intake associated with solid fats and added sugars. *Source for measuring indicator:* NHANES

Process Indicators

- The federal government's expansion of its healthy vending/concession guidelines to include all federal government-owned, -operated, and -occupied buildings, worksites, and facilities. *Sources for measuring indicator:* GSA and HHS

- Increase in the proportion of states and municipalities that adopt and implement policies designed to ensure that foods/beverages sold and served in government-owned and -operated buildings, worksites, and facilities and other public places where foods and beverages are sold/served are aligned with the recommendations of the Dietary Guidelines for Americans. *Source needed for measurement of indicator.*

- Increase in the proportion of public places where foods and beverages are sold that offer a range of affordable and healthy food and beverage options. *Source needed for measurement of indicator.*

- Assurance of age-appropriate portion sizes and increase in quality of foods and beverages offered in government-owned and/or -operated child care programs. *Source for measuring indicator:* USDA program monitoring/reporting for funded programs

Foundational Indicator

- Adoption of healthy vending and food/beverage standards by members of the business community selling foods/beverages for public consumption. *Source needed for measurement of indicator.*

NOTE: GSA = U.S. General Services Administration; HHS = U.S. Department of Health and Human Services; NHANES = National Health and Nutrition Examination Survey; USDA = U.S. Department of Agriculture.

Strategy 2-4: Introduce, Modify, and Utilize Health-Promoting Food and Beverage Retailing and Distribution Policies

States and localities should utilize financial incentives such as flexible financing or tax credits, streamlined permitting processes, and zoning strategies, as well as cross-sectoral collaborations (e.g., among industry, philanthropic organizations, government, and the community) to enhance the quality of local food environments, particularly in low-income communities. These efforts should include encouraging or attracting retailers and distributors of healthy food (e.g., supermarkets) to locate in underserved areas and limiting the concentration of unhealthy food venues (e.g., fast-food restaurants, convenience stores). Incentives should be linked to public health goals in ways that give priority to stores that also commit to health-promoting retail strategies (e.g., through placement, promotion, and pricing).

Potential actions include

- states creating cross-agency teams to analyze and streamline regulatory processes and create tax incentives for retailing of healthy foods in underserved neighborhoods;
- states and localities creating cross-sectoral collaborations among the food and beverage industry, philanthropy, the finance and banking sector, the real estate sector, and the community to develop private funding to facilitate the development of healthy food retailing in underserved areas; and

- localities utilizing incentive tools to attract retailing of healthy foods (e.g., supermarkets and grocery stores) to underserved neighborhoods, such as through flexible financing or tax credits, streamlined permitting processes, zoning strategies, grant and loan programs, small business/economic development programs, and other economic incentives.

Context

As noted earlier, there is a positive relationship between access to healthy foods and eating behaviors (Larson et al., 2009; Treuhaft and Karpyn, 2010). Studies have found that individuals with access to a greater abundance of healthy foods consume more fresh produce and other healthful items (Lopez, 2007; Morland et al., 2006; Powell et al., 2007; Treuhaft and Karpyn, 2010). Yet many neighborhoods in the United States are without any type of grocery store or supermarket (Powell, 2009). Rural areas have fewer food retailers of any type than urban areas (controlling for population density) (Morton and Blanchard, 2007). Neighborhoods that are predominantly black, Hispanic, and low-income have disproportionately limited access and have seen the greatest decrease in the introduction of new food stores compared with predominantly Caucasian and higher-income neighborhoods (Powell, 2009; Treuhaft and Karpyn, 2010). Even when supermarkets are available in the former neighborhoods, healthier food items are less available (Krukowski et al., 2010; Treuhaft and Karpyn, 2010).

Additionally, greater access to convenience stores and fast-food restaurants, where healthy choices may not be readily available and may cost more, has been associated with a greater likelihood of lower dietary quality (Boone-Heinonen et al., 2011; Hickson et al., 2011; Larson et al., 2009). The availability of fast-food restaurants, convenience stores, and calorie-dense foods is greater in lower-income and minority neighborhoods (Baker et al., 2006; Larson et al., 2009).

Local food environments influence the choices made by children, families, and community members (IOM, 2009). Emerging evidence indicates that community strategies designed to reduce obesity by modifying the local food environment must take a comprehensive approach that is designed both to increase the availability of and access to healthy food options and to limit the concentration of and access to unhealthy food options (Boone-Heinonen et al., 2011). The relative balance of healthy and unhealthy food options may be more important than the presence or absence of any given food resource. Additionally, strategies that actively promote the selection and purchase of healthy food options (e.g., in-store promotions/placement, favorable display locations) may be critical to optimizing the benefits of healthy food resources.

Evidence

Since 2005 a number of expert committees have recommended that communities improve access to healthy foods, particularly in low-income and underserved areas, through a variety of evidence-based strategies in order to improve healthy eating (IOM, 2005, 2009; Khan et al., 2009; Lee et al., 2008; RWJF, 2009; White House Task Force on Childhood Obesity, 2010). The IOM report *Local Government Actions to Prevent Childhood Obesity* (IOM, 2009), in addition to recommending strategies for improving access to healthy foods, recommends strategies designed to discourage unhealthy local foods and resources.

In general, these strategies are supported by research indicating that consuming a diet rich in fruits and vegetables (in conjunction with other behaviors) tends to be associated with reduced weight gain and lower prevalence of obesity (or weight gain); however, the relationship of fruit and vegetable intake and eating behaviors to adiposity (i.e., BMI) in children is not clear (Alinia et al., 2009; Jago et al., 2007; Kahn et al., 1997; Ledoux et al., 2010; Muller et al., 1999). Evidence as to whether the availability of a specific type of food resource is associated with dietary consumption patterns or obesity rates is mixed, although it appears to be stronger for low-income males (Boone-Heinonen et al., 2011). Still, research suggests that individuals with greater access to retail venues that sell healthy foods (e.g., supermarkets) and limited access to those where healthy choices may not be available and cost more (e.g., fast-food restaurants, convenience stores) tend to have a lower risk of obesity or reduced weight gain (Giskes et al., 2011; Jilcott et al., 2011; Larson et al., 2009; Lopez, 2007; Morland and Evenson, 2009; Morland et al., 2006; Powell et al., 2007). More specifically, greater access to supermarkets can positively influence fruit and vegetable intake, dietary intake, consumption patterns, and diet quality compared with limited access, and for adolescents has been associated with lower BMI (Auld and Powell, 2009; Mikkelsen and Chehimi, 2007; Morland et al., 2002; Powell et al., 2007, 2010; Rose and Richards, 2004; Zenk et al., 2005). For example, Supplemental Nutrition Assistance Program (SNAP) participants who do not shop at supermarkets purchase fewer fresh fruits and vegetables and less milk than those who shop at supermarkets (ERS, 2009).

Evidence is mixed, however, on the influence of the availability and proximity of supermarkets on dietary quality, fruit and vegetable intake, and prevalence of obesity (Boone-Heinonen et al., 2011; Michimi and Wimberly, 2010). This mixed evidence suggests that the impact of supermarkets on food intake and obesity is mediated by what happens inside the store—other factors such as food prices and promotion/retailing practices. Access to affordable healthy foods does not necessarily mean that consumers will purchase and consume them. Building a store is the first step toward increasing availability of healthy foods, but complementary strategies to promote dietary behavior change must be included in such initiatives. Although research is limited, Glanz and Yaroch (2004) found that point-of-purchase information; reduced prices and coupons; increased availability, variety, and convenience; and promotion and advertising in supermarkets were moderately effective in influencing purchasing behavior. Major food retailers likewise have stated that in-store retailing practices are an essential influence on their customers' purchasing decisions (Rogers, 2011; Thomas, 2011).

As noted earlier, poor food environments often include an abundance of fast-food restaurants and convenience stores selling high-calorie, high-fat meals at relatively low prices (Lewis et al., 2005), as is disproportionately the case in lower-income and minority neighborhoods. Fast-food consumption and availability are related among low-income individuals (Boone-Heinonen et al., 2011). Adolescents who live and attend school in areas with more fast-food restaurants and convenience stores than food outlets with healthier selections, such as grocery stores, are more likely to consume soda and fast food than those who live and attend school in areas with healthier food environments (Babey et al., 2011). For example, fast-food availability may contribute to greater energy intake in younger black Americans (Hickson et al., 2011).

Despite the growing evidence base linking the concentration of fast-food restaurants to the consumption of calorie-dense food, community-level strategies to limit access to or reduce the concentration of fast-food restaurants are limited. Moratoriums on such restaurants and other strategies designed to limit the concentration of certain restaurant types are relatively new and as yet unproven. Given the emerging evidence implicating the concentration of fast-food restaurants in unhealthy eating, such strategies may prove beneficial in enhancing the quality of local food environments, particularly in low-income communities.

Implementation

A number of efforts have been undertaken to support and implement the sentiment of this recommended strategy by developing programs, initiatives, and legislation through public and private partnerships. The introduction of supermarkets in neighborhoods where they are lacking has yielded some initial positive economic results (see Box 6-5 for an example of supermarket initiatives and support programs).

Given the disproportionate lack of access to affordable healthy foods for a large number of Americans, the use of financial incentives, zoning, and cross-sectoral collaborations can attract healthy food retailing and distribution (e.g., supermarkets) to underserved areas and limit the concentration of unhealthy

---

BOX 6-5
Supermarket Programs, Initiatives, and Legislation

- The Food Trust's Supermarket Campaign[a]

- Pennsylvania Fresh Food Financing Initiative[b]

- Food Retail Expansion Support Health in New York City[c]

- New Orleans Fresh Food Retailer Initiative[d]

- Louisiana Healthy Food Retail Act[e]

- TransForm Baltimore[f]

- California FreshWorks Fund[g]

- Re/Store Nashville[h]

- Federal Incentive Programs (USDA, HHS, HUD, EPA, US Treasury)[i]

---

[a]The Food Trust, 2011.
[b]The Reinvestment Fund, 2010.
[c]New York City Government, 2009.
[d]The City of New Orleans, 2011.
[e]*Healthy Food Retail Act 2009.* No. 252, §1.
[f]TransForm Baltimore, 2011.
[g]California FreshWorks Fund, 2011.
[h]Get Out. Be Active., 2011.
[i]Summarized in ERS, 2009, p. 105.

food venues (e.g., fast food). Preliminary economic impact assessments of such initiatives have found that they have a significant impact on estate prices, employment, and earnings, and they are expected to significantly increase access to healthy foods for millions of households and communities that are currently underserved (The Reinvestment Fund, 2010; Treuhaft and Karpyn, 2010). Yet while a large number of initiatives and investments are already being implemented in some localities, it is clear that further work is needed to provide access to healthy foods for everyone. In 2011, leaders from major retailers, foundations, and small businesses announced commitments to provide access to healthy, affordable food for millions of people in underserved communities (Partnership for a Healthier America, 2011). As part of the retail industry's focus on healthy food initiatives, some of these same retailers have reported undertaking large-scale efforts to encourage healthier food purchases by understanding their customers and meeting their needs through the use of pricing strategies (e.g., coupons, daily specials), simple labeling or endorsements of healthier food products, in-store cooking demonstrations and recipes, and reorganization of the supermarket itself (customers must walk through the produce area to get to other sections of the store) (Rogers, 2011; Thomas, 2011).

In sum, the committee believes this recommended strategy would likely have a direct effect on the availability and accessibility of healthy and unhealthy foods in targeted neighborhoods and could encourage consumers to purchase foods that would help them meet the Dietary Guidelines for Americans. In particular, this strategy has the potential to reduce disparities in obesity rates for consumers who have no or limited access to retailers of healthy foods (e.g., supermarkets) and are exposed to a large number of retailers of unhealthy food. These include residents of neighborhoods that are predominantly black, Hispanic, low-income, and rural, as well as individuals lacking transportation.

Indicators for Assessing Progress in Obesity Prevention for Strategy 2-4

Process Indicators

- Increase in the proportion of Americans who have access to a food retail outlet that sells a variety of foods recommended by the Dietary Guidelines for Americans.
  Source needed for measurement of indicator.

- Adoption and achievement of the grocery industry standard of 3 square feet of retail space per capita by all grocery retailers.*
  Source needed for measurement of indicator.

Foundational Indicator

- Development and implementation by municipal governments of incentive programs for new and/or existing food retailers to increase access to healthier food and beverage options in underserved areas.
  Source needed for measurement of indicator.

---

*Three square feet of space per person is a measure of demand for grocery retail service in a defined area commonly used by grocery retailers (International Council of Shopping Centers, 2008).

Strategy 2-5: Broaden the Examination and Development of U.S. Agriculture Policy and Research to Include Implications for the American Diet

Congress, the Administration, and federal agencies should examine the implications of U.S. agriculture policy for obesity, and should ensure that such policy includes understanding and implementing, as appropriate, an optimal mix of crops and farming methods for meeting the Dietary Guidelines for Americans.

Potential actions include

- the President appointing a Task Force on Agriculture Policy and Obesity Prevention to evaluate the evidence on the relationship between agriculture policies and the American diet, and to develop recommendations for policy options and future policy-related research, specifically on the impact of farm subsidies and the management of commodities on food prices, access, affordability, and consumption;
- Congress and the Administration establishing a process by which federal food, agriculture, and health officials would review and report on the possible implications of U.S. agriculture policy for obesity prevention to ensure that this issue will be fully taken into account when policy makers consider the Farm Bill;
- Congress and the U.S. Department of Agriculture (USDA) developing policy options for promoting increased domestic production of foods recommended for a healthy diet that are generally underconsumed, including fruits and vegetables and dairy products, by reviewing incentives and disincentives that exist in current policy;
- as part of its agricultural research agenda, USDA exploring the optimal mix of crops and farming methods for meeting the current Dietary Guidelines for Americans, including an examination of the possible impact of smaller-scale agriculture, of regional agricultural product distribution chains, and of various agricultural models from small to large scale, as well as other efforts to ensure a sustainable, sufficient, and affordable supply of fresh fruits and vegetables; and
- Congress and the Administration ensuring that there is adequate public funding for agricultural research and extension so that the research agenda can include a greater focus on supporting the production of foods Americans need to consume in greater quantities according to the Dietary Guidelines for Americans.

Context

U.S. agriculture policy is a complex system that has evolved over many decades. The impact that farm policy has on the nation's food supply and diet reflects not only current policies but also the long history of agriculture policies. Whether and how farm policy is related to the obesity epidemic are questions research has only recently begun to explore, and a definitive evidence base has not yet emerged. But a consensus does appear to be developing around two key points: first, blunt approaches such as eliminating farm subsidies are unlikely to offer a quick fix to the obesity epidemic; and second, there are real opportunities to adjust farm policies in meaningful ways to better support the nation's changing food and nutrition needs.

The current farm system does not produce sufficient fruits and vegetables and dairy products to support a substantial increase in the availability of healthier food and beverage options at affordable, competitive prices. Indeed, even including imports, the supply of fresh fruits and vegetables would be inadequate if all Americans adopted a diet consistent with the Dietary Guidelines for Americans (Buzby et al., 2006). This imbalance is a result of decades of farm policies and will take time to address.

Because considerable time will be required for the changes to agriculture policy that could positively impact obesity prevention to be implemented and translate to weight outcomes, action must be taken now to move policy toward a constructive long-term approach. The committee believes the nation can no longer ignore the need to address the potential role of farm policies in preventing obesity. This means giving priority to ensuring that U.S. farm and trade policies promote healthy eating and do not undermine obesity prevention, and applying that perspective to the evaluation of current policies and the development of policy alternatives. American farmers can and should be important allies in the fight against obesity, but they will assume that role only if agriculture policies support them in doing so.

Evidence

The impact of U.S. agriculture policies on obesity has received increasing attention over the past decade. In particular, concern has been raised about the impact of farm subsidies, check-off programs, marketing orders, and land use rules. Relative to the role of other sectors in the causes of obesity, the contribution of U.S. agriculture policies has received less scholarly analysis. This is one reason the committee is recommending an acceleration of both agriculture- and policy-focused research and deliberation.

Previous IOM committees have made similar recommendations, but without delineating specific implementing actions. A 2005 IOM report suggests that government agencies at all levels need to reexamine their existing policies and initiatives that may hinder progress toward prevention of childhood obesity, including agriculture policies. It suggests that a review of agriculture policies could identify unintended effects of U.S. agriculture subsidies on human health, noting that further investigation of the possible relationships among agriculture policies (such as corn subsidies and the production and use of high fructose corn syrup in the U.S. food supply), the obesity epidemic (Bray et al., 2004), and the marked increase in type 2 diabetes (Gross et al., 2004; Schulze et al., 2004) is warranted. Specifically, the report recommends that the federal government undertake an independent assessment of federal nutrition assistance programs and agriculture policies to ensure that they promote healthful dietary intake for all children and adolescents. It also recommends that policies and programs be revised as necessary to promote a U.S. food system that supports energy balance at a healthy weight.

In assessing progress made toward this recommendation, a 2007 IOM report notes that there have been limited analyses examining the relationships among U.S. food supply-related agricultural, industrial, and economic policies (or the environments resulting from these policies) and consumer demand-driven nutrition policies (e.g., dietary guidance) (IOM, 2007b; Tillotson, 2004). The report suggests that future efforts to improve the U.S. food and agriculture system will need to forge connections among health, food, and farm policies that support the 2005 Dietary Guidelines for Americans. It also identifies the Farm Bill as an opportunity to foster changes that both support healthier diets and strengthen agricultural economies. The Institute for Agriculture and Trade Policy has drawn similar conclusions (Schoonover and Muller, 2006).

International health organizations likewise have called on member nations to step up efforts to ensure consistency between farm and health policies. The World Health Organization's (WHO's) *Global Strategy on Diet, Physical Activity, and Health* (WHO, 2004, p. 8) states that "national food and agriculture policies should be consistent with the promotion and protection of public health" and directs member states to consider "healthy nutrition" in their agriculture policies. The International Obesity Task Force recommends a three-pronged strategy: include nutritional criteria in agriculture policies, undertake health impact assessments of such policies, and provide support for agriculture programs aimed at meeting WHO's dietary guidelines (Hawkes, 2007). The International Assessment of Agricultural Knowledge, Science and Technology for Development considers "improving nutrition and human health" as one of the goals in its framework for making decisions on international agriculture policies (McIntyre et al., 2009). The Chicago Council on Global Affairs and the UK Government Office of Science provided further support on connecting future farm policies with obesity (Foresight, 2011; The Chicago Council on Global Affairs, 2011).

Documenting the relationship between specific agriculture policies and public health outcomes is difficult because as noted, there is likely to be a time lag between agricultural cause and dietary effect (Hawkes, 2007), and a number of variables could mask or amplify the causal relationships (Muller et al., 2009). U.S. agriculture policy includes a complex set of programs that affect production costs, production, commodity prices, and farm incomes. Furthermore, farm outputs often go through several processing steps before reaching consumers, making it difficult to quantify the effect of a given policy on obesity. Consequently, the effects of agriculture policies on dietary intake and obesity are not well understood (Alston et al., 2006).

Implementation

Farm subsidies Existing examinations of the issues outlined above are limited, and researchers have reached differing conclusions. Some in the health professions believe that agriculture policies—particularly farm subsidies—have decreased the price of obesogenic foods, presumably leading to overconsumption of these foods and thereby contributing to the increase in obesity prevalence (e.g., Pollan, 2003; Schoonover and Muller, 2006; Tillotson, 2003). Others, including some in the agricultural economics community, conclude that farm subsidies bear little responsibility for lower food prices, increased consumption of obesogenic foods, and increased obesity prevalence (e.g., Alston et al., 2006, 2008; Miller and Coble, 2008; Schaffer et al., 2007).

Some analysts argue that farm subsidies have contributed to obesity because they decrease the prices of corn, soybeans, and other commodity crops. Food processors therefore can purchase these commodities at lower prices and thus are encouraged to use them as ingredients. Such ingredients (e.g., high fructose corn syrup and partially hydrogenated vegetable oils) often are found in low-nutrient, energy-dense (obesogenic) foods. The reasoning continues that because of the low input costs, such foods can be sold at low prices that encourage consumers to purchase and consume more of these foods, contributing to weight gain (Schaffer et al., 2007; Schoonover and Muller, 2006; Wallinga et al., 2009). Cawley and Kirwan (2011) use estimates and assumptions about the relationships among subsidies, food prices, and BMI to estimate that agriculture subsidies increase youth BMI by 0.08 percent. They also point out that the USDA's commodity distribution program donates agriculture commodities to schools and maintain that in most cases, these commodities—cheese, milk, beef, pork, and oils—are energy dense. They estimate that the risk of obesity among children and adolescents who consume school lunches is raised by 0.14 percentage points because of the commodity distribution program.

Wallinga and colleagues (2009) suggest that the relatively low prices for obesogenic foods have caused them to proliferate in the U.S. diet and have placed healthier foods, such as fruits and vegetables, at a competitive disadvantage. They also speculate that low commodity prices help maintain high profit margins on foods that make liberal use of these commodity inputs, consequently driving interest in the marketing of these foods.

Taking a different perspective, a number of papers and presentations on this topic were developed as part of a 4-year project undertaken by the University of California, Davis and Iowa State University, funded under a National Research Initiative Grant from the USDA National Institute for Food and Agriculture.[18] The project team concluded that U.S. farm subsidy programs—namely, price and income supports for commodities—have had negligible effects on commodity prices and that eliminating or reversing commodity subsidy policies would be unlikely to affect consumer dietary behaviors such that obesity rates would be meaningfully reduced (Alston, 2010; Alston et al., 2006, 2007, 2008). First, they cite evidence that subsidies have had mixed and only modest effects on the availability and prices of commodities, particularly those that are ingredients in obesogenic foods. Second, they report that the magnitude of the effect of changes in commodity prices on retail prices depends on the cost share of the commodity in retail prices. Because food commodities represent about 20 percent of the current cost of food in the United States (and less for products such as soda and meals away from home), changes in the prices of commodities used in high-calorie foods may not translate into perceptible changes in the price of high-calorie food products. Cawley and Kirwan (2011) concur that the cost of farm commodities typically represents a small percentage of food's retail price. Furthermore, Alston and colleagues (2006, 2008; Alston, 2010) maintain that even if subsidy policies affect food prices, food consumption patterns are relatively unresponsive to changes in market prices.

Production of foods recommended for a healthy diet While the evidence regarding the relationship between subsidies and obesity is mixed, what is clearer is that the current agriculture system fails to produce the mix and quantity of foods necessary for Americans to consume diets recommended by the Dietary Guidelines for Americans. A 2006 Economic Research Service report examining the implications for U.S. agriculture if Americans consumed the recommended fruits, vegetables,

---

[18]See http://aic.ucdavis.edu/obesity/papers.htm (accessed October 19, 2011).

and whole grains concludes that an additional 7.4 million acres of cropland would need to be harvested per year, and that meeting the dairy guidelines would require the production of an additional 108 billion pounds of dairy products domestically (Buzby et al., 2006).

Buzby and colleagues (2006) found that the average American is eating too much food made with refined grains, but would need to increase whole-grain consumption by more than 200 percent to meet the recommendations of the Dietary Guidelines for Americans (see Figure 6-1 earlier in this chapter). Overall, this means that Americans would need to reduce consumption of total grains by 27 percent. Because it takes less raw wheat to produce a whole-grain product than a similar refined-grain product, the overall drop in demand could translate to 5.6 million fewer acres of wheat each year. Additionally, Buzby and colleagues (2006) point out that an increase in dairy demand (of roughly 65 percent) would likely require an increase in the number of dairy cows, an increase in the volume of feed grains needed, and possibly an increase in the acreage devoted to dairy production. Still, producers of whole grains and dairy have existing mechanisms in place to aid in the availability and affordability of these products. Whole grains are a commodity crop, which provides price and income support, and dairy has an organized pricing, marketing, and support system (and can be subsidized) (Manchester and Blayney, 2001).

However, fruit and vegetable consumption is influenced by several factors, including domestic production, convenience, cost, palatability and personal preference, the desire to cultivate a healthy lifestyle, and the availability and diversity of products procured through trade (Pollack, 2001). Their consumption is positively correlated with income, as well as per capita supply. In the current agriculture policy environment, farmers may be dissuaded from producing fruits and vegetables for a number of reasons, including planting restrictions under commodity programs, financial concerns (e.g., difficulty accessing credit or securing sufficient crop insurance, higher risk, high startup costs, higher production costs), complex production practices, the need for specialized equipment and sufficient labor for harvesting, and agronomic constraints (e.g., limited season, water) (Johnson et al., 2006; Krueger et al., 2010).

Most harvested cropland in the United States is enrolled in the primary commodity payment program, which makes price and income support payments to farmers in proportion to the acreage on which traditional program crops (wheat, feed grains, cotton, rice, oilseeds) are grown. In general, farmers are prohibited from planting and harvesting fruits and vegetables on acres enrolled in the commodity payment program. An Economic Research Service analysis found that eliminating planting restrictions would likely have a small market effect, but could have a significant effect on individual producers depending on the costs and returns for producing a particular crop, which vary across regions and over time (Johnson et al., 2006).

Farmers may be deterred from producing fruits and vegetables because of the relative difficulty (compared with other crops) of obtaining loan approval to plant them (Krueger et al., 2010). USDA has collected a body of data on historical yields and prices for the covered commodity crops grown on restricted acres. Such data do not exist for fruits and vegetables, making it difficult for farmers of those crops to project their income in order to obtain loan approval, while the federal government and private entities can more confidently offer loans and financing to producers of commodity crops that are supported by more data.

Price and yield data also are used to determine insurance coverage, which fruit and vegetable farmers rely on to protect against losses. Many fruit and vegetable crops are highly sensitive to weather perturbations, and crop insurance is the primary tool for managing climate-related risks. The lack of data is a factor in the lack of individual crop insurance policies for many fruits and vegetables, leaving farmers to rely on catastrophic coverage under the Non-insured Crop Disaster Assistance Program, which covers about 28 percent of the value of a total loss (Krueger et al., 2010). In an Institute for Agriculture and Trade Policy webinar[19] about the challenges to growing healthy foods, fruit and vegetable farmers stated that it was difficult to obtain insurance for growing fruits and vegetables, in part because banks are increasingly risk-averse and perceive those crops to be relatively risky. Krueger and colleagues (2010) offer policy change recommendations designed to remedy the dearth of crop price and yield data.

Local food systems Although local food systems remain a small share of total U.S. agriculture sales, interest has increased in these systems as part of food and agriculture policy. In relation to obesity prevention, the benefits of local food markets remain largely unstudied. In a recent review of local food systems, USDA's Economic Research Service cites a number of potential benefits, including reducing safety risks, developing social capital, improving environmental quality, reducing energy use, and fostering local economic development. It is unclear what direct role local food systems have in consumer or dietary choices as opposed to

---

[19]See http://healthyfoodaction.org/?q=hero/what-it-takes-grow-healthy-food-views-farm (accessed December 12, 2011).

Accelerating Progress in Obesity Prevention

availability and access in general (Martinez et al., 2010). Additionally, the precise role of local food systems in improving food security in areas with limited access to fresh foods is difficult to assess (Martinez et al., 2010). Furthermore, prices of local foods depend on the market dynamics in particular locations and may be comparable to or lower or higher than prices of other products or in other markets (Pirog and McCann, 2009).

Agricultural research Cawley and Kirwan (2011, p. 8) maintain that publicly funded agricultural research is "the agricultural policy with potentially the greatest impact on food prices and consumption." According to Alston and colleagues (2006, 2008), agricultural research and development (R&D) policies are a reason that farm commodity prices have fallen so substantially. Agricultural R&D contributes to lower production and processing costs, increasing farm productivity and thereby making agricultural commodities much less expensive and more abundant than they would otherwise be. One study (Miller and Coble, 2007) that econometrically modeled farm productivity showed that agricultural technology gains have increased food affordability across food groups. Faulkner and colleagues (2010) concur that agricultural R&D has had an impact on consumption and obesity through increased agricultural output and lower farm commodity prices. Alston and Okrent (2009) conclude that compared with farm subsidies, public agricultural research policy has had much larger long-term effects on food prices and consumption.

In summary, this strategy and the associated potential implementing actions address a gap in the current arsenal of obesity prevention strategies. According to Muller and colleagues (2009), food and agriculture issues usually are discussed in silos, without consideration of their effect on public health or other aspects of the food system. Lock and colleagues (2010) note that neither sector considers the complex interactions among agritrade, food consumption patterns, health, and development. This strategy encourages stakeholders to view food and agriculture issues from a broader perspective as the foundation of the nation's food supply, which in turn impacts consumption behaviors and energy intake. The reach of this strategy is broad and would affect every American.

Indicators for Assessing Progress in Obesity Prevention for Strategy 2-5

Foundational Indicators

- Encouragement and promotion of increased consumption of fresh fruits and vegetables by policy makers, other governmental decision makers, and the business community through competitive pricing and increased availability and production to enable all Americans to consume the amounts of fruits and vegetables recommended by the Dietary Guidelines for Americans.
  Source needed for measurement of indicator.

- Formation of a task force to examine the relationships between U.S. agriculture policy and obesity prevention.
  Source needed for measurement of indicator.

- Issuance of a government report on the obesity-related implications of the Farm Bill.
  Source needed for measurement of indicator.

- Occurrence of congressional hearings on the relationship between U.S. agriculture policy and obesity to inform future agriculture policy.
  Source needed for measurement of indicator.

- Establishment of a process for obesity-related review of the Farm Bill.
  Source needed for measurement of indicator.

- Introduction of legislative and regulatory policies to increase domestic production of fruits and vegetables.
  Source needed for measurement of indicator.

- Maintenance of or increases in funding budgets for USDA research and Land Grant universities.
  Source needed for measurement of indicator.

NOTE: USDA = U.S. Department of Agriculture.

INTEGRATION OF STRATEGIES FOR ACCELERATING PROGRESS IN OBESITY PREVENTION

The strategies included in this chapter have one goal: to make the healthy option the routine and affordable option. Increasing access to healthy food and beverage options recommended by the Dietary Guidelines for Americans (HHS/USDA, 2010) and decreasing consumption of solid fats and added sugars (e.g., sugar-sweetened beverages), in particular, are critical steps toward achieving energy balance when implemented in concert with achieving recommended levels of physical activity (Chapter 5). However, adherence to the food patterns recommended by the Dietary Guidelines for Americans is no easy task and will take time. The current obesogenic environment provides unhealthy options that are often more affordable and available than healthy options. For this situation to change, a concerted effort will be required on the part of governments, industry, restaurants and other food service providers, schools and child care providers, and members of the business community/private sector operating places frequented by the public to change the types of foods and beverages sold or offered to consumers such that they provide a range of competitively priced options.

Governments, in particular, have a critical role to play in this effort. Through their policy-making authority, governments (at all levels) can incentivize the purchase of healthier food and beverage options or impose taxes on unhealthy options (e.g., sugar-sweetened beverages). State and local governments also can remove regulatory barriers to and create incentives for retailing of healthy foods, particularly in underserved neighborhoods without ready access to healthy food options. Governments should support the work of community groups and coalitions in their efforts to create healthy food environments in the nation's communities. And the federal government should examine the extent to which U.S. farm policy can support production of the optimal mix of crops and the farming methods necessary to meet the food patterns recommended in the Dietary Guidelines for Americans.

In short, the strategies presented in this chapter are intended to support the evidence-based recommendations included in the Dietary Guidelines for Americans. Taken in isolation, the individual strategies included in this chapter likely will be insufficient to accelerate progress in obesity prevention. Taken together, however, in concert with comparable changes in physical activity levels, in school environments, in messaging, in health care and worksite environments, and in critical community supports, these strategies can go a long way toward helping Americans meet the food patterns recommended by the Dietary Guidelines for Americans and, in turn, accelerate progress in obesity prevention.

REFERENCES

AAP (American Academy of Pediatrics). 2011. Sports drinks and energy drinks for children and adolescents: Are they appropriate? *Pediatrics* 127(6):1182-1189.

AAP Committee on Nutrition. 2001. The use and misuse of fruit juice in pediatrics. *Pediatrics* 107(5):1210-1213.

AAP Section on Pediatric Dentistry and Oral Health. 2008. Preventive oral health intervention for pediatricians. *Pediatrics* 122(6):1387-1394.

AAPD (American Academy of Pediatric Dentistry). 2010. Policy on vending machines in schools. *Reference Manual: Oral Health Policies* 33(6):55-56.

ABA (American Beverage Association). 2010. *Alliances school beverage guidelines final progress report.* http://www.ameribev.org/files/240_School%20Beverage%20 Guidelines%20Final%20Progress%20Report.pdf (accessed December 5, 2011).

Alinia, S., O. Hels, and I. Tetens. 2009. The potential association between fruit intake and body weight—a review. *Obesity Reviews* 10(6):639-647.

Alliance for a Healthier Generation. 2006. *School beverage and competitive foods guidelines.* http://www.healthiergeneration.org/companies.aspx?id=5691 (accessed October 19, 2011).

Alston, J. M. 2010. Farm subsidies, agricultural R&D, and obesity. Presented at the Workshop on Farm and Food Policy and Obesity, May 21-22, 2010, Davis, CA.

Alston, J. M, and A. Okrent. 2009. *Farm commodity policy and obesity.* Paper presented at Pre-Conference Workshop, Diet and Obesity: Role of Prices and Policies, August 16, 2009, Beijing, China.

Alston, J. M., D. A. Sumner, and S. A. Vosti. 2006. Are agricultural policies making us fat? Likely links between agricultural policies and human nutrition and obesity, and their policy implications. *Review of Agricultural Economics* 28(3):313-322.

Alston, J. M., J. C. Beghin, H. H. Jensen, L. Kaiser, D. A. Sumner, and S. A. Vosti. 2007. *Effects of agricultural policies on human nutrition and obesity.* Paper presented at USDA-NRI Human Nutrition and Obesity Project Directors' Workshop, June 26-28, 2007, Washington, DC.

Alston, J. M., D. A. Sumner, and S. A. Vosti. 2008. Farm subsidies and obesity in the United States: National evidence and international comparisons. *Food Policy* 33(6):470-479.

AMA (American Medical Association). 2007. *Childhood obesity: American Medical Association policy and guidelines.* http://www.ama-assn.org/ama1/pub/upload/ mm/433/ama-policies-childhood-obesity.pdf (accessed November 13, 2011).

AMC Entertainment. 2011. *AMC Theatres® raises the curtain on AMC smart movie snacks & trade.* http://www.investor.amctheaters.com/releasedetail. cfm?ReleaseID=561642 (accessed September 16, 2011).

American Dental Association. 2005. *Food marketing to kids workshop—comment (project no. P034519)*. http://ada.org/sections/advocacy/pdfs/nutrition_letter_ftc.pdf (accessed October 21, 2011).

Anderson, L. M., T. A. Quinn, K. Glanz, G. Ramirez, L. C. Kahwati, D. B. Johnson, L. R. Buchanan, W. R. Archer, S. Chattopadhyay, G. P. Kalra, and D. L. Katz. 2009. The effectiveness of worksite nutrition and physical activity interventions for controlling employee overweight and obesity: A systematic review. *American Journal of Preventive Medicine* 37(4):340-357.

Andreyeva, T., M. W. Long, and K. D. Brownell. 2010. The impact of food prices on consumption: A systematic review of research on the price elasticity of demand for food. *American Journal of Public Health* 100(2):216-222.

Andreyeva, T., F. J. Chaloupka, and K. D. Brownell. 2011. Estimating the potential of taxes on sugar-sweetened beverages to reduce consumption and generate revenue. *Preventive Medicine* 52(6):413-416.

Auld, M. C., and L. M. Powell. 2009. Economics of food energy density and adolescent body weight. *Economica* 76(304):719-740.

Babey, S. H., J. Wolstein, and A. L. Diamant. 2011. Food environments near home and school related to consumption of soda and fast food. *Policy Brief UCLA Center for Health Policy Research* (PB2011-6):1-8.

Baker, E. A., M. Schootman, E. Barnidge, and C. Kelly. 2006. The role of race and poverty in access to foods that enable individuals to adhere to dietary guidelines. *Preventing Chronic Disease* 3(3):A76.

Ball, S. C., S. E. Benjamin, and D. S. Ward. 2008. Dietary intakes in North Carolina child-care centers: Are children meeting current recommendations? *Journal of the American Dietetic Association* 108(4):718-721.

Befort, C., H. Kaur, N. Nollen, D. K. Sullivan, N. Nazir, W. S. Choi, L. Hornberger, and J. S. Ahluwalia. 2006. Fruit, vegetable, and fat intake among non-Hispanic black and non-Hispanic white adolescents: Associations with home availability and food consumption settings. *Journal of the American Dietetic Association* 106(3):367-373.

Bellisle, F., and M. F. Rolland-Cachera. 2001. How sugar-containing drinks might increase adiposity in children. *Lancet* 357(9255):490-491.

Blumenthal, D. M., and M. S. Gold. 2010. Neurobiology of food addiction. *Current Opinion in Clinical Nutrition & Metabolic Care* 13(4):359.

Boone-Heinonen, J., P. Gordon-Larsen, C. I. Kiefe, J. M. Shikany, C. E. Lewis, and B. M. Popkin. 2011. Fast food restaurants and food stores: Longitudinal associations with diet in young to middle-aged adults: The CARDIA study. *Archives of Internal Medicine* 171(13):1162-1170.

Boutelle, K. N., J. A. Fulkerson, D. Neumark-Sztainer, M. Story, and S. A. French. 2004. Fast food for family meals: Relationships with parent and adolescent food intake, home food availability and weight status. *Public Health Nutrition* 10:16-23.

Bowman, S. A., S. L. Gortmaker, C. B. Ebbeling, M. A. Pereira, and D. S. Ludwig. 2004. Effects of fast-food consumption on energy intake and diet quality among children in a national household survey. *Pediatrics* 113(1 Pt 1):112-118.

Bray, G. A., S. J. Nielsen, and B. M. Popkin. 2004. Consumption of high-fructose corn syrup in beverages may play a role in the epidemic of obesity. *American Journal of Clinical Nutrition* 79(4):537-543.

Bridging the Gap Program. 2011. *State sales taxes on regular, sugar-sweetened soda and snacks, 1997-2011.* http://www.bridgingthegapresearch.org (accessed December 6, 2011).

Briefel, R. R., and C. L. Johnson. 2004. Secular trends in dietary intake in the United States. *Annual Review of Nutrition* 24:401-431.

Briefel, R. R., M. K. Crepinsek, C. Cabili, A. Wilson, and P. M. Gleason. 2009a. School food environments and practices affect dietary behaviors of U.S. public school children. *Journal of the American Dietetic Association* 109(2):S91-S107.

Briefel, R. R., A. Wilson, and P. M. Gleason. 2009b. Consumption of low-nutrient, energy-dense foods and beverages at school, home, and other locations among school lunch participants and nonparticipants. *Journal of the American Dietetic Association* 109(2):579-590.

Brownell, K. D., and D. S. Ludwig. 2011. The supplemental nutrition assistance program, soda, and USDA policy: Who benefits? *Journal of the American Medical Association* 306(12):1370-1371.

Brownell, K. D., T. Farley, W. C. Willett, B. M. Popkin, F. J. Chaloupka, J. W. Thompson, and D. S. Ludwig. 2009. The public health and economic benefits of taxing sugar-sweetened beverages. *New England Journal of Medicine* 361(16):1599-1605.

Buzby, J. C., H. F. Wells, and G. Vocke. 2006. *Possible implications for U.S. agriculture from adoption of select dietary guidelines.* Economic Research Report No. 31. Washington, DC: USDA, ERS.

California Food Policy Advocates. 2011. *Why water?* http://www.waterinschools.org/whywater.shtml (accessed October 18, 2011).

California FreshWorks Fund. 2011. *Freshworks.* http://www.cafreshworks.com/ (accessed October 21, 2011).

Carollo, K. 2011. *Movie theatres to sell healthy snacks.* http://abcnews.go.com/Health/movie-theatres-sell-healthy-snack-pack-amc-sells/story?id=13311986 (accessed September 16, 2011).

Cawley, J., and B. Kirwan. 2011. Agricultural policy and childhood obesity. In *Handbook of the social science of obesity*, edited by J. Cawley. New York: Oxford University Press.

CDC (Centers for Disease Control and Prevention). 2010. *The CDC guide to strategies for reducing consumption of sugar-sweetened beverages.* http://www.cdph.ca.gov/SiteCollectionDocuments/StratstoReduce_Sugar_Sweetened_Bevs.pdf (accessed November 13, 2011).

CDC. 2011. *Health and sustainability guidelines for federal concessions and vending operations*. http://www.cdc.gov/chronicdisease/resources/guidelines/food-service-guidelines.htm (accessed October 19, 2011).

CFBAI (Children's Food and Beverage Advertising Initiative). 2011. *Category-specific uniform nutrition criteria*. http://www.bbb.org/us/storage/16/documents/cfbai/CFBAI-Category-Specific-Uniform-Nutrition-Criteria.pdf (accessed August 9, 2011).

Chaloupka, F. J., L. M. Powell, and J. F. Chriqui. 2011a. Sugar-sweetened beverages and obesity prevention: Policy recommendations. *Journal of Policy Analysis and Management* 30(3):662-664.

Chaloupka, F. J., Y. C. Wang, L. M. Powell, T. Andreyeva, J. F. Chriqui, and L. M. Rimkus. 2011b. *Estimating the potential impact of sugar-sweetened and other beverage excise taxes in Illinois*. Report to the Illinois State Legislature.

Chriqui, J. F., L. Schneider, F. J. Chaloupka, C. Gourdet, A. Bruursema, K. Ide, and O. Pugach. 2010. *School district wellness policies: Evaluating progress and potential for improving children's health three years after the federal mandate: School years 2006-07, 2007-08 and 2008-09, volume 2*. Chicago, IL: Bridging the Gap Program, Health Policy Center, Institute for Health Research and Policy, University of Illinois.

Citizens' Committee for Children of New York, Inc. 2008. *Public opinion poll conducted by Beck Research, LLC. Voter preferences for closing the New York State budget gap*. http://www.cccnewyork.org/publications/12-12-08CCCPoll.pdf (accessed July 6, 2011).

Cradock, A. L., A. McHugh, H. Mont-Ferguson, L. Grant, J. L. Barrett, C. Wang, and S. L. Gortmaker. 2011. Effect of school district policy change on consumption of sugar-sweetened beverages among high school students, Boston, Massachusetts, 2004-2006. *Preventing Chronic Disease* 8(4):A74.

CSPI (Center for Science in the Public Interest). 2010. *Coke to fleece America by charging more for less, says CSPI*. http://www.cspinet.org/new/201001291.html (accessed October 28, 2011).

CSPI. 2011. *Life's sweeter with fewer sugary drinks*. http://www.aapd.org/media/Policies_Guidelines/P_VendingMachines.pdf (accessed September 21, 2011).

Daniels, M. C., and B. M. Popkin. 2010. Impact of water intake on energy intake and weight status: A systematic review. *Nutrition Reviews* 68(9):505-521.

Defense Logistics Agency. 2011. *Subsistence*. http://www.dscp.dla.mil/subs/ (accessed October 19, 2011).

Defense Manpower Media Center. 2011. *Active duty military personnel strengths by regional area and by country (309a)*. http://media.hotnews.ro/media_server1/document-2011-05-11-8614257-0-numarul-total-soldati-americani-desfasurati-nivel-mondial.pdf (accessed October 19, 2011).

Delaware State Parks. 2011. *Healthy eating initiative*. http://www.destateparks.com/general_info/healthy-eating.asp (accessed October 21, 2011).

Dennis, E. A., A. L. Dengo, D. L. Comber, K. D. Flack, J. Savla, K. P. Davy, and B. M. Davy. 2010. Water consumption increases weight loss during a hypocaloric diet intervention in middle-aged and older adults. *Obesity* 18(2):300-307.

DGAC (Dietary Guidelines Advisory Committee). 2010. *Report of the Dietary Guidelines Advisory Committee on the Dietary Guidelines for Americans, 2010, to the Secretary of Agriculture and the Secretary of Health and Human Services.* Washington, DC: USDA, ERS.

Dharmasena, S., and O. Capps. 2011. Intended and unintended consequences of a proposed national tax on sugar-sweetened beverages to combat the U.S. obesity problem. *Health Economics.*

DiMeglio, D. P., and R. D. Mattes. 2000. Liquid versus solid carbohydrate: Effects on food intake and body weight. *International Journal of Obesity* 24(6):794-800.

Dodgers. 2010. *Dodgers and Levy Restaurants to unveil new menus at Dodger Stadium on opening day. The Picante Dog will be reintroduced this season.* http://mlb.mlb.com/news/press_releases/press_release.jsp?ymd=20100409&content_id=9174090&vkey=pr_la&fext=.jsp&c_id=la (accessed September 16, 2011).

Epstein, L. H., E. A. Handley, K. K. Dearing, D. D. Cho, J. N. Roemmich, R. A. Paluch, S. Raja, Y. Pak, and B. Spring. 2006. Purchases of food in youth: Influence of price and income. *Psychological Science* 17(1):82-89.

Epstein, L. H., K. K. Dearing, R. A. Paluch, J. N. Roemmich, and D. Cho. 2007. Price and maternal obesity influence purchasing of low- and high-energy-dense foods. *American Journal of Clinical Nutrition* 86(4):914-922.

ERS (Economic Research Service). 2004. *Diet quality and food consumption: Daily food consumption at different locations: All individuals ages 2 and older.* http://www.ers.usda.gov/briefing/DietQuality/data/foods/table5.htm (accessed December 12, 2011).

ERS. 2009. *Access to affordable and nutritious food: Measuring and understanding food deserts and their consequences.* Report to Congress. Washington, DC: ERS.

ERS. 2011a. *Food CPI and expenditures: Table 3t—food away from home: Total expenditures.* http://www.ers.usda.gov/Briefing/CPIFoodAndExpenditures/Data/Expenditures_Tables/table3.htm (accessed October 19, 2011).

ERS. 2011b. *Food CPI and expenditures: Table 10—food away from home as a share of food expenditures.* http://www.ers.usda.gov/Briefing/CPIFoodAndExpenditures/Data/Expenditures_tables/table10.htm (accessed October 19, 2011).

Faulkner, G., P. Grootendorst, V. H. Nguyen, R. Ferrence, R. Mendelson, P. Donnelly, and K. Arbour-Nicitopoulos. 2010. *Economic policy, obesity and health: A scoping review. Final report submitted to the Heart and Stroke Foundation of Canada.* Toronto, Ontario: Exercise Psychology Unit.

Finkelstein, E. A., C. Zhen, J. Nonnemaker, and J. E. Todd. 2010. Impact of targeted beverage taxes on higher- and lower-income households. *Archives of Internal Medicine* 170(22):2028-2034.

Fletcher, J. M., D. E. Frisvold, and N. Tefft. 2011a. Are soft drink taxes an effective mechanism for reducing obesity? *Journal of Policy Analysis and Management* 30(3):655-662.

Fletcher, J. M., D. E. Frisvold, and N. Tefft. 2011b. The proof is in the pudding: Response to Chaloupka, Powell, and Chriqui. *Journal of Policy Analysis and Management* 30(3):664-665.

FNS (Food and Nutrition Service). 2011a. *Healthier U.S. school challenge.* http://www.fns.usda.gov/tn/healthierus/index.html (accessed November 13, 2011).

FNS. 2011b. *Nutrition assistance programs.* http://www.fns.usda.gov/fns/ (accessed October 19, 2011).

Foresight. 2011. *The future of food and farming. Final project report.* London: The Government Office for Science.

Fox, M. K., A. Gordon, R. Nogales, and A. Wilson. 2009. Availability and consumption of competitive foods in the U.S. public schools. *Journal of the American Dietetic Association* 109(2):S57-S66.

French, S. A. 2003. Pricing effects on food choices. *Journal of Nutrition* 133(3):841S-843S.

French, S. A., R. W. Jeffery, M. Story, P. Hannan, and M. P. Snyder. 1997. A pricing strategy to promote low-fat snack choices through vending machines. *American Journal of Public Health* 87(5):849-851.

French, S. A., R. W. Jeffery, M. Story, K. K. Breitlow, J. S. Baxter, P. Hannan, and M. P. Snyder. 2001a. Pricing and promotion effects on low-fat vending snack purchases: The CHIPS Study. *American Journal of Public Health* 91(1):112-117.

French, S. A., M. Story, D. Neumark-Sztainer, J. A. Fulkerson, and P. Hannan. 2001b. Fast food restaurant use among adolescents: Associations with nutrient intake, food choices and behavioral and psychosocial variables. *International Journal of Obesity and Related Metabolic Disorders* 25(12):1823-1833.

Gable, L. 2011. *Healthy Weight Commitment Foundation triples membership in first year, launches program in all of its priority areas.* http://www.healthyweightcommit.org/news/healthy_weight_commitment_foundation_triples_membership_in_first_year/ (accessed January 30, 2012).

GAO (Government Accountability Office). 2000. *Food and commodities: Federal purchases and major regulations that potentially affect prices paid.* Washington, DC: GAO.

Garber, A. K., and R. H. Lustig. 2011. Is fast food addictive? *Current Drug Abuse Reviews* 4(3):146-162.

Gearhardt, A. N., S. Yokum, P. T. Orr, E. Stice, W. R. Corbin, and K. D. Brownell. 2011. Neural correlates of food addiction. *Archives of General Psychiatry* 68(8):808-816.

Get Out. Be Active. 2011. *Re/store Nashville.* http://nashville.getoutbeactive.com/2011/02/21/restore-nashville/ (accessed October 21, 2011).

Gidding, S. S., B. A. Dennison, L. L. Birch, S. R. Daniels, M. W. Gillman, A. H. Lichtenstein, K. T. Rattay, J. Steinberger, N. Stettler, and L. Van Horn. 2006. Dietary recommendations for children and adolescents: A guide for practitioners. *Pediatrics* 117(2):544-559.

Giskes, K., F. van Lenthe, M. Avendano-Pabon, and J. Brug. 2011. A systematic review of environmental factors and obesogenic dietary intakes among adults: Are we getting closer to understanding obesogenic environments? *Obesity Reviews* 12(5):e95-e106.

Glanz, K., and A. L. Yaroch. 2004. Strategies for increasing fruit and vegetable intake in grocery stores and communities: Policy, pricing, and environmental change. *Preventive Medicine* 39(Suppl. 2):S75-S80.

Greenwood, M. R. C., P. B. Crawford, and R. M. Ortiz. 2009. *Legislative Task Force on Diabetes and Obesity: Report to the California legislature*. Santa Clara, CA: Offices of Santa Clara County Supervisors.

Gross, L. S., L. Li, E. S. Ford, and S. Liu. 2004. Increased consumption of refined carbohydrates and the epidemic of type 2 diabetes in the United States: An ecologic assessment. *American Journal of Clinical Nutrition* 79(5):774-779.

Harris, J. L., M. B. Schwartz, K. D. Brownell, V. Sarda, A. Ustjanauskas, M. Javadizadeh, M. Weinberg, C. Munsell, S. Speers, E. Bukofzer, A. Cheyne, P. Gonzalez, J. Reshetnyak, H. Agnew, and P. Ohri-Vachaspati. 2010. *Fast food facts: Evaluating fast food nutrition and marketing to youth*. New Haven, CT: Yale Rudd Center for Food Policy and Obesity.

Hawkes, C. 2007. Promoting healthy diets and tackling obesity and diet-related chronic diseases: What are the agricultural policy levers? *Food and Nutrition Bulletin* 28(Suppl. 2):S312-S322.

Healthy Weight Commitment Foundation. 2011. *Healthy Weight Commitment Foundation 2010 annual report*. Washington, DC: Healthy Weight Commitment Foundation.

HHS/USDA (U.S. Department of Health and Human Services/U.S. Department of Agriculture). 2010. *Dietary Guidelines for Americans*. Washington, DC: U.S. Government Printing Office.

Hickson, D., A. Diez Roux, A. Smith, K. Tucker, L. Gore, L. Zhang, and S. Wyatt. 2011. Associations of fast food restaurant availability with dietary intake and weight among African Americans in the Jackson Heart Study, 2000-2004. *American Journal of Public Health* 101(Suppl.):S301-S309.

Ifland, J. R., H. G. Preuss, M. T. Marcus, K. M. Rourke, W. C. Taylor, K. Burau, W. S. Jacobs, W. Kadish, and G. Manso. 2009. Refined food addiction: A classic substance use disorder. *Medical Hypotheses* 72(5):518-526.

International Council of Shopping Centers. 2008. *Inside site selection: Retailers' search for strategic business locations.* http://www.icsc.org/srch/government/briefs/200805_insidesite.pdf (accessed January 3, 2012).

IOM (Institute of Medicine). 2002. *Dietary reference intakes for energy, carbohydrate, fiber, fat, fatty acids, cholesterol, protein, and amino acids.* Washington, DC: The National Academies Press.

IOM. 2005. *Preventing childhood obesity: Health in the balance*, edited by J. P. Koplan, C. T. Liverman, and V. A. Kraak. Washington, DC: The National Academies Press.

IOM. 2006a. *Dietary reference intakes: The essential guide to nutrient requirements.* Washington, DC: The National Academies Press.

IOM. 2006b. *Food marketing to children and youth: Threat or opportunity?*, edited by J. M. McGinnis, J. Gootman, and V. I. Kraak. Washington, DC: The National Academies Press.

IOM. 2007a. *Nutrition standards for foods in schools: Leading the way toward healthier youth.* Washington, DC: The National Academies Press.

IOM. 2007b. *Progress in preventing childhood obesity: How do we measure up?* Washington, DC: The National Academies Press.

IOM. 2009. *Local government actions to prevent childhood obesity.* Washington, DC: The National Academies Press.

IOM. 2010. *Strategies to reduce sodium intake in the United States.* Washington, DC: The National Academies Press.

IOM. 2011. *Hunger and obesity: Understanding a food insecurity paradigm: Workshop summary*, edited by L. M. Troy, E. A. Miller, and S. Olson. Washington, DC: The National Academies Press.

Jago, R., T. Baranowski, J. C. Baranowski, K. W. Cullen, and D. Thompson. 2007. Distance to food stores and adolescent male fruit and vegetable consumption: Mediation effects. *International Journal of Behavioral Nutrition and Physical Activity* 4:35.

James, A. 2010. *Forget popcorn; executive demands healthy treats at movie theatres.* http://www.popeater.com/2010/03/17/healthy-food-movie-theater/ (accessed September 16, 2011).

Jilcott, S. B., T. Keyserling, T. Crawford, J. T. McGuirt, and A. S. Ammerman. 2011. Examining associations among obesity and per capita farmers' markets, grocery stores/supermarkets, and supercenters in US counties. *Journal of the American Dietetic Association* 111(4):567-572.

Johnson, D., B. Krissoff, E. Young, L. Hoffman, G. Lucier, and V. Breneman. 2006. *Eliminating fruit and vegetable planting restrictions: How would markets be affected?* Economic Research Report No. 40. Washington, DC: USDA, ERS.

Johnson, R. K., L. J. Appel, M. Brands, B. V. Howard, M. Lefevre, R. H. Lustig, F. Sacks, A. Steffen, and J. Wylie-Rosett. 2009. Dietary sugars intake and cardiovascular health: A scientific statement from the American Heart Association. *Circulation* 120:1011-1020.

Kahn, H. S., L. M. Tatham, C. Rodriguez, E. E. Calle, M. J. Thun, and C. W. Heath, Jr. 1997. Stable behaviors associated with adults' 10-year change in body mass index and likelihood of gain at the waist. *American Journal of Public Health* 87(5):747-754.

Kant, A. K., and B. I. Graubard. 2004. Eating out in America, 1987-2000: Trends and nutritional correlates. *Preventive Medicine* 38(2):243-249.

Keystone Forum. 2006. *The Keystone Forum on away-from home foods: Opportunities for preventing weight gain and obesity.* Washington, DC: The Keystone Center.

Khan, L. K., K. Sobush, D. Keener, K. Goodman, A. Lowry, J. Kakietek, and S. Zaro. 2009. Recommended community strategies and measurements to prevent obesity in the United States. *Morbidity and Mortality Weekly Report* 58(RR-7):1-26.

Kim, D., and I. Kawachi. 2006. Food taxation and pricing strategies to "thin out" the obesity epidemic. *American Journal of Preventive Medicine* 30(5):430-437.

Kraak, V. I., M. Story, E. A. Wartella, and J. Ginter. 2011. Industry progress to market a healthful diet to American children and adolescents. *American Journal of Preventive Medicine* 41(3):322-333.

Krueger, J. E., K. R. Krub, and L. A. Hayes. 2010. *Planting the seeds for public health: How the farm bill can help farmers to produce and distribute healthy foods.* St. Paul, MN: Farmers' Legal Action Group, Inc.

Krukowski, R. A., D. S. West, J. Harvey-Berino, and T. Elaine Prewitt. 2010. Neighborhood impact on healthy food availability and pricing in food stores. *Journal of Community Health* 35(3):315-320.

Larson, N. I., M. T. Story, and M. C. Nelson. 2009. Neighborhood environments: Disparities in access to healthy foods in the U.S. *American Journal of Preventive Medicine* 36(1):74-81.

Ledoux, T. A., M. D. Hingle, and T. Baranowski. 2010. Relationship of fruit and vegetable intake with adiposity: A systematic review. *Obesity Reviews* 12(5):e143-e150.

Lee, V., L. Mikkelsen, J. Srikantharajah, and L. Cohen. 2008. *Promising strategies for creating healthy eating and active living environments.* Oakland, CA: Prevention Institute, Healthy Eating Active Living Convergence Partnership, and PolicyLink.

Lenoir, M., F. Serre, L. Cantin, and S. H. Ahmed. 2007. Intense sweetness surpasses cocaine reward. *PLoS One* 2(8):e698.

Levy, D. T., K. B. Friend, and Y. C. Wang. 2011. A review of the literature on policies directed at the youth consumption of sugar-sweetened beverages. *Advances in Nutrition: An International Review Journal* 2(2):182S-200S.

Lewis, L. B., D. C. Sloane, L. M. Nascimento, A. L. Diamant, J. J. Guinyard, A. K. Yancey, and G. Flynn. 2005. African Americans' access to healthy food options in south Los Angeles restaurants. *American Journal of Public Health* 95(4):668-673.

Lin, B. H., J. Guthrie, and E. Frazao. 1999. *Away-from-home foods increasingly important to quality of American diet.* Washington, DC: ERS.

Lock, K., R. D. D. Smith, A. D. Dangour, M. Keogh-Brown, G. Pigatto, C. Hawkes, R. M. Fisberg, and Z. Chalabi. 2010. Health, agricultural, and economic effects of adoption of healthy diet recommendations. *The Lancet* 376(9753):1699-1709.

Lopez, R. P. 2007. Neighborhood risk factors for obesity. *Obesity (Silver Spring)* 15(8):2111-2119.

Ludwig, D. S. 2011. Technology, diet, and the burden of chronic disease. *Journal of the American Medical Association* 305(13):1352-1353.

Manchester, A. C., and D. P. Blayney. 2001. *Milk pricing in the United States. Agriculture information bulletin no. 761.* Washington, DC: USDA, ERS.

Martinez, S., M. Hand, M. Da Pra, S. Pollack, K. Ralston, T. Smith, S. Vogel, S. Clark, L. Lohr, S. Low, and C. Newman. 2010. *Local food systems: Concepts, impacts, and issues. Report no# 97.* Washington, DC: USDA, ERS.

Massachusetts Department of Public Health. 2007. *Healthy meeting and event guide.* http://www.mass.gov/Eeohhs2/docs/dph/com_health/nutrition_phys_activity/healthy_meeting_event_guide.pdf (accessed December 1, 2011).

Mattes, R. D. 1996. Dietary compensation by humans for supplemental energy provided as ethanol or carbohydrate in fluids. *Physiology and Behavior* 59(1):179-187.

McDonald's. 2011. *McDonald's announces commitments to offer improved nutrition choices.* http://www.aboutmcdonalds.com/mcd/media_center/recent_news/corporate/commitments_to_offer_improved_nutrition_choices.html (accessed August 10, 2011).

McIntyre, B. D., H. R. Herren, J. Wakhungu, and R. T. Watson. 2009. *Agriculture at a crossroads. Washington, DC: International assessment of agriculture knowledge, science, and technology for development.* http://www.agassessment.org/reports/IAASTD/EN/Agriculture%20at%20a%20Crossroads_Global%20Report%20(English).pdf (accessed December 12, 2011).

Michels, K. B., B. R. Bloom, P. Riccardi, B. A. Rosner, and W. C. Willett. 2008. A study of the importance of education and cost incentives on individual food choices at the Harvard School of Public Health cafeteria. *Journal of the American College of Nutrition* 27(1):6-11.

Michimi, A., and M. C. Wimberly. 2010. Associations of supermarket accessibility with obesity and fruit and vegetable consumption in the conterminous United States. *International Journal of Health Geographics* 9:49.

Mikkelsen, L., and S. Chehimi. 2007. *The links between the neighborhood food environment and childhood nutrition.* Princeton, NJ: RWJF.

Miller, J. C., and K. H. Coble. 2007. Cheap food policy: Fact or rhetoric? *Food Policy* 32(1):98-111.

Miller, J. C., and K. H. Coble. 2008. An international comparison of the effect of government agricultural support on food budget shares. *Journal of Agricultural and Applied Economics* 40(2):551-558.

Morland, K. B., and K. R. Evenson. 2009. Obesity prevalence and the local food environment. *Health Place* 15(2):491-495.

Morland, K. B., S. Wing, and A. Diez Roux. 2002. The contextual effect of the local food environment on residents' diets: The atherosclerosis risk in communities study. *American Journal of Public Health* 92(11):1761-1767.

Morland, K. B., A. V. Diez Roux, and S. Wing. 2006. Supermarkets, other food stores, and obesity: The atherosclerosis risk in communities study. *American Journal of Preventive Medicine* 30(4):333-339.

Morton, L. W., and T. C. Blanchard. 2007. Starved for access: Life in rural America's food deserts. *Rural Realities* 1(4).

Motion Picture Association of America. 2010. *Theatrical market statistics*. http://www.mpaa.org/Resources/93bbeb16-0e4d-4b7e-b085-3f41c459f9ac.pdf (accessed December 1, 2011).

Muckelbauer, R., L. Libuda, K. Clausen, A. M. Toschke, T. Reinehr, and M. Kersting. 2009. Promotion and provision of drinking water in schools for overweight prevention: Randomized, controlled cluster trial. *Pediatrics* 123(4):e661-e667.

Mulheron, J., and K. Vonasek. 2009. *Shaping a healthier generation: Successful state strategies to prevent childhood obesity*. Washington, DC: National Governors Association, Center for Best Practices.

Muller, M. J., I. Koertzinger, M. Mast, K. Langnase, and A. Grund. 1999. Physical activity and diet in 5 to 7 years old children. *Public Health Nutrition* 2(3A):443-444.

Muller, M., A. Tagtow, S. L. Roberts, and M. Erin. 2009. Aligning food systems policies to advance public health. *Journal of Hunger and Environmental Nutrition* 4(3-4):225-240.

NACCHO (National Association of County and City Health Officials). 2010. *Statement of policy, comprehensive obesity prevention*. Washington, DC: NACCHO.

National Association of Local Boards of Health. 2010. *Position statement: Nutrition, physical activity and obesity*. Washington, DC: National Association of Local Boards of Health.

National Prevention Council. 2011. *National prevention strategy. America's plan for better health and wellness*. Rockville, MD: Office of the Surgeon General, HHS.

NCES (National Center for Education Statistics). 2010. *Table 52. Enrollment of 3-, 4-, and 5-year-old children in preprimary programs, by level of program, control of program, and attendance status: Selected years, 1965 through 2009*. http://nces.ed.gov/programs/digest/d10/tables/dt10_052.asp (accessed October 19, 2011).

NCES. 2011. *Fast facts*. http://nces.ed.gov/fastfacts/display.asp?id=65 (accessed October 19, 2011).

NCI (National Cancer Institute). 2010a. *Mean intake of added sugars & percentage contribution of various foods among U.S. population, by age, NHANES 2005-2006*. http://riskfactor.cancer.gov/diet/foodsources/added_sugars/table5a.html (accessed December 19, 2011).

NCI. 2010b. *Mean intake of energy and mean contribution (kcal) of various foods among U.S. population, by age, NHANES 2005-06*. http://riskfactor.cancer.gov/diet/foodsources/energy/table1b.html (accessed December 19, 2011).

Neumark-Sztainer, D., P. J. Hannan, M. Story, J. Croll, and C. Perry. 2003. Family meal patterns: Associations with sociodemographic characteristics and improved dietary intake among adolescents. *Journal of the American Dietetic Association* 103(3):317-322.

New York City Department of Health and Mental Hygiene. 2011. *New York City food standards*. http://www.nyc.gov/html/doh/html/cardio/cardio-vend-nutrition-standard.shtml (accessed October 19, 2011).

New York City Government. 2009. *Food retail expansion to support health*. http://www.nyc.gov/html/misc/html/2009/fresh.shtml (accessed December 1, 2011).

Ni Mhurchu, C., T. Blakely, Y. Jiang, H. C. Eyles, and A. Rodgers. 2010. Effects of price discounts and tailored nutrition education on supermarket purchases: A randomized controlled trial. *American Journal of Clinical Nutrition* 91(3):736-747.

Nielsen, S. J., A. M. Siega-Riz, and B. M. Popkin. 2002. Trends in energy intake in US between 1977 and 1996: Similar shifts seen across age groups. *Obesity Research* 10(5):370-378.

Niemeier, H. M., H. A. Raynor, E. E. Lloyd-Richardson, M. L. Rogers, and R. R. Wing. 2006. Fast food consumption and breakfast skipping: Predictors of weight gain from adolescence to adulthood in a nationally representative sample. *Journal of Adolescent Health* 39(6):842-849.

NRA (National Restaurant Association). 2011. *Kids LiveWell: About*. http://www.restaurant.org/foodhealthyliving/kidslivewell/about/ (accessed August 10, 2011).

O'Donnell, S. I., S. L. Hoerr, J. A. Mendoza, and E. T. Goh. 2008. Nutrient quality of fast food kids meals. *American Journal of Clinical Nutrition* 88(5):1388-1395.

Ogden, C. L., B. K. Kit, M. D. Carroll, and S. Park. 2011. *Consumption of sugar drinks in the United States, 2005–2008*. Data brief no. 71. Hyattsville, MD: National Center for Health Statistics.

Padget, A., and M. E. Briley. 2005. Dietary intakes at child-care centers in central Texas fail to meet food guide pyramid recommendations. *Journal of the American Dietetic Association* 105(5):790-793.

Paeratakul, S., D. P. Ferdinand, C. M. Champagne, D. H. Ryan, and G. A. Bray. 2003. Fast-food consumption among US adults and children: Dietary and nutrient intake profile. *Journal of the American Dietetic Association* 103(10):1332-1338.

Partnership for a Healthier America. 2011. *News and information.* http://www. ahealthieramerica.org/#!/news-and-information (accessed October 19, 2011).

Pearson, N., A. Timperio, J. Salmon, D. Crawford, and S. J. Biddle. 2009. Family influences on children's physical activity and fruit and vegetable consumption. *The International Journal of Behavioral Nutrition and Physical Activity* 6:34.

Pirog, R., and N. McCann. 2009. *Is local food more expensive? A consumer price perspective on local and non-local foods purchased in Iowa.* Ames, IA: Leopold Center for Sustainable Agriculture.

Pollack, S. 2001. Consumer demand for fruit and vegetables: The US example. In *Changing structure of global food consumption and trade,* edited by A. Regmi. Washington, DC: USDA, ERS. Pp. 49-54.

Pollan, M. 2003. The (agri)cultural contradictions of obesity. *The New York Times,* October 12.

Popkin, B. M., and K. J. Duffey. 2010. Sugar and artificial sweeteners: Seeking the sweet truth. In *Nutrition and health: Nutrition guide for physicians,* edited by T. Wilson, G. A. Bray, N. J. Temple, and M. B. Struble. New York: Humana Press.

Poti, J. M., and B. M. Popkin. 2011. Trends in energy intake among U.S. children by eating location and food source, 1977-2006. *Journal of the American Dietetic Association* 111(8):1156-1164.

Powell, L. M. 2009. Fast food costs and adolescent body mass index: Evidence from panel data. *Journal of Health Economics* 28(5):963-970.

Powell, L. M., and F. J. Chaloupka. 2009. Food prices and obesity: Evidence and policy implications for taxes and subsidies. *Milbank Quarterly* 87(1):229-257.

Powell, L. M., and J. F. Chriqui. 2011. Food taxes and subsidies: Evidence and policies for obesity prevention. In *The Oxford handbook of the social science of obesity,* edited by J. Cawley. Pp. 639-664.

Powell, L. M., M. C. Auld, F. J. Chaloupka, P. M. O'Malley, and L. D. Johnston. 2007. Associations between access to food stores and adolescent body mass index. *American Journal of Preventive Medicine* 33(Suppl. 4):S301-S307.

Powell, L. M., J. Chriqui, and F. J. Chaloupka. 2009. Associations between state-level soda taxes and adolescent body mass index. *Journal of Adolescent Health* 45(Suppl. 3):S57-S63.

Powell, L. M., E. Han, and F. J. Chaloupka. 2010. Economic contextual factors, food consumption, and obesity among U.S. adolescents. *Journal of Nutrition* 140(6):1175-1180.

Randolph, W., and K. Viswanath. 2004. Lessons learned from public health mass media campaigns: Marketing health in a crowded media world. *Annual Review of Public Health* 25:419-437.

Reedy, J., and S. M. Krebs-Smith. 2010. Dietary sources of energy, solid fats, and added sugars among children and adolescents in the United States. *Journal of the American Dietetic Association* 110(10):1477-1484.

Ritchie, L. D., S. Whaley, K. Hecht, K. Chandran, M. Boyle, P. Spector, S. Samuels, and P. Crawford. 2012. Participation in the Child and Adult Care Food Program is associated with more nutritious foods and beverages in childcare. *Childhood Obesity*. In press.

Rogers, K. 2011. Accelerating progress in obesity prevention. Presented at the Farm and Food Policy: Relationship to Obesity Prevention, May 19, 2011, Washington, DC.

Rose, D., and R. Richards. 2004. Food store access and household fruit and vegetable use among participants in the US food stamp program. *Public Health Nutrition* 7(8):1081-1088.

Rudd Center for Food Policy and Obesity. 2010. *Public opinion data.* http://www.yaleruddcenter.org/what_we_do.aspx?id=273 (accessed July 19, 2011).

Rudd Center for Food Policy and Obesity. 2011. *Sugar-sweetened beverage taxes and sugar intake: Policy statements, endorsements, and recommendations.* New Haven, CT: Yale University Rudd Center on Food Policy and Obesity Prevention.

RWJF (Robert Wood Johnson Foundation). 2009. *Action strategies toolkit: A guide for local and state leaders working to create healthy communities and prevent childhood obesity.* Princeton, NJ: RWJF.

RWJF. 2011. Summary of food marketing research roundtable. Presented at the RWJF Food Marketing Research Roundtable, April 4-5, 2011, Washington, DC.

Schaffer, H., D. B. Hunt, and D. E. Ray. 2007. *US agricultural commodity policy and its relationship to obesity.* Background paper developed for the Wingspread Conference on Childhood Obesity, Healthy Eating & Agriculture Policy. Knoxville, TN: Agricultural Policy Analysis Center, University of Tennessee.

Schmidt, M., S. G. Affenito, R. Striegel-Moore, P. R. Khoury, B. Barton, P. Crawford, S. Kronsberg, G. Schreiber, E. Obarzanek, and S. Daniels. 2005. Fast-food intake and diet quality in black and white girls: The National Heart, Lung, and Blood Institute Growth and Health Study. *Archives of Pediatrics and Adolescent Medicine* 159(7):626-631.

Schoonover, H., and M. Muller. 2006. *Food without thought: How U.S. farm policy contributes to obesity.* Minneapolis, MN: The Institute for Agriculture and Trade Policy.

Schulze, M. B., J. E. Manson, D. S. Ludwig, G. A. Colditz, M. J. Stampfer, W. C. Willett, and F. B. Hu. 2004. Sugar-sweetened beverages, weight gain, and incidence of type 2 diabetes in young and middle-aged women. *Journal of the American Medical Association* 292(8):927-934.

Sharma, L. L., S. P. Teret, and K. D. Brownell. 2010. The food industry and self-regulation: Standards to promote success and to avoid public health failures. *American Journal of Public Health* 100(2):240-246.

Smith, T. A., B. Lin, and J. Lee. 2010. *Taxing caloric sweetened beverages: Potential effects on beverage consumption, calorie intake, and obesity.* Economic Research Report No. 100. Washington, DC: USDA, ERS.

Stein, J. 2009. *A Dodger Dog with a side of yogurt?* http://articles.latimes.com/2009/apr/12/science/sci-stadiumfare12 (accessed December 1, 2011).

Stookey, J. D., F. Constant, C. D. Gardner, and B. M. Popkin. 2007. Replacing sweetened caloric beverages with drinking water is associated with lower energy intake. *Obesity* 15(12):3013-3022.

Stookey, J. D., F. Constant, B. M. Popkin, and C. D. Gardner. 2008. Drinking water is associated with weight loss in overweight dieting women independent of diet and activity. *Obesity* 16(11):2481-2488.

Story, M., K. M. Kaphingst, and S. French. 2006. The role of child care settings in obesity prevention. *Future of Children* 16(1):143-168.

Story, M., K. M. Kaphingst, R. Robinson-O'Brien, and K. Glanz. 2008. Creating healthy food and eating environments: Policy and environmental approaches. *Annual Review of Public Health* 29:253-272.

Sturm, R., L. M. Powell, J. F. Chriqui, and F. J. Chaloupka. 2010. Soda taxes, soft drink consumption, and children's body mass index. *Health Affairs* 29(5):1052-1058.

Taber, D. R., J. F. Chriqui, L. M. Powell, and F. J. Chaloupka. 2011. Banning all sugar-sweetened beverages in middle schools: Reduction of in-school access and purchasing but not overall consumption. *Archives of Pediatrics and Adolescent Medicine* [epub ahead of print].

The Chicago Council on Global Affairs. 2011. *Bringing agriculture to the table.* Chicago, IL: The Council on Global Affairs.

The City of New Orleans. 2011. *Fresh food retailer initiative.* http://www.nola.gov/HOME/FreshFoodRetailersInitiative (accessed December 12, 2011).

The Food Trust. 2011. *Supermarket campaign.* http://www.thefoodtrust.org/php/programs/super.market.campaign.php (accessed July 15, 2011).

The Reinvestment Fund. 2010. *Pennsylvania fresh food financing initiative.* http://www.trfund.com/resource/downloads/Fresh_Food_Financing_Initiative_Comprehensive.pdf (accessed November 13, 2011).

The Walt Disney Company. 2011. *Promoting healthy lifestyles.* http://corporate.disney.go.com/citizenship2010/familyentertainment/overview/promotinghealthylifestyles/ (accessed January 27, 2012).

Thomas, A. 2011. Healthier food initiative. Presented at the Farm and Food Policy: Relationship to Obesity Prevention, May 19, 2011, Washington, DC.

Thompson, O., C. Ballew, K. Resnicow, A. Must, L. G. Bandini, H. Cyr, and W. H. Dietz. 2004. Food purchased away from home as a predictor of change in BMI Z-score among girls. *International Journal of Obesity* 28:282-289.

Tillotson, J. E. 2003. Pandemic obesity: Agriculture's cheap food policy is a bad bargain. *Nutrition Today* 38:186.

Tillotson, J. E. 2004. America's obesity: Conflicting public policies, industrial economic development, and unintended human consequences. *Annual Review of Nutrition* 24(1):617-643.

TransForm Baltimore. 2011. *Transform Baltimore: The zoning code rewrite.* http://www.transformbaltimore.net/portal/ (accessed October 21, 2011).

Treuhaft, S., and A. Karpyn. 2010. *The grocery gap: Who has access to healthy food and why it matters.* Oakland, CA and Philadelphia, PA: PolicyLink and The Food Trust.

Trust for America's Health and RWJF. 2011. *F as in fat: How obesity threatens America's future*, edited by J. Levi, L. M. Segal, R. St. Laurent and D. Kohn. Washington, DC: Trust for America's Health.

Turner, L., and F. J. Chaloupka. 2010. Wide availability of high-calorie beverages in U.S. elementary schools. *Archives of Pediatrics and Adolescent Medicine* 165(3):223-228.

UNC Carolina Population Center. 2011. *Evaluation of food industry initiatives to reduce obesity.* http://www.cpc.unc.edu/projects/nutrans/policy/food-industry-eval (accessed January 3, 2012).

U.S. Census Bureau. 2007. *Census of government employment. Table 1. Summary of public employment and payrolls by type of government: March 2007.* http://www2.census.gov/govs/apes/emp_compendium.pdf (accessed October 21, 2011).

U.S. Census Bureau. 2011. *S2601b. Characteristics of the group quarters population by group quarters type data set: 2005-2009 American community survey 5-year estimates.* http://factfinder.census.gov/servlet/STTable?_bm=y&-geo_id=01000US&-qr_name=ACS_2009_5YR_G00_S2601B&-ds_name=ACS_2009_5YR_G00_&-redoLog=false (accessed October 19, 2011).

U.S. Surgeon General. 2010. *The Surgeon General's vision for a healthy and fit nation.* Washington, DC: HHS.

Wakefield, M. A., B. Loken, and R. C. Hornik. 2010. Use of mass media campaigns to change health behaviour. *The Lancet* 376(9748):1261-1271.

Wallinga, D., H. Schoonover, and M. Muller. 2009. Considering the contribution of US agricultural policy to the obesity epidemic: Overview and opportunities. *Journal of Hunger and Environmental Nutrition* 4(1):3-19.

Wang, Y. C., D. S. Ludwig, K. Sonneville, and S. L. Gortmaker. 2009. Impact of change in sweetened caloric beverage consumption on energy intake among children and adolescents. *Archives of Pediatrics and Adolescent Medicine* 163(4):336-343.

Wang, Y. C., P. Coxson, Y.-M. Shen, L. Goldman, and K. Bibbins-Domingo. 2012. A penny-per-ounce tax on sugar-sweetened beverages would cut health and cost burdens of diabetes. *Health Affairs* 31(1):199-207.

Welsh, J. A., A. J. Sharma, L. Grellinger, and M. B. Vos. 2011. Consumption of added sugars is decreasing in the United States. *American Journal of Clinical Nutrition* 94(3):726-734

Wendt, M., and J. E. Todd. 2011. *The effect of food and beverage prices on children's weights.* Economic Research Report No. 118. Washington, DC: USDA, ERS.

White House Task Force on Childhood Obesity. 2010. *Solving the problem of childhood obesity within a generation: White House Task Force on Childhood Obesity report to the President.* Washington, DC: Executive Office of the President of the United States.

WHO (World Health Organization). 2004. *Global strategy on diet, physical activity, and health.* Geneva, Switzerland: WHO.

Wiecha, J. L., D. Finkelstein, P. J. Troped, M. Fragala, and K. E. Peterson. 2006. School vending machine use and fast-food restaurant use are associated with sugar-sweetened beverage intake in youth. *Journal of the American Dietetic Association* 106(10):1624-1630.

Woodward-Lopez, G., J. Kao, and L. Ritchie. 2010. To what extent have sweetened beverages contributed to the obesity epidemic? *Public Health Nutrition* 1-11.

Wootan, M. G., A. Batada, and E. Marchlewicz. 2008. *Kids meals. Obesity on the menu.* Washington, DC: Center for Science in the Public Interest.

Zenk, S. N., A. J. Schulz, B. A. Israel, S. A. James, S. Bao, and M. L. Wilson. 2005. Neighborhood racial composition, neighborhood poverty, and the spatial accessibility of supermarkets in metropolitan Detroit. *American Journal of Public Health* 95(4):660-667.

Zoumas-Morse, C., C. L. Rock, E. J. Sobo, and M. L. Neuhouser. 2001. Children's patterns of macronutrient intake and associations with restaurant and home eating. *Journal of the American Dietetic Association* 101(8):923-925.

7

Message Environments

Message Environments:
Goal, Recommendation, Strategies, and Actions for
Implementation

Goal: Transform messages about physical activity and
nutrition.

Recommendation 3: Industry, educators, and governments
should act quickly, aggressively, and in a sustained manner
on many levels to transform the environment that sur-
rounds Americans with messages about physical activity,
food, and nutrition.

Strategy 3-1: Develop and support a sustained, targeted physical activity
and nutrition social marketing program. Congress, the Administration, other
federal policy makers, and foundations should dedicate substantial funding
and support to the development and implementation of a robust and sustained
social marketing program on physical activity and nutrition. This program
should encompass carefully targeted, culturally appropriate messages aimed at
specific audiences (e.g., tweens, new parents, mothers); clear behavior-change
goals (e.g., take a daily walk, reduce consumption of sugar-sweetened beverages among adolescents, introduce infants to vegetables, make use of the new
front-of-package nutrition labels); and related environmental change goals
(e.g., improve physical environments, offer better food choices in public places,
increase the availability of healthy food retailing).

For **Congress, the Administration, and other federal policy makers, working with entertainment media,** potential actions include

- providing a sustained source of funding for a major national social marketing program on physical activity and nutrition; and

- designating a lead agency to guide and oversee the federal program and appointing a small advisory group of physical activity, nutrition, and marketing experts to recommend message and audience priorities for the program; ensuring that the program includes a balance of messages on physical activity and nutrition, and on both individual behavior change and related environmental change goals; and exploring all forms of marketing, including message placement in popular entertainment, viral and social marketing, and multiplatform advertising—including online, outdoor, radio, television, and print.

For **foundations, working with state, local, and national organizations and the news media,** potential actions include

- enhancing the social marketing program by encouraging and supporting the news media's coverage of obesity prevention policies through the development of local and national media programs that engage individuals in the civic debate about local, state, and national-level environmental and policy changes, including such steps as providing resources to enable journalists to cover these issues and enhancing the expertise of local, state, and national organizations in engaging the news media on these issues.

Strategy 3-2: Implement common standards for marketing foods and beverages to children and adolescents. The food, beverage, restaurant, and media industries should take broad, common, and urgent voluntary action to make substantial improvements in their marketing aimed directly at children and adolescents aged 2-17. All foods and beverages marketed to this age group should support a diet that accords with the Dietary Guidelines for Americans in order to prevent obesity and risk factors associated with chronic disease risk. Children and adolescents should be encouraged to avoid calories from foods that they generally overconsume (e.g., products high in sugar, fat, and sodium) and to replace them with foods they generally underconsume (e.g., fruits, vegetables, and whole grains).

The standards set for foods and beverages marketed to children and adolescents should be widely publicized and easily available to parents and other consumers. They should cover foods and beverages marketed to children and adolescents aged 2-17 and should apply to a broad range of marketing and advertising practices, including digital marketing and the use of licensed characters and toy premiums. If such marketing standards have not been adopted within 2 years by a substantial majority of food, beverage, restaurant, and media companies that market foods and beverages to children and adolescents, policy makers at the local, state, and federal levels should consider setting mandatory nutritional standards for marketing to this age group to ensure that such standards are implemented.

Potential actions include

- all food and beverage companies, including chain and quick-service restaurants, adopting and implementing voluntary nutrition standards for foods and beverages marketed to children and adolescents;

- the Children's Food and Beverage Advertising Initiative and National Restaurant Association Initiative, as major self-regulatory marketing efforts, adopting common marketing standards for all member companies, and actively recruiting additional members to increase the impact of improved food marketing to children and adolescents;

- media companies adopting nutrition standards for all foods they market to young people; and

- the Federal Trade Commission regularly tracking the marketing standards adopted by food and beverage companies, restaurants, and media companies.

Strategy 3-3: Ensure consistent nutrition labeling for the front of packages, retail store shelves, and menus and menu boards that encourages healthier food choices. The Food and Drug Administration (FDA) and the U.S.

Department of Agriculture (USDA) should implement a standard system of nutrition labeling for the front of packages and retail store shelves that is harmonious with the Nutrition Facts panel, and restaurants should provide calorie labeling on all menus and menu boards.

Potential actions include

- the FDA and USDA adopting a single standard nutrition labeling system for all fronts of packages and retail store shelves, the FDA and USDA considering making this system mandatory to enable consumers to compare products on a standard nutrition profile, and the guidelines provided by the Institute of Medicine (2011a) being used for implementation; and

- restaurants implementing the FDA regulations that require restaurants with 20 or more locations to provide calorie labeling on their menus and menu boards, and the FDA/USDA monitoring industry for compliance with this policy.

Strategy 3-4: Adopt consistent nutrition education policies for federal programs with nutrition education components. USDA should update the policies for Special Supplemental Nutrition Assistance Program Education (SNAP-Ed) and the policies for other federal programs with nutrition education components to explicitly encourage the provision of advice about types of foods to reduce in the diet, consistent with the Dietary Guidelines for Americans.

Potential actions include

- removing the restrictions on the types of information that can be included in SNAP-Ed programs and encouraging advice about types of foods to reduce;

- disseminating, immediately and effectively, notification of the revised regulations, along with authoritative guidance on how to align federally funded nutrition education programs with the Dietary Guidelines; and

- ensuring that such full alignment of nutrition education with the Dietary Guidelines applies to all federal programs with a nutrition education component, particularly programs that target primary food shoppers in low-income families (e.g., the Expanded Food and Nutrition Education Program and the Special Supplemental Nutrition Program for Women, Infants, and Children [WIC]).

NOTE: Instruction in food and nutrition for children and adolescents in schools is covered in Chapter 9, on school environments.

Each day, Americans of all ages are surrounded by an environment replete with messages about physical activity and food: advertising on television, billboards, and cell phones; product placements in movies and video games; product packaging at grocery stores and on the kitchen table; public service campaigns; and nutrition and physical activity classes provided through schools and government programs. Some messages are explicit, making direct appeals (e.g., soft drink ads or public service messages), and some are implicit, operating more on a subconscious level (e.g., when people pass a familiar fast-food chain every day on the way to school or come to expect the local sports team to be sponsored by a chain restaurant). Indeed, the food and beverage and restaurant industries have invested heavily in extensive research into understanding complex, deep-seated motivation.

As discussed in the preceding chapters, what is available in people's daily environment circumscribes their choices: for example, whether there are safe playgrounds within walking distance or which drinks are in the vending machine. But what is *promoted* in people's daily environment influences their choices as well. It is the message environments in which people live (highlighted in Figure 7-1) that help create the expectation that a "treat" involves a fast-food outlet or that drinking a particular soda is a sign of a hip or active lifestyle. This chapter addresses these message environments, including marketing and the provision of nutrition education within federal programs with nutrition education components; Chapter 9 covers instruction in food and nutrition for children and adolescents in schools.

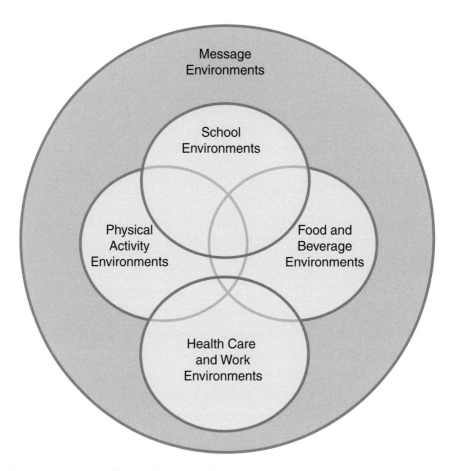

FIGURE 7-1 Five areas of focus of the Committee on Accelerating Progress in Obesity Prevention.
NOTE: The area addressed in this chapter is highlighted.

RECOMMENDATION 3

Industry, educators, and governments should act quickly, aggressively, and in a sustained manner on many levels to transform the environment that surrounds Americans with messages about physical activity, food, and nutrition.

While changing the physical environment is critical to accelerating progress in preventing obesity—whether by expanding bike paths or building more grocery stores—equally important is changing the message environments in which people function every day. These environments take many forms: advergames on popular children's websites; brand ambassadors sent to offer free products to students on their first day of college; public service campaigns on billboards and bus shelters; product placements in video games or reality television shows; health messages embedded in children's educational television shows; nutrition labeling on food packages and menu boards; physical activity and eating behaviors modeled on popular sitcoms; the products that are placed at children's eye level in grocery stores; the brand icons, celebrity endorsements, and character tie-ins featured on product packages; the mobile ads texted to teenagers; the information provided in school health classes or in education programs for those receiving public assistance; and what a doctor does or does not say about physical activity and diet during an annual checkup.

Many different actors influence these message environments. Exerting this influence on a large scale costs money, and most of those who make that investment do so not because they care about the health outcomes they may be influencing but because they have a financial stake in the choices people make: whether a young boy chooses to play a video game with friends online instead of a softball game with his neighbors, or whether a young mother decides that the best reward for her daughter's good grades at school is a meal at her favorite fast-food restaurant instead of a home-cooked dinner.

The committee therefore recommends that actors at all levels—the food and beverage industry, the entertainment and sports industries, educators, and government at all levels—do their part to contribute to the transformation of the message environments that is needed to accelerate progress in obesity prevention. Four strategies and potential actions for implementing this recommendation are provided. These strategies and actions are detailed in the remainder of this chapter. (As noted above, the strategy of providing food literacy in schools, along with potential actions for implementing this strategy, is included in Chapter 9.) Indicators for measuring progress toward the implementation of each strategy, organized according to the scheme presented in Chapter 4 (primary, process, foundational) are presented in a box following the discussion of that strategy.

STRATEGIES AND ACTIONS FOR IMPLEMENTATION

Strategy 3-1: Develop and Support a Sustained, Targeted Physical Activity and Nutrition Social Marketing Program

Congress, the Administration, other federal policy makers, and foundations should dedicate substantial funding and support to the development and implementation of a robust and sustained social marketing program on physical activity and nutrition. This program should encompass carefully targeted, culturally appropriate messages aimed at specific audiences (e.g., tweens, new parents, mothers); clear behavior-change goals (e.g., take a daily walk, reduce consumption of sugar-sweetened beverages among adolescents, introduce infants to vegetables, make use of the new front-of-package nutrition labels); and related environmental change goals (e.g., improve physical environments, offer better food choices in public places, increase the availability of healthy food retailing).

For **Congress, the Administration, and other federal policy makers, working with entertainment media,** potential actions include

- providing a sustained source of funding for a major national social marketing program on physical activity and nutrition; and
- designating a lead agency to guide and oversee the federal program and appointing a small advisory group of physical activity, nutrition, and marketing experts to recommend message and audience priorities for the program; ensuring that the program includes a balance of messages on physical activity and nutrition, and on both individual behavior change and related environmental change goals; and exploring all forms of marketing, including message placement in popular entertainment, viral and social marketing, and multiplatform advertising—including online, outdoor, radio, television, and print.

For **foundations, working with state, local, and national organizations and the news media,** potential actions include

- enhancing the social marketing program by encouraging and supporting the news media's coverage of obesity prevention policies through the development of local and national media programs that engage individuals in the civic debate about local, state, and national-level environmental and policy changes, including such steps as providing resources to enable journalists to cover these issues and enhancing the expertise of local, state, and national organizations in engaging the news media on these issues.

Context

Americans of all ages, including children and adolescents, are exposed to a tremendous amount of well-financed and expertly crafted marketing and advertising messages designed to encourage food and beverage consumption (Cheyne et al., 2011; FTC, 2008; Harris et al., 2009, 2010). The most frequently marketed foods and beverages are often of lower nutritional value and tend to be from the food groups Americans are already overconsuming (Cheyne et al., 2011; Grotto and Zied, 2010; Harris et al., 2010; Harrison and Marske, 2005; IOM, 2006). For example, a 2009 study found that approximately 87 percent of the 7.9 food and beverage ads seen by children aged 6-11 on television each day were for products high in saturated fat, sugar, or sodium (Powell et al., 2011). Moreover, many of these advertisements include incentives such as premiums, sweepstakes, and contests to induce purchases and consumption. One study, for example, found that 14 percent of fast-food ads and 17 percent of dine-in and delivery restaurant messages targeting children included at least one premium offer (Gantz et al., 2007). In addition, American consumers are exposed to a vast amount of marketing that promotes sedentary activities (such as television viewing). For example, Gantz and colleagues (2007) found that children aged 8-12 viewed approximately 8,400 promotions for upcoming television shows and approximately 5,000 ads for entertainment media products each year.

The news media also are a key part of the message environments that surround Americans. A recent survey found that 83 percent of Americans watch local or national television news, read a newspaper, listen to news radio, or visit an online news site daily (Pew Research Center for the People and the Press, 2010). The national broadcast network evening news programs together attract approximately 21.6 million viewers per night (Guskin et al., 2011). News media continue to play an essential role in highlighting the issues that are seen as legitimate or important for public consideration and in informing citizens on those topics. In describing the potential role of the news media in public health issues, a previous Institute of Medicine (IOM) committee concluded that "the more coverage a topic receives in the news, the more likely it is to be a concern of the public. Conversely, issues not mentioned by the media are likely to be ignored or to receive little attention" (IOM, 2002, p. 308). Too often, however, news coverage of physical activity and nutrition focuses on strategies for individuals to eat better and move more. This focus on the individual can obscure the importance of broader environment or policy changes (Lawrence, 2004; Woodruff et al., 2003).

Foods, beverages, and entertainment media are marketed to children, adolescents, and adults because for-profit entities stand to benefit financially from the investment in advertising. No similar investments are made in marketing messages about fitness and nutrition, in part because there are no entities with a similarly clear financial stake in promoting those messages (Gantz et al., 2007). For example, in 2005 children aged 8-12 saw an average of 158 public service announcements (PSAs) on fitness or nutrition in that one year compared with 7,609 ads for foods and beverages, or about 1 hour and 15 minutes of messages about fitness or nutrition compared with more than 50 hours of messages promoting food and beverage consumption (Gantz et al., 2007). Across the television landscape, a total of just 17 seconds per hour is donated to PSAs on all topics combined—the equivalent of less than one-half of 1 percent of air time—compared with the 21 percent of air time that is devoted to paid commercial advertising (Gantz et al., 2008).

Evidence

Social marketing is broadly defined as the application of commercial marketing principles to benefit society and the intended audience rather than the marketer. Social marketing applies the techniques of commercial advertising and marketing to the marketing of healthful or prosocial behaviors. Instead of simply providing the consumer with information about public health issues, social marketing often focuses on behavior change, sometimes includes broader environmental and policy goals, and generally uses the insights and avenues of modern product marketing (Grier and Bryant, 2005). For example, the well-regarded "truth" antitobacco youth campaign did not focus on imparting factual information about the health risks of smoking; instead, it focused on fostering a sense of rebellion against corporate tobacco companies, using popular youth media outlets and an edgy youth-oriented visual style to convey its messages and empower the targeted youth. A campaign evaluation concluded that from 1999 to 2002, the "truth" campaign resulted in 300,000 fewer youth smokers (Farrelly et al., 2005).

Because many health-based social marketing campaigns are insufficiently funded, assessing their effectiveness accurately is difficult. However, evidence from carefully designed studies indicates that media campaigns can have a positive impact on health behaviors if they are carefully crafted, well tested, fully funded, highly targeted (in terms of audience and behavior), and sustained over a long period of time (Wakefield et al., 2010).

Social marketing has been used to impact a variety of health and risk behaviors among children, adolescents, and adults. A comprehensive review of mass media campaigns and effects on behavior published by Wakefield et al. (2010) found "strong evidence for benefit" from the majority of antismoking campaigns, and moderate evidence for campaigns to promote physical activity (especially among motivated individuals who received prompts at decision-making moments) and nutrition (when specific healthy food choices were promoted) (Stead et al., 2007; Wakefield et al., 2010). On the other hand, campaigns to combat drug abuse have had mixed results, and those to reduce alcohol consumption have had little success (Wakefield et al., 2010).

Many health-based social marketing campaigns target parents, who can address the home health environment and talk to their children about specific health behaviors. To initiate health behavior change, many of these campaigns take a multifaceted approach, utilizing community outreach as well as mass media (Evans et al., 2010). One example of a social marketing campaign targeting parents was the Centers for Disease Control and Prevention's (CDC's) VERB™ campaign, a well-funded, carefully planned, and highly focused campaign aimed at promoting physical activity among 9- to 13-year-olds (tweens) (Wong et al., 2004). The multi-ethnic campaign was notable for its use of tailored messages aimed at specific audience segments, which included white, black, Hispanic, American Indian, and Asian American tweens (Berkowitz et al., 2008; Huhman et al., 2008; Wong et al., 2004). An evaluation revealed increases in physical activity among important subgroups of youth exposed to the campaign (e.g., 9- to 10-year-olds, girls, children living in urban areas of high density, children from households with annual incomes between $25,000 and $50,000, and children who were low-active at baseline), and also indicated that as tween exposure to the campaign messages increased, more physical activity sessions were reported (a dose-response relationship) (Huhman et al., 2005, 2010). The VERB™ campaign provided evidence that the development of a national media campaign with social marketing messages for young people can help address a significant public health issue such as physical activity (Asbury et al., 2008; Banspach, 2008; Huhman et al., 2010).

In addition to the "truth" campaign referenced above, other youth anti-smoking campaigns have had an impact on behaviors (Bauer et al., 1999; Biglan et al., 2000; Flynn et al., 1994, 1997; Wakefield et al., 2003). Some of these successful campaigns have included engaging teens and parents in supporting community-level social changes to help prevent adolescent tobacco use (Biglan et al., 2000; Wakefield et al., 2003).

Social marketing also has been found effective in promoting safer sexual behaviors (Zimmerman et al., 2007). One such experiment used extensive formative research to select high-performing ads, targeted a well-defined audience (high-sensation-seeking youth, who were most at risk of unprotected sex), and purchased an extensive inventory of well-targeted air time (Zimmerman et al., 2007). Previous safe sex campaigns not using such techniques generally had yielded modest results.

Implementation

Changing behavior through social marketing campaigns is not easy in the best of circumstances, and most campaigns are waged under less than ideal conditions. Many campaigns are highly underfunded and forced to rely on and settle for infrequent and untargeted donated media time. Often there are few, if any, funds for formative message development and testing, which would allow for the identification of approaches that would garner attention, resonate with the target audience, and be most effective in changing behavior. Adding to these challenges, many social marketing campaigns are not sustained over significant periods of time (Randolph and Viswanath, 2004; Wakefield et al., 2010).

Even when well funded and designed, social marketing programs can be challenging. Most of these campaigns are aimed at behaviors that are difficult to change because of the ubiquitous marketing of foods and beverages that generally are overconsumed according to national dietary guidelines. Further, Cohen (2008) identifies biological (neural) pathways that can lead to food choices that are subconscious, reflexive, or uncontrollable, including responses to food images, cues, and smells and imitation of the eating behaviors of others without awareness of doing so.

To help overcome these challenges, the committee recommends—as is reflected in its recommended potential actions for implementing this strategy—that the proposed new social marketing campaign

- identify a specific set of narrowly targeted audiences;
- focus on a specific set of narrowly defined goals for behavior change among each audience;
- craft tailored messages for each audience;
- sustain each message/audience focus over a period of several years;
- use multiple media platforms, including television, online, print, mobile, and social media platforms;
- enlist support from and develop partnerships with communities, nongovernmental organizations, and for-profit companies to help broaden and sustain the campaign; and
- be sufficiently funded to conduct extensive message-testing research, secure high-quality creative communication experts, and purchase advertising space in media that are highly rated among the target audience, rather than having to rely on donated placements.

A social marketing campaign such as that proposed here can be supported through media advocacy, defined as "strategic use of the mass media to support community organizing to advance a social or public policy initiative." Media advocacy helps people "understand the importance and reach of news coverage, the need to participate actively in shaping such coverage, and the methods to do so effectively" (Dorfman and Gonzalez, 2011). It is seen as part of a broader strategy of health communication that supports community organizing and policy development and advancement. Additionally, it can support a social marketing campaign's focus on changing individual health habits by promoting environmental and policy changes required to effect social change (Wallack et al., 1993). This is accomplished by engaging individuals in advocating for larger issues by targeting those in power who can affect these larger community changes (Wallack and Dorfman, 1996). For example, Wallack and Dorfman (2000) describe a local 5-a-Day social marketing campaign with a goal of increasing consumption of fruits and vegetables for pregnant teens in a specific inner-city neighborhood. Before individual behaviors could be expected to change, economic conditions had to change (i.e., the availability and affordability of fruits and vegetables had to be improved). Accomplishing the latter changes involved mobilizing teens to demand the return of grocers, initiate community gardens, and advocate for environmental changes that would make it easier for them and their families to make healthy choices (IOM, 2002).

Basic concepts, tools, planning, and lessons from other media advocacy campaign are detailed elsewhere (Gardner et al., 2010; Wallack and Dorfman, 1996; Wallack et al., 1993), but in this era of reduced resources for journalism, news outlets often lack the resources necessary for the more challenging reporting needed to cover these issues from this broader, societal-level perspective. In addition, it often takes sustained advocacy from health organizations to persuade journalists of the importance of this broader focus. Developing the communication skills of health organizations and supporting journalism education programs can help contribute to a more balanced message environment and promote citizen engagement in the critical policy issues that affect individual behavior change.

Too often, social marketing campaigns are paid lip service by policy makers and expert committees. Ambitious health goals are identified, but the scope and scale of the marketing effort are incommensurate with the goals. A 2006 Government Accountability Office (GAO) report identified 105 PSA campaigns in seven federal agencies from fiscal year (FY) 2003 through the first half of FY 2005 (GAO, 2006). Total funding varied dramatically, including $22,250 for a campaign against human trafficking, approximately $2.3 million for a campaign to promote adoption, $6,400 for a campaign aimed at "all Americans" on aspirin therapy for cardiac health, $550,000 for a long-term care campaign, approximately $184,000 to raise awareness about Head Start in the Hispanic community, and $1,100 for a campaign on the safe use of medicines and supplements during pregnancy (GAO, 2006).

Costs associated with an effective long-term social marketing program will be significant, but represent only a small fraction of the increasing health care costs associated with obesity each year. The use of lower-cost digital media as an important part of the program will help limit expenses and make the program more effective and responsive. However, young people spend much less time with these media than with more expensive outlets, such as television. In 2009, 8- to 18-year-olds spent an average of nearly 4.5 hours a day watching television on a television set, compared with 22 minutes a day using social networking sites (Rideout et al., 2010). To achieve the kind of campaign exposure that will be necessary to effect behavior change, television likely will need to be an important platform.

Indicators for Assessing Progress in Obesity Prevention for Strategy 3-1

Primary Indicators

- Increase in the proportion of children, adolescents, and adults in the target audience meeting the Physical Activity Guidelines for Americans.*
  Source needed for measurement of indicator.

- Increase in the proportion of children, adolescents, and adults in the target audience meeting the Dietary Guidelines for Americans.*
  Source needed for measurement of indicator.

Accelerating Progress in Obesity Prevention

Process Indicators

- Successful implementation of a targeted social marketing program.
  Sources for measuring indicator: Nielsen (global marketing and advertising research company) and other commercial data

- Documentation of purchases of advertising time and exposure of the target audience to the messages.
  Sources for measuring indicator: Nielsen (global marketing and advertising research company) and other commercial data

- Changes in knowledge and attitudes on obesity, physical activity, and nutrition in the target audience from each phase of the campaign.
  Source needed for measurement of indicator.

Foundational Indicator

- Provision of funding for the campaign and designation of a lead agency to oversee it.
  Sources for measuring indicator: Federal budget and appropriations legislation

---

*See Box B-1 in Appendix B.

Strategy 3-2: Implement Common Standards for Marketing Foods and Beverages to Children and Adolescents

The food, beverage, restaurant, and media industries should take broad, common, and urgent voluntary action to make substantial improvements in their marketing aimed directly at children and adolescents aged 2-17. All foods and beverages marketed to this age group should support a diet that accords with the Dietary Guidelines for Americans in order to prevent obesity and risk factors associated with chronic disease risk. Children and adolescents should be encouraged to avoid calories from foods that they generally overconsume (e.g., products high in sugar, fat, and sodium) and to replace them with foods they generally undercon-sume (e.g., fruits, vegetables, and whole grains).

The standards set for foods and beverages marketed to children and adolescents should be widely publicized and easily available to parents and other consumers. They should cover foods and beverages marketed to children and adolescents aged 2-17 and should apply to a broad range of marketing and advertising practices, including digital marketing and the use of licensed characters and toy premiums. If such marketing standards have not been adopted within 2 years by a substantial majority of food, beverage, restaurant, and media companies that market foods and beverages to children and adolescents, policy makers at the local, state, and federal levels should consider setting mandatory nutritional standards for marketing to this age group to ensure that such standards are implemented.

Potential actions include

- all food and beverage companies, including chain and quick-service restau-rants, adopting and implementing voluntary nutrition standards for foods and beverages marketed to children and adolescents;
- the Children's Food and Beverage Advertising Initiative (CFBAI) and National Restaurant Association Initiative, as major self-regulatory market-ing efforts, adopting common marketing standards for all member compa-nies, and actively recruiting additional members to increase the impact of improved food marketing to children and adolescents;
- media companies adopting nutrition standards for all foods they market to young people; and
- the Federal Trade Commission (FTC) regularly tracking the marketing standards adopted by food and beverage companies, restaurants, and media companies.

Context

Children and adolescents are a specific target for food and beverage marketing within societywide message environments including media and packaging. As previ-ously mentioned, food and beverage messaging targeting children and adolescents is much like their diet—mostly high in sugars, fat, sodium, and calories and very low in fruits, vegetables, whole grains, and dairy products (Cheyne et al., 2011; Grotto and Zied, 2010; Harris et al., 2010; Harrison and Marske, 2005; IOM, 2006). The media messaging environment surrounding children and adolescents is ubiquitous and occupies more of their waking time than any other daily activity, including school. Average daily media use by 8- to 18-year-olds is more than 7.5 hours, more than one-fourth of which is spent using multiple media (Rideout et al., 2010). One study estimates that in 2009, 2- to 11-year-olds saw 11-13 television food and beverage–related ads per day (Powell et al., 2011). In another study, Kunkel and colleagues (2009) estimate that children viewing children's programming saw on average 7.5 food and beverage advertisements per hour. Black children and adolescents view significantly more television than their peers and consequently are exposed to more food and beverage and restaurant advertisements on television—36 percent more food and beverage product advertisements and 21 percent more restaurant advertisements (Harris et al., 2010).

The message environments directly targeting children and adolescents show year-to-year variations in product mix, dollars spent, and media mix in food and beverage marketing. For example, food advertising on television has declined somewhat, while less expensive digital marketing is growing rapidly. Nevertheless, foods marketed to children and adolescents continue to be nutrition poor and high in fat, sugars, and sodium (FTC, 2008; Harris et al., 2010, 2011; IOM, 2006; Powell et al., 2011).

Furthermore, the above estimates regarding foods marketed to children and adolescents generally do not include product placement on television or in digital media (e.g., the Internet, mobile devices). Nontraditional marketing, such as Internet-based advergames featuring brands or product avatars, virtual environments, couponing on cell phones, or stealth marketing on social networks (e.g., an individual child's 8-minute engagement with a brand or product in an advergame), is not easily measured by dollars spent, and exposure can be difficult to "count" (Chester and Montgomery, 2011; Cheyne et al., 2011). An estimated 85 percent of child-oriented brands from food companies that advertise heavily to children on television also have a website with content for children (Moore and Rideout, 2007). Minority children and adolescents (i.e., Hispanic, Asian, black) are especially attractive market segments for digital media and product placement because, on average, they spend significantly more time using computers and video games than their white counterparts, are increasingly targeted for low-cost and low-nutrition foods and beverages, and have more favorable attitudes toward marketing efforts targeting them (Aaker et al., 2000; Grier and Brumbauch, 1999; Grier and Kumanyika, 2008; Rideout et al., 2011). Chester and Montgomery (2007) describe how the rapid expansion of digital marketing requires the participation of various stakeholders, such as the food and media industries, and suggest that the paucity of research regarding nontraditional marketing practices warrants a new set of food and beverage regulations encompassing these practices as well as traditional advertising.

In short, there is good evidence that children and adolescents consume too much sugar, fat, and sodium and insufficient amounts of fruits, vegetables, and whole grains; that food marketing targeting children and adolescents is heavily for products high in sugar, fat, and sodium; and that marketing is ubiquitous in the message environments of children and adolescents.

Evidence

Marketing—including marketing targeting children and adolescents—works. A systematic review of peer-reviewed research documents evidence of a causal relationship between television advertising and the food and beverage preferences, purchase requests, and short-term consumption of children aged 2-11 (IOM, 2006). Additionally, a body of evidence documents an association of food and beverage television advertising with the adiposity (body fatness) of children and adolescents aged 2-18, although the literature is insufficient to convincingly rule out other explanations (IOM, 2006). Because food marketing reaches children and adolescents regularly through multiple media channels, short-term consumption can become regular consumption. In short, marketing works effectively to cause children to prefer, request, and consume sugary, fatty, and salty foods marketed to them.

Although there is agreement among researchers that children aged 8 and younger do not effectively comprehend the persuasive intent of marketing messages (IOM, 2006), reviews of basic research on adolescent development in the fields of neuroscience, physiology, and marketing find evidence that adolescents (aged 12-17) are more impulsive and self-conscious than adults—unable to resist acting on urges and relying on positive images to gain self-worth (Pechmann et al., 2005). This and other emerging research (Dosenbach et al., 2010; Luna, 2009; Steinberg, 2010) continues to support the protection of adolescents from exposure to advertising and promotions "for high-risk, addictive products, especially if impulsive behaviors or image benefits are depicted" (Pechmann et al., 2005, p. 202).

As a result of these findings, the landmark 2006 IOM report on food marketing to children and youth recommends that "the food, beverage, restaurant and marketing industries should work with government, scientific, public health and consumer groups to establish and enforce the highest standards of marketing of foods, beverages and meals to children and youth" (p. 12). The report also calls on industry to reformulate products to be "substantially lower in fats, salt and added sugars, and higher in nutrient content" (p. 11). Finally, the report recommends that the Secretary of the Department of Health and Human Services (HHS) report to Congress within 2 years on the progress made and additional actions necessary to accelerate progress (IOM, 2006).

Implementation

Some food and beverage companies, including some fast-food restaurants, have taken steps that acknowledge their responsibility to help protect some children and adolescents from marketing of less healthy foods.

Following publication of the 2006 IOM report on food marketing to children and youth, the Council of Better Business Bureaus and the Children's Advertising Review Unit organized a self-regulatory initiative of 10 major food and beverage companies—CFBAI—to limit their food and beverage marketing (mostly television advertising) to children under age 12 to "better for you" products. The initiative encompasses the use of licensed characters, movie tie-ins, and celebrity use. The television marketing requirements also restrict the use of paid product placements in child-directed programming. In 2008, the FTC presented a report to Congress regarding food marketing to children and adolescents that described significant progress such as the establishment of the CFBAI and outlined necessary future actions for the food and beverage industry and entertainment and media industries (FTC, 2008). In 2010, the CFBAI was extended to include aspects of digital marketing (Kolish, 2011). Definitions of "better for you" were determined individually by each participating company (Peeler et al., 2010). In 2011, the CFBAI reported having 17 member companies representing 79 percent of food, beverage, and restaurant television advertisements and 73 percent of products promoted on children's televisions programming; the initiative's representation in media other than television (i.e., radio, the Internet) has not been reported (Kolish, 2011). CFBAI reports have shown nearly total compliance by members with their individual marketing standards; however, compliance in media other than television has not yet been reported (Kolish, 2011).

Independent researchers, using uniform and more stringent nutrition standards of independent authorities such as the HHS "Go-Slow-Whoa" food rating system or recommended school meal standards, have found that since the CFBAI began, most advertisements directly targeting children have continued to be for products high in calories, fats, sugars, and sodium and low in other nutrients underrepresented in children's diets—a reported 72 percent of all food and beverage advertisements for children's programming and 86 percent of food and beverage advertisements seen by children (Kraak et al., 2011; Kunkel et al., 2009; Powell et al., 2011). A recent analysis found that exposure to advertisements for "sugary drinks and energy drinks" increased from 2008 to 2010 for preschoolers (4 percent), children (8 percent), and teens (18 percent) (Harris et al., 2011). In addition, a significant proportion—about 25 percent—of television food ads targeting children are by non-CFBAI companies and are for products of poorer nutritional quality than those of CFBAI members (Kunkel et al., 2009). In 2011, the FTC released the voluntary nutrition principles of the federal Interagency Working Group on Food Marketed to Children for foods and beverages marketed to children and adolescents aged 2-17 (Interagency Working Group on Food Marketed to Children, 2011). After the proposed principles were published, they were rejected in public comments from the food and beverage industry, the fast-food industry, media companies, and the U.S. Chamber of Commerce on the grounds of their potential to have a significant economic impact (i.e., job and sales losses) and to lead to interference with companies' First Amendment rights to free speech (Bachman, 2011; Layton and Eggen, 2011). Additionally, the food and beverage industry claimed that the proposed principles were extremely limiting and could prohibit marketing of healthy foods, an argument that was refuted by researchers analyzing CFBAI-approved products[1] (GMA, 2011b; Wootan, 2011).

Furthermore, the public health community is concerned about the potential for overfortification of foods with nutrients that are encouraged by the Dietary Guidelines for Americans. Unless rules are put in place to prevent it, manufacturers could choose to fortify products to allow them to be marketed to children and adolescents. As summarized in a recent IOM report (2010), overfortification could result in deceptive or misleading claims or could encourage the addition of nutrients to food products in which the nutrient is unstable or biologically unavailable (counter to the Food and Drug Administration's [FDA's] fortification policy).

Since the CFBAI began, a number of new food, beverage, and restaurant industry initiatives have been announced, including additional self-regulatory efforts regarding marketing of products to children aged 2-12, as well as product reformulations. Among these initiatives are uniform nutritional standards for marketing in the CFBAI; a new initiative from the National Restaurant Association, which was adopted by 19 large restaurant chains; and a commitment by several major quick-service restaurants and large food manufacturers and distributors regarding nutritional formulation of some child and adult meals and food products (CFBAI, 2011; McDonald's, 2011; NRA, 2011; Walmart, 2011). The committee welcomes such

---

[1]Researchers used CFBAI standards as of March 2011.

steps toward reducing marketing of unhealthy foods to some children and adolescents and improving the nutritional quality of some foods intended for children, as well as recognition by several companies and industry associations of the need to protect children from marketing of unhealthy foods.

In sum, changing the current message environments to market healthy foods for children and adolescents and eliminating marketing of foods that could negatively impact their health and weight, thereby reducing their overall exposure to marketing of such foods, will accelerate obesity prevention because of the documented effects of food marketing on this population's preferences, purchase requests, and consumption. Adoption of uniform guidelines developed around a central goal of healthy dietary patterns and covering all foods and beverages marketed to children and adolescents will help all families and their children prefer, request, and consume healthier foods and meals. The recent activity of the food and beverage manufacturing and restaurant industries to this end is welcome and encouraging, but food marketing targeting children and adolescents continues to heavily promote products high in sugar, fat, and sodium. Implementing a common set of guidelines that includes all forms of marketing and extending these guidelines to the age of 17 will accelerate reductions in the consumption of nutrients that are currently overconsumed relative to the 2010 Dietary Guidelines for Americans and may increase the consumption of nutrients that support a healthy diet and are currently underconsumed. These actions also may help reduce disparities in obesity rates for those youth who have greater exposure to media, including black, Hispanic, and Asian youth.

Indicators for Assessing Progress in Obesity Prevention for Strategy 3-2

Primary Indicator

- Reduction in the proportion of solid fats and added sugars consumed by children aged 2 and older as recommended by the Dietary Guidelines for Americans.*
  Source for measuring indicator: NHANES

Process Indicators

- Increase in the proportion of companies that adopt marketing standards substantially similar to the committee's recommendation.
  Sources for measuring indicator: CFBAI reports or other trade organization tracking report

- Increase in the market share of products marketed to children and adolescents that are consistent with the marketing standards recommended in this report.
  Sources for measuring indicator: CFBAI reports or other trade organization tracking report

- Increase in the proportion of healthy foods marketed to children and adolescents (i.e., as defined by the marketing standards recommended in this report) across all media.
  Source needed for measurement of indicator.

- Increase in the proportion of foods and beverages marketed to children and adolescents that are recommended by the Dietary Guidelines for Americans.*
  Source for measuring indicator: NHANES

- Increase in the proportion of food and beverage and media companies that establish common nutritional requirements for foods and beverages marketed to children and adolescents.
  Sources for measuring indicator: CFBAI reports or other industry-related tracking reports

Foundational Indicators

- Promulgation by self-regulation or government of marketing standards for children and adolescents substantially similar to the committee's recommendation.
  Sources for measuring indicator: CFBAI reports or other industry-related tracking reports

- Continued monitoring of food marketing to children and adolescents by the FTC.
  Source for measuring indicator: FTC follow-up study

- Development of appropriate exposure measures covering digital marketing as well as traditional ads.
  Source needed for measurement of indicator.

NOTE: CFBAI = Children's Food and Beverage Advertising Initiative; FTC = Federal Trade Commission; NHANES = National Health and Nutrition Examination Survey.

---

*See Box B-1 in Appendix B.

Strategy 3-3: Ensure Consistent Nutrition Labeling for the Front of Packages, Retail Store Shelves, and Menus and Menu Boards That Encourages Healthier Food Choices

The FDA and the U.S. Department of Agriculture (USDA) should implement a standard system of nutrition labeling for the front of packages and retail store shelves that is harmonious with the Nutrition Facts panel, and restaurants should provide calorie labeling on all menus and menu boards.

Potential actions include

- The FDA and USDA adopting a single standard nutrition labeling system for all fronts of packages and retail store shelves, the FDA and USDA considering making this system mandatory to enable consumers to compare products on a standard nutrition profile, and the guidelines provided by the Institute of Medicine (2011a) being used for implementation; and
- restaurants implementing the FDA regulations that require restaurants with 20 or more locations to provide calorie labeling on their menus and menu boards, and the FDA/USDA monitoring industry for compliance with this policy.

Context

Americans may intend to eat more healthfully, but this intention does not necessarily reflect their behavior. Consumer research based on self-reports suggests that 75 percent of adults are actively trying to make healthier choices, but the number reporting certain eating behaviors (e.g., attempts to limit calories, trans fats, or sodium) in accord with those intentions is about 50 percent (FDA, 2008). Nutrition labeling, one marketing technique, is intended to be used as a tool to help consumers to eat healthier diets and meet dietary recommendations.

Consumers generally are unaware of, or inaccurately estimate, the number of calories in restaurant foods (Elbel, 2011). Even if the caloric values of menu items are displayed in restaurants, consumers have difficulty placing this information in context with their total daily caloric intake. Such limitations in comprehension resulting from, for example, displaying calorie values without providing an anchor of recommended meal or daily caloric intake, can limit the effect of the information provided (Roberto et al., 2010).

Additionally, detailed nutrition labeling on prepackaged foods generally is misinterpreted or difficult to understand for consumers (Morestin et al., 2011). Consumers have difficulty interpreting the amount of calories and nutrients that is appropriate for them to consume, and some of the information presented on food packaging can be misleading. The variety of logos and criteria currently being used for nutrient content claims and health claims—about 20 different systems are in use by food manufacturers—is confusing to the consumer (IOM, 2010; Kelly et al., 2009; Lobstein and Davies, 2009; Louie et al., 2008) and sometimes requires interpretation. This situation is counterproductive to the goal of nutrition labeling given that consumers tend to make buying decisions in seconds (Hoyer, 1984) and do not take time to analyze nutritional information that is presented (Higginson et al., 2002; Scott and Worsley, 1997).

Evidence gathered since the introduction of the standardized food label in 1994 on the influence of food labels on purchasing behavior and thereby on nutrient intake and dietary patterns is encouraging but limited (Blitstein and Evans, 2006; Kim et al., 2001; Lin et al., 2004; Neuhouser et al., 1999; Ollberding et al., 2010; Satia et al., 2005). Nonetheless, it is known that significant disparities exist in the use of food labels across many demographic characteristics. Disparities have consistently been found by sex, education, income, language, length of residency in the United States for those foreign born, and race (Bender and Derby, 1992; Blitstein and Evans, 2006; Guthrie et al., 1995; Kim et al., 2001; Lin et al., 2004; Nayga, 2000; Neuhouser et al., 1999; Ollberding et al., 2010; Satia et al., 2005).

Despite the potential of food and menu labeling to encourage healthier food purchases and dietary patterns, the consistently low rates of label use, especially among particular populations that also are disproportionately at risk of over-weight and obesity, suggest it may be necessary to modify existing food labels or restaurant labeling to achieve a greater impact on the population. A standard system for fronts of packages, retail shelving, and menu labeling at restaurants would help simplify consumers' choices and enable them to have more information when they make these choices outside the home.

Evidence

Restaurant menu labeling Prior expert committees have made recommendations similar to those offered here for posting calorie content on menus and menu boards (IOM, 2005, 2006, 2009; Keystone Forum, 2006; Lee et al., 2008; RWJF, 2009). These recommendations are supported by the fact that consumers over-estimate the healthfulness of restaurant items, and recent research has shown that calorie and nutrition information provided at the point of purchase may influence their food choices, even prompting them to purchase menu items that lower their overall caloric intake. Indeed, a number of localities have begun to institute such menu labeling policies (IOM, 2009; Morrison et al., 2011; RWJF, 2009).

Front-of-package nutrition labeling Front-of-package labeling is designed to help customers identify products that support healthy diets for themselves and their families by providing useful information at the point of purchase (IOM, 2010). An IOM committee recommended implementing a common front-of-package labeling system on prepackaged foods in 2005, and this recommendation was reinforced by another IOM committee in 2010 (IOM, 2005, 2010; White House Task Force on Childhood Obesity, 2010).

Nationally, a number of front-of-package systems currently are being used on prepackaged foods, and there has been some preliminary evaluation of their impact. Compared with detailed nutrition labeling, more positive evidence has been gathered on the impact of front-of-package labeling on consumer comprehension and healthier food purchases, although some of the evidence in this regard is mixed (Larsson et al., 1999; Morestin et al., 2011; Sacks et al., 2011; Sutherland et al., 2010). A recent review concluded that consumers are able to understand certain front-of-package logos quickly and use them to correctly differentiate healthy and less healthy foods (Borgmeier and Westenhoefer, 2009; Feunekes et al., 2008; Grunert and Wills, 2007; Kelly et al., 2009).

Effects on product reformulation Nutrition labeling has been hypothesized and observed to have an effect on the manufacturing of food (Morestin et al., 2011). Researchers have proposed that displaying the nutritional value on a food product can raise awareness of its nutritional quality and lead to increased consumer demand for healthier products, thus motivating manufacturers to make their products healthier. A recent review cites numerous studies finding that nutrition labeling (including front-of-package systems and menu labeling in restaurants) has motivated food producers and restaurants to make healthier products (Morestin et al., 2011). Additionally, it has been observed that the reformulation of food products benefits all consumers, not just those who use nutritional information to influence their purchases, because it automatically improves the nutritional value of products in the food supply (Golan et al., 2007). For example, a federal trans fat labeling requirement led to a dramatic increase in products claiming "no trans fat" (Golan et al., 2007; Morrison et al., 2011) and a 50 percent reduction in partially hydrogenated oils in foods in North America (Watkins, 2008). Similarly, when the 2005 Dietary Guidelines for Americans recommended that half of the grains people consume be whole grains, the number of new whole-grain products dramatically increased. This dramatic increase in whole grains in the food supply resulted in an increase in sales of healthier foods containing these grains (Morrison et al., 2011).

Implementation

Nutrition labeling in restaurants with 20 or more locations is set to be implemented through FDA regulations (preempting state and local policies), providing calorie information on standard menu items in certain chain restaurants and similar retail food establishments (FDA, 2011). These provisions also include posting a statement describing the recommended daily caloric intake as an anchor for the posted calorie information. These requirements may encourage other restaurants not already covered by the regulations to take similar actions (FDA, 2011).

Detailed labeling of prepackaged foods, meat, poultry, and egg products, including nutrition information and the ingredients list, is required by regulations of the FDA and USDA. Additionally, food packages must include the Nutrition Facts panel and can include nutrient content claims (e.g., "low fat") and health claims to characterize the food's relationship to a disease or health condition (e.g., "may reduce the risk of heart disease") (FDA, 2009). Two IOM reports (2010, 2011a) provide insight on how front-of-package systems should be used as a tool in the future, their target audience, nutrient information that would be most useful to include, and criteria that would be useful in determining which systems and symbols are most helpful.

Internationally, some steps have been taken toward developing national guidance for a front-of-package labeling system, including use of the keyhole symbol and the "traffic-light" system (National Food Administration, 2011; NHS, 2011). Both of these systems are voluntary. In January 2011, leading food and beverage manufacturers and retailers launched a voluntary front-of-package labeling system to help consumers make informed choices in the United States (GMA, 2011a). This *Facts Up Front* system adheres to current FDA nutrition labeling regulations and guidelines and provides information about calories and three nutrients to limit (saturated fats, sodium, and sugars); there is also an option to include up to two nutrients to encourage (e.g., fiber, potassium). This labeling system was intended to complement the American Beverage Association's "Clear on Calories" labeling system, launched in February 2011, whereby all beverages 20 ounces in size or smaller will be labeled with the total calories per container on the front of the package (ABA, 2011). Because implementation of the *Facts Up Front* labeling system has only just begun, its effect on consumer choice is unknown; however, researchers have begun to question the science base for and the possibly confusing nature of the consumer approach taken with this system (Brownell and Koplan, 2011).

Finally, a number of food manufacturers and restaurants have already begun to reformulate products, reduce portion sizes, or use more healthy ingredients (Bernstein, 2011; Rogers, 2011; Walmart, 2011). Although forthcoming federal nutrition labeling regulations have not always been directly cited as the impetus for such actions, others have hypothesized that they are having this effect (Golan et al., 2007; Morrison et al., 2011).

In sum, given the proliferation of front-of-package labeling systems and logos for prepackaged foods and restaurant menu labeling policies, a common labeling system in stores and restaurants that can be easily understood by the general population will help optimize opportunities for children, adolescents, parents, and other adults to identify and encourage purchases of healthier foods. Although a number of menu labeling policies have been introduced and implemented over the past decade, a majority of the population is not impacted by these policies. Additionally, although recent actions of the food and beverage industry are encouraging, the recently developed voluntary front-of-package system may not be easily understood by all consumers or maximize the opportunity for them to make healthier food choices. Implementing a common system for prepackaged foods and restaurant menu labels could also continue to move the industry to reformulate or repackage foods, thereby altering the food supply and encouraging consumers to purchase healthier foods. This recommendation may have the added benefit of reducing disparities in obesity rates for consumers who are less likely to use the more detailed (existing) label on prepackaged foods and are at an increased risk of obesity, including individuals with lower education and income levels, racial and ethnic minority groups, and those with limited English language proficiency.

Indicators for Assessing Progress in Obesity Prevention for Strategy 3-3

Process Indicators

- Increase in the percentage of food manufacturers that voluntarily agree to market only healthy foods to children and adolescents.
  Sources for measuring indicator: Government, trade, and advocate organizations

- Increase in the proportion of restaurants with 20 or more locations that meet the menu and menu board calorie labeling regulations.
  Sources for measuring indicator: Government, trade, and advocate organizations

- Increase in the proportion of consumers who purchase and consume foods recommended by the Dietary Guidelines for Americans.*
  Sources for measuring indicator: BRFSS and YRBSS

- Increase in the number of new products that help children, adolescents, and adults meet the Dietary Guidelines for Americans.
  Sources needed for measurement of indicator, such as follow-up reports from government and academics, corporate social responsibility reports by food manufacturers.

- Increase in purchases of reformulated foods that meet the definition in the Dietary Guidelines for Americans of foods people should consume in greater quantities.
  Source for measuring indicator: Nielsen Home scan data

Strategy 3-4: Adopt Consistent Nutrition Education Policies for Federal Programs with Nutrition Education Components

USDA should update the policies for Supplemental Nutrition Assistance Program Education (SNAP-Ed) and the policies for other federal programs with nutrition education components to explicitly encourage the provision of advice about types of foods to reduce in the diet, consistent with the Dietary Guidelines for Americans.

Potential actions include

- removing the restrictions on the types of information that can be included in SNAP-Ed programs and encouraging advice about types of foods to reduce;
- disseminating, immediately and effectively, notification of the revised regulations, along with authoritative guidance on how to align federally funded nutrition education programs with the Dietary Guidelines; and
- ensuring that such full alignment of nutrition education with the Dietary Guidelines applies to all federal programs with a nutrition education component, particularly programs that target primary food shoppers in low-

income families (e.g., the Expanded Food and Nutrition Education Program and the Special Supplemental Nutrition Program for Women, Infants, and Children [WIC]).

Context

This strategy leverages the extensive reach of the largest federally funded nutrition assistance program, SNAP, to address disparities in obesity. When specific recommendations to accelerate progress in obesity prevention are being considered, including strategies involving SNAP is essential in light of the scale, reach, and federal dollar investment of this program. The committee viewed the context for making SNAP-related recommendations as particularly complex given the program's reach to a large segment of the low-income population, the potentially far-reaching effects of any changes to the program, and an ongoing public debate concerning ethical and practical questions about strategies that will be most fair and effective (Barnhill, 2011; Brownell and Ludwig, 2011; Hartline-Grafton et al., 2011; Shenkin and Jacobson, 2010). The committee considered various options, including extant proposals for restrictions on purchases of sugar-sweetened beverages and incentives for purchases of healthy foods such as fruits and vegetables.

Viewed in its historical and nutrition policy context as a food security program operating as a cash transfer to low-income families, the overarching aim of SNAP has been and continues to be to ensure that low-income households have enough food to eat based on a market basket of foods determined to meet nutrient needs and the Dietary Guidelines for Americans. Over time, as evidence has accumulated about the role of diet in chronic disease development, interest in the quality of foods allowable for purchase with SNAP benefits has increased. This interest was reflected in the renaming of the program (from the Food Stamp Program) in 2008 (USDA/FNS, 2011b). Nutritional goals other than the ability to afford an adequate diet are not explicit in the SNAP regulations, which permit purchases of a wide range of foods (USDA, 2011c). In contrast, the WIC has always targeted pregnant and lactating women and infants and children up to age 5, and participants may use its financial assistance to purchase only pre-approved food items that have been deemed most nutritionally beneficial.[2]

SNAP targets low-income populations in which poorer dietary quality and higher-than-average risks of diet-related diseases are observed relative to higher-income groups (IOM, 2011b). Theoretically, specific strategies to promote healthful food choices among SNAP participants—such as incentives for healthy food

---

[2]These pre-approved food items make up a portion of the diet, but do not comprise a complete diet.

purchases and restrictions on the types of foods and beverages permissible for purchase with SNAP benefits—could help address these disparities. Sugar-sweetened beverages have been the most widely discussed products to target for restrictions as a way of both reducing their consumption and freeing SNAP dollars for purchases of products that contribute to a nutritionally adequate diet.

Advocates of restricting sugar-sweetened beverage purchases with SNAP benefits argue that they deteriorate diet quality and promote chronic disease (see Chapter 6, Strategy 2-1), with the costs of treating such diseases falling primarily to taxpayers (Brownell and Ludwig, 2011; Shenkin and Jacobson, 2010). In addition, members of the SNAP-eligible population are heavily targeted by sugar-sweetened beverage marketers (Grier and Kumanyika, 2008), and a USDA study found that SNAP participants were more likely than higher-income (ineligible for SNAP) nonparticipants to consume regular (nondiet) soda (Cole and Fox, 2008). Market-oriented arguments also are advanced to support restrictions on foods eligible for SNAP purchases (Alston et al., 2009). For example, SNAP benefit expenditures totaled approximately $50.4 billion in 2009 (the 2011 figure is $71.8 billion) (USDA, 2011d), and because 84 percent of total benefits in 2009 were redeemed in supermarkets/supercenters (USDA/FNS, 2011a), changes to SNAP regulations could provide an indirect stimulus for changes in the behavior of the retail food industry in terms of what products are stocked and promoted (Alston et al., 2009).

On the other hand, restrictions raise both practical and economic concerns. Practical concerns relate to implementation and program administration. Current implementation approaches for SNAP heavily prioritize a transactional process that encourages (or at least does not discourage) program participation through ease of use at the point of purchase and the absence of stigma, and is relatively easy to implement at the retail level. Arguments against restriction include that it may be difficult for policy makers, food retailers, and SNAP participants to distinguish which products are eligible for purchase with SNAP dollars, and purchasing restrictions could cause stigma and confusion at checkout counters, potentially decreasing SNAP participation (Barnhill, 2011; Cook, 2011; Hartline-Grafton et al., 2011; USDA, 2007). Economic analysts raise cautions about the difficulty of estimating with certainty the health or economic outcomes that would result from various perturbations of such a complex system. Simulations of possible effects require multiple assumptions about how both SNAP participants and the retail food market would react—for example, respectively, the types of trade-offs SNAP participants would make with respect to use of their other sources of income, and effects on demand curves and supplies for certain products (Alston et al., 2009).

Restrictions also raise ethical and social justice concerns related to potential infringement on freedom of choice of SNAP participants. From this perspective, limiting food choices for SNAP recipients may be viewed as patronizing and discriminatory to low-income consumers (Barnhill, 2011; Hartline-Grafton et al., 2011; USDA, 2007). It is also expected that efforts to reform SNAP purchasing regulations would be difficult, given the strong bipartisan support for the program as currently formulated and the strong opposition to restrictive changes from those interested in protecting the role of SNAP in addressing potential hunger and food insecurity for all people at risk.

Support for testing an alternative SNAP reform strategy—providing incentives for healthy food choices—has been more forthcoming than support for trials of restrictions. In August 2011, USDA rejected New York City's request to pilot a program that would have restricted the purchase of selected sugar-sweetened beverages with SNAP dollars (USDA, 2011a), and requests from other states to implement similar pilot programs have not been approved. USDA is currently testing an incentive strategy for its effects on the purchasing behaviors and diet quality of SNAP participants. The 2008 Farm Bill authorized $20 million to pilot test and rigorously evaluate the impact on the diet quality of SNAP participants of financial incentives at the point of sale for the purchase of fruits, vegetables, or other healthful foods. This Healthy Incentives pilot will run for 15 months during 2011-2013, with key outcomes of interest including changes in the amount of fruits and vegetables consumed and whether additional calories consumed from fruits and vegetables displace calories consumed from other food groups. Several smaller-scale programs incentivizing the purchase of fruits and vegetables are under way in localities such as New York City, Boston, and Philadelphia (Food Fit Philly, 2011; New York City Department of Health and Mental Hygiene, 2010; The Food Project, 2011).

Given the current absence of firm evidence to indicate which, if either, approach to reform of SNAP regulations related to food purchases—restrictions or incentives—would meet standards for feasibility, equity, and impact, the committee identified strategies to improve the marketing and information environment in which SNAP participants purchase foods as an important and viable mechanism with predictable positive effects in accelerating obesity prevention. The USDA Food and Nutrition Service encourages states to provide nutrition education to SNAP participants and eligibles as part of their program operations. The objective is to provide clear and effective messages for SNAP participants and eligibles about how to make healthy food choices within a limited budget and prevent excess weight gain.

However, current regulations for the SNAP education component (SNAP-Ed) are ambiguous and restrictive in a way that deprives SNAP participants of clear nutrition education, exacerbating existing disparities and undermining the SNAP goals related to overall dietary quality. Although the regulatory language indicates that states should ensure that all nutrition messages conveyed as a part of SNAP-Ed are consistent with the Dietary Guidelines for Americans, it also stipulates that "SNAP-Ed funds may not be used to convey negative written, visual, or verbal expressions about any specific foods, beverages, or commodities. This includes messages of belittlement or derogation of such items, as well as any suggestion that such foods, beverages, or commodities should never be consumed" (USDA, 2011b, p. 18). An appendix to the SNAP-Ed guidance (USDA, 2011b, p. 72) states that nutrition education messages and social marketing campaigns that convey negative messages or disparage specific foods, beverages, or commodities are not allowed. Yet "foods to reduce" are the subject of an entire chapter in the Dietary Guidelines (Chapter 3), along with the chapter devoted to "foods to increase" (Chapter 4). In effect, SNAP participants are allowed to receive only half the message. SNAP regulations place few constraints on the types of foods that can be purchased with program benefits (USDA, 2011c), and this flexibility is inconsistent with the constraints on the content of nutrition guidance that can be provided in SNAP-Ed programs. For example, Shenkin and Jacobson (2010) report that according to the federal guidance, health agencies and organizations in four states were required to stop using SNAP-Ed funds to discourage soft drink consumption.

While motivated SNAP-Ed providers may identify ways to work around this limitation, clarification of USDA regulations is required to address this apparent policy conflict. Addressing this problem in ways that explicitly reduced the purchase and consumption of foods identified in the Dietary Guidelines as conducive to obesity and chronic disease development could stimulate the purchase of healthier foods among SNAP participants, who numbered more than 40.3 million in 2010, corresponding to $64.7 billion in benefits for that year (USDA, 2011d). While this strategy refers primarily to SNAP-Ed, it has implications for ensuring that other federal nutrition programs with a nutrition education component (e.g., the Expanded Food and Nutrition Education Program [EFNEP] and WIC) convey the full scope of advice in the Dietary Guidelines.

Evidence

SNAP, and therefore SNAP-Ed, have extensive reach to populations at a higher-than-average risk of obesity. Eligibility for SNAP requires a family income that is at or below 130 percent of the federal poverty level (Leftin et al., 2010). At some point in their lives, about half of adults (between the ages of 20 and 65) and children in the American population participate in SNAP (Rank and Hirschl, 2003). Approximately half of participants are children, and about a third of participating households are single-adult households with children (VerPloeg and Ralston, 2008).

In absolute numbers, most U.S. adults and children who are obese are in the middle- or high-income range. Relative to adults with higher incomes, however, the prevalence of obesity is higher among low-income women and lower-income children of both sexes (Ogden et al., 2010a,b). In addition, non-Hispanic black and Hispanic adults have higher obesity prevalence than non-Hispanic whites of the same ages (Flegal et al., 2010), and a greater percentage of these populations were below the poverty level in 2009 (25.8 percent of blacks and 25.3 percent of Hispanics, compared with 12.3 percent of whites) (DeNavas-Walt et al., 2010).

Some studies have suggested a positive relationship between SNAP participation and obesity among women. Based on an extensive review by Ver Ploeg and Ralston (2008), some evidence suggests that long-term SNAP participation may contribute to weight gain in women. Nevertheless, the nature of the available data and the differences between characteristics of SNAP participants and income-eligible as well as other nonparticipants make it difficult to confirm a causal relationship (Ver Ploeg and Ralston, 2008). For example, Ver Ploeg and colleagues (2007) report that black women who participated in SNAP had weight levels similar to those of income-eligible black women who did not participate in the program (Ver Ploeg et al., 2007). Food insecurity also has been linked to overweight and obesity in women (Adams et al., 2003; Basiotis and Lino, 2003; Jilcott et al., 2011; Olson, 1999; Townsend et al., 2001). This is important to note given that SNAP was designed to address food insecurity, and SNAP participants are more likely than nonparticipants to experience food insecurity (Cohen et al., 1999; Jensen, 2002; Wilde and Nord, 2005). In other words, as discussed at a 2010 IOM workshop on food insecurity and obesity, it becomes difficult to infer a causal relationship between SNAP participation and obesity because of the many other variables that can influence the likelihood of obesity (IOM, 2011b).

Whether the association between being overweight and the characteristics of those who participate in SNAP is causal or coincidental, this association justifies an intensified focus on providing guidance to SNAP participants about prevention of excess weight gain. This justification is supported by evidence based on comparisons of the dietary intake of adult SNAP participants with that of income-eligible nonparticipants and higher-income individuals in national survey data. Diets of adult SNAP participants are comparable to those of the other two groups with respect to nutrient adequacy, but contain higher amounts of calories from solid fats and added sugars and reflect a greater frequency of consuming foods recommended for only occasional consumption (Cole and Fox, 2008).

The other compelling considerations that justify actions to update federal nutrition education policies relate to food marketing environments. The fact that high-calorie, low-nutrition foods are convenient and often less expensive than healthier alternatives makes them particularly attractive to people with limited resources (Drewnowski and Specter, 2004; Monsivais et al., 2010). In addition, SNAP participants make their food choices in a marketing environment that is less favorable with respect to promotion of healthy food relative to higher-income and nonminority communities (Grier, 2009; Grier and Kumanyika, 2008). Moreover, the demographics of low-income and ethnic minority populations represented in the SNAP population are associated with lower availability of food stores that offer a range of healthy food choices—numerous studies and reviews have concluded that healthy food is less available in low-income and predominantly black neighborhoods (Grier and Kumanyika, 2008; Larson et al., 2009; Powell et al., 2007a; see also Chapter 6). Accessing healthy food also requires more time, inconvenience, awareness, and motivation than accessing less healthy food, and food advertising may bias motivation and awareness in the opposite direction. Low-income and ethnic minority households are disproportionately exposed to promotions for high-calorie, low-nutrition foods and beverages through television, in-store, and outdoor advertising (Grier and Kumanyika, 2008; Henderson and Kelly, 2005; Tirodkar and Jain, 2003; Yancey et al., 2009). Exposure to television ads is generally higher in both low-income and minority communities because of more hours of television use (Powell et al., 2007b; Rideout et al., 2010).

While the committee does not believe that at this time there is enough evidence on the impact on obesity prevention of a particular program to incentivize or restrict purchases of certain foods and beverages with SNAP dollars, it believes that research on such programs should continue in order to inform any future SNAP reform. It believes further that potential SNAP reforms should take a broad view, for example, reconsidering the current restrictions on using SNAP benefits to purchase hot prepared foods in supermarkets. Should reform of SNAP be undertaken, researchers and policy makers must consider the political and practical feasibility, as well as the effectiveness and any unintended consequences, of particular strategies. Pilot programs that test incentives and restrictions may be an appropriate way to evaluate effects of changes in SNAP participants' food purchase patterns and overall dietary intakes, food retailing patterns within stores where SNAP benefits are redeemed, potential stigmatization of participants, and program participation levels. Furthermore, it will be necessary to predict whether the American food system will be able to meet the demand for incentivized foods.

Implementation

SNAP-Ed regulations explicitly prohibit offering advice to discourage consumption of any particular food or type of food, even though advice to reduce consumption of certain foods and beverages is fundamental to the 2010 Dietary Guidelines for Americans. The committee suggests a number of actions to implement its recommendation to update the policies of federal nutrition education programs to explicitly encourage the provision of advice about the types of foods to reduce in the diet, consistent with the Dietary Guidelines. These actions include disseminating, immediately and effectively, notification of the revised regulations, along with authoritative guidance on how to align federally funded nutrition education programs with the Dietary Guidelines, and ensuring that such alignment applies to all federal programs with a nutrition education component, particularly programs that target primary food shoppers in low-income families (e.g., EFNEP and WIC).

Successful implementation of this recommendation will be dependent on the effectiveness of implementation of other recommendations in this report. People cannot choose or favor foods that are out of reach, geographically or financially. The committee believes that approaches to increase access to healthy foods for SNAP recipients are critical, and such changes are recommended under Strategy 2-4 (Chapter 6), which is intended to attract healthy food retailing and distribution outlets into underserved areas and limit the concentration of unhealthy food venues. And Strategy 2-1 (also in Chapter 6) focuses on reducing overconsumption of sugar-sweetened beverages through a variety of actions, including a social marketing campaign and greater availability of healthier beverages that are affordably priced. As described in Appendix B, the committee expects that the synergy among recommendations in the system will enhance the effect of any individual recommendation.

Indicators for Assessing Progress in Obesity Prevention for Strategy 3-4

Process Indicators

- Increase in the proportion of states that adopt SNAP-Ed curricula that address the foods and beverages to increase (i.e., those recommended by the Dietary Guidelines for Americans*) and those to decrease (e.g., solid fats and added sugars).
  Sources for measuring indicator: State SNAP-Ed plans

- Increase in the proportion of foods and beverages purchased by SNAP participants that are recommended by the Dietary Guidelines for Americans.*
  Sources for measuring indicator: NHANES and HomeScan

Foundational Indicator

- USDA's revision of the SNAP regulations to remove any prohibitions on the types of messages that can be delivered and reinforce that the intent is to convey the full picture of advice reflected in the 2010* and subsequent Dietary Guidelines for Americans.
  Source for measuring indicator: USDA regulations

NOTE: NHANES = National Health and Nutrition Examination Survey; SNAP = Supplemental Nutrition Assistance Program; SNAP-Ed = Supplemental Nutrition Assistance Program Education; USDA = U.S. Department of Agriculture.

---

*See Box B-1 in Appendix B.

INTEGRATION OF STRATEGIES FOR ACCELERATING PROGRESS IN OBESITY PREVENTION

Just as many disparate elements make up the message environments that surround Americans, many different actors must be involved in transforming those environments to support and encourage healthier decision making about physical activity and nutrition. A large-scale, sustained social marketing campaign will need to enter the national consciousness through multiple media streams; industry will need to set high standards for the healthfulness of the foods and beverages it markets to children and adolescents; nutrition information will need to move front and center on product packaging and menus; and schools and government programs will need to greatly enhance nutrition education.

On their own, any one of these actions might help accelerate progress in obesity prevention, but together, their effect would be reinforced, amplified, and maximized. A social marketing campaign on its own, without a decrease in young people's exposure to food and beverage marketing, would be less effective. Likewise, a shift in food and beverage marketing would be more powerful when accompanied by a vigorous social marketing campaign. Changing front-of-package nutrition labels and adding calorie counts to menus would be more useful if accompanied by a social marketing campaign to raise awareness about how to interpret the new labels or about total daily calorie requirements. And changes in federal nutrition education messages would be more effective in reaching populations at high risk of overweight and obesity if food and beverage marketing practices reflected the same messages targeting the same populations. Such a combined approach can shift the overall tone of messaging environments to one that facilitates and encourages healthy living and helps individuals meet the Dietary Guidelines for Americans.

REFERENCES

Aaker, J., A. Brumbaugh, and S. Grier. 2000. Non-target markets and viewer distinctiveness: The impact of target marketing on advertising. *Journal of Consumer Psychology* 9(3):127-140.

ABA (American Beverage Association). 2011. *New calorie labels on front of beverages arrives in stores.* http://www.ameribev.org/news--media/news-releases--statements/more/235/ (accessed August 3, 2011).

Adams, E. J., L. Grummer-Strawn, and G. Chavez. 2003. Food insecurity is associated with increased risk of obesity in California women. *Journal of Nutrition* 133(4):1070-1074.

Alston, J. M., C. C. Mullally, D. A. Sumner, M. Townsend, and S. A. Vosti. 2009. Likely effects on obesity from proposed changes to the US food stamp program. *Food Policy* 34(2):176-184

Asbury, L. D., F. L. Wong, S. M. Price, and M. J. Nolin. 2008. The VERB campaign: Applying a branding strategy in public health. *American Journal of Preventive Medicine* 34(Suppl. 6):S183-S187.

Bachman, K. 2011. Industry group: Feds would muzzle advertising of popular foods. Lobby keeps pressure on government to change guidelines. *AdWeek*, August 4.

Banspach, S. W. 2008. The VERB campaign. *American Journal of Preventive Medicine* 34(Suppl. 6):S275.

Barnhill, A. 2011. Impact and ethics of excluding sweetened beverages from the SNAP program. *American Journal of Public Health* 101(11):2037-2043.

Basiotis, P. P., and M. Lino. 2003. Food insufficiency and prevalence of overweight among adult women. *Family Economics & Nutrition Review* 15(2):55-57.

Bauer, U., T. Johnson, J. Pallentino, R. Hopkins, W. McDaniel, and R. Brooks. 1999. Tobacco use among middle and high school students—Florida, 1998 and 1999. *Morbidity and Mortality Weekly Report* 48:248-253.

Bender, M. M., and B. M. Derby. 1992. Prevalence of reading nutrition and ingredient information on food labels among adult Americans: 1982-1988. *Journal of Nutrition Education* 24(6):292-297.

Berkowitz, J. M., M. Huhman, C. D. Heitzler, L. D. Potter, M. J. Nolin, and S. W. Banspach. 2008. Overview of formative, process, and outcome evaluation methods used in the VERB™ campaign. *American Journal of Preventive Medicine* 34(6):S222-S229.

Bernstein, S. 2011. Restaurants revamping menus in response to calorie count rules. *Los Angeles Times*, June 22, 2011.

Biglan, A., D. V. Ary, K. Smolkowski, T. Duncan, and C. Black. 2000. A randomised controlled trial of a community intervention to prevent adolescent tobacco use. *Tobacco Control* 9(1):24.

Blitstein, J. L., and W. D. Evans. 2006. Use of nutrition facts panels among adults who make household food purchasing decisions. *Journal of Nutrition Education and Behavior* 38(6):360-364.

Borgmeier, I., and J. Westenhoefer. 2009. Impact of different food label formats on healthiness evaluation and food choice of consumers: A randomized-controlled study. *BMC Public Health* 9:184.

Brownell, K. D., and J. P. Koplan. 2011. Front-of-package nutrition labeling— an abuse of trust by the food industry? *New England Journal of Medicine* 364(25):2373-2375.

Brownell, K. D., and D. S. Ludwig. 2011. The Supplemental Nutrition Assistance Program, soda, and USDA policy: who benefits? *Journal of the American Medical Association* 306(12):1370-1371.

CFBAI (Children's Food and Beverage Advertising Initiative). 2011. *Category-specific uniform nutrition criteria.* http://www.bbb.org/us/storage/16/documents/cfbai/CFBAI-Category-Specific-Uniform-Nutrition-Criteria.pdf (accessed August 9, 2011).

Chester, J., and K. Montgomery. 2007. *Interactive food and beverage marketing: Targeting children and youth in the digital age.* http://digitalads.org/ (accessed January 26, 2012).

Chester, J., and K. Montgomery. 2011. Recent trends in digital food marketing. Presented at the Presentation to the IOM Committee on Accelerating Progress in Obesity Prevention, January 13, Irvine, CA.

Cheyne, A., L. Dorfman, P. Gonzalez, and P. Mejia. 2011. *Food and beverage marketing to children and adolescents: An environment at odds with good health. A research synthesis.* Healthy Eating Research. Princeton, NJ: RWJF.

Cohen, B., J. Ohls, M. Andrews, M. Ponza, L. Moreno, A. Zambrowski, and R. Cohen. 1999. *Food stamp participants' food security and nutrient availability: Final report.* Princeton, NJ: Mathematica Policy Research.

Cohen, D. A. 2008. Neurophysiological pathways to obesity: Below awareness and beyond individual control. *Diabetes* 57(7):1768-1773.

Cole, N., and M. K. Fox. 2008. *Diet quality of Americans by food stamp participation status: Data from the National Health and Nutrition Examination Survey, 1999-2004.* Alexandria, VA: USDA/FNS.

Cook, J. 2011. Sugar-sweetened beverages in the Supplemental Nutrition Assistance Program (letter). *Journal of the American Medical Association* 306(24):2670.

DeNavas-Walt, C., D. Proctor, and J. Smith. 2010. *Income, poverty, and health insurance coverage in the United States: 2009.* Current Population Reports, P60-238. Washington, DC: U.S. Census Bureau.

Dorfman, L., and P. Gonzalez. 2011. *Media advocacy.* http://www.oxfordbibliographiesonline.com/view/document/obo-9780199756797/obo-9780199756797-0111.xml;jsessionid=B34DE260FA7B3788D5D0950881343316#obo-9780199756797-0111-div1-0002 (accessed December 29, 2011).

Dosenbach, N. U., B. Nardos, A. L. Cohen, D. A. Fair, J. D. Power, J. A. Church, S. M. Nelson, G. S. Wig, A. C. Vogel, C. N. Lessov-Schlaggar, K. A. Barnes, J. W. Dubis, E. Feczko, R. S. Coalson, J. R. Pruett, Jr., D. M. Barch, S. E. Petersen, and B. L. Schlaggar. 2010. Prediction of individual brain maturity using fMRI. *Science* 329(5997):1358-1361.

Drewnowski, A., and S. Specter. 2004. Poverty and obesity: The role of energy density and energy costs. *The American Journal of Clinical Nutrition* 79(1):6-16.

Elbel, B. 2011. Consumer estimation of recommended and actual calories at fast food restaurants. *Obesity (Silver Spring)* 19(10):1971-1978.

Evans, W. D., K. K. Christoffel, J. W. Necheles, and A. B. Becker. 2010. Social marketing as a childhood obesity prevention strategy. *Obesity (Silver Spring)* 18(Suppl. 1):S23-S26.

Farrelly, M. C., K. C. Davis, M. L. Haviland, P. Messeri, and C. G. Healton. 2005. Evidence of a dose-response relationship between "truth" antismoking ads and youth smoking prevalence. *American Journal of Public Health* 95(3):425.

FDA (U.S. Food and Drug Administration). 2008. *Health and diet survey: Dietary guidelines supplement. Report of findings (2004 & 2005).* http://www.fda.gov/food/scienceresearch/researchareas/consumerresearch/ucm080331.htm (accessed July 29, 2011).

FDA. 2009. *Guidance for industry: A food labeling guide.* http://www.fda.gov/Food/GuidanceComplianceRegulatoryInformation/GuidanceDocuments/FoodLabelingNutrition/FoodLabelingGuide/default.htm (accessed July 28, 2011).

FDA. 2011. *Food labeling; nutrition labeling of standard menu items in restaurants and similar retail food establishments; proposed rule.* http://edocket.access.gpo.gov/2011/2011-7940.htm (accessed August 3, 2011).

Feunekes, G. I., I. A. Gortemaker, A. A. Willems, R. Lion, and M. van den Kommer. 2008. Front-of-pack nutrition labelling: Testing effectiveness of different nutrition labelling formats front-of-pack in four European countries. *Appetite* 50(1):57-70.

Flegal, K. M., M. D. Carroll, C. L. Ogden, and L. R. Curtin. 2010. Prevalence and trends in obesity among U.S. adults, 1999-2008. *Journal of the American Medical Association* 303(3):235-241.

Flynn, B. S., J. K. Worden, R. H. Secker-Walker, P. L. Pirie, G. J. Badger, J. H. Carpenter, and B. M. Geller. 1994. Mass media and school interventions for cigarette smoking prevention: Effects 2 years after completion. *American Journal of Public Health* 84(7):1148.

Flynn, B. S., J. K. Worden, R. H. Secker-Walker, P. L. Pirie, G. J. Badger, and J. H. Carpenter. 1997. Long-term responses of higher and lower risk youths to smoking prevention interventions. *Preventive Medicine* 26(3):389-394.

Food Fit Philly. 2011. *Philly food bucks: Helping people who use access cards/food stamps to buy fresh produce.* http://foodfitphilly.org/eat-healthy/philly-food-bucks/ (accessed January 4, 2012).

FTC (Federal Trade Commission). 2008. *Marketing food to children and adolescents: A review of industry expenditures, activities, and self-regulation.* Washington, DC: FTC.

Gantz, W., N. Schwartz, J. R. Angelini, and V. Rideout. 2007. *Food for thought: Television food advertising to children in the United States.* Menlo Park, CA: Kaiser Family Foundation.

Gantz, W., N. Schwarts, J. R. Agngelini, and V. Rideout. 2008. *Shouting to be heard (2): Public service advertising in a changing television world.* Menlo Park, CA: Kaiser Family Foundation.

GAO (Government Accountability Office). 2006. *Public service announcements campaign: Activities and financial obligations for seven federal departments.* Washington, DC: U.S. Government Printing Office.

Gardner, A., S. Geierstanger, C. Brindis, and C. McConnel. 2010. Clinic consortia media advocacy capacity: Partnering with the media and increasing policymaker awareness. *Journal of Health Communication* 15(3):293-306.

GMA (Grocery Manufacturers Association). 2011a. *Facts up front.* http://www.factsupfront.org (accessed March 8, 2012).

GMA. 2011b. *Fact sheet on IWG food marketing restrictions.* http://www.gmaonline.org/file-manager/Health_Nutrition/IWGFactSheet.doc (accessed August 10, 2011).

Golan, E., F. Kuchler, and B. Krissof. 2007. Do food labels make a difference? . . . Sometimes. *Amber Waves* 5(5):10-17, http://www.ers.usda.gov/AmberWaves/November07/PDF/FoodLabels.pdf (accessed August 3, 2011).

Grier, S. A. 2009. *African American & Hispanic youth vulnerability to target marketing: Implications for understanding the effects of digital marketing.* Memo prepared for the Second NPLAN/BMSG Meeting on Digital Media and Marketing to Children. Berkeley, CA: NPLAN and Berkeley Media Studies Group.

Grier, S. A., and A. M. Brumbaugh. 1999. Noticing cultural differences: Ad meanings created by target and non-target markets. *Journal of Advertising* 18(1):79-93.

Grier, S. A., and C. A. Bryant. 2005. Social marketing in public health. *Annual Review of Public Health* 26:319-339.

Grier, S. A., and S. K. Kumanyika. 2008. The context for choice: Health implications of targeted food and beverage marketing to African Americans. *American Journal of Public Health* 98(9):1616-1629.

Grotto, D., and E. Zied. 2010. The standard American diet and its relationship to the health status of Americans. *Nutrition in Clinical Practice* 25(6):603-612.

Grunert, K. G., and J. M. Wills. 2007. A review of European research on consumer response to nutrition information on food labels. *Journal of Public Health* 15(5):385-399.

Guskin, E., T. Rosenstiel, and P. Moore. 2011. *Network: By the numbers.* Washington, DC: Pew Research Center.

Guthrie, J. F., J. J. Fox, L. E. Cleveland, and S. Welsh. 1995. Who uses nutrition labeling, and what effects does label use have on diet quality. *Journal of Nutrition Education* 27(4):163-172.

Harris, J. L., J. L. Pomeranz, T. Lobstein, and K. D. Brownell. 2009. A crisis in the marketplace: How food marketing contributes to childhood obesity and what can be done. *Annual Review of Public Health* 30:211-225.

Harris, J. L., M. E. Weinberg, M. B. Schwartz, C. Ross, J. Ostroffa, and K. D. Brownell. 2010. *Trends in television food advertising: Progress in reducing unhealthy marketing to young people?* New Haven, CT: Rudd Center for Food Policy and Obesity.

Harris, J. L., M. B. Schwartz, K. B. Brownell, J. Javadizadeh, M. Weinberg, V. Sarda, C. Munsell, C. Shin, F. F. Milici, A. Ustjanauskas, R. Gross, S. Speers, A. Cheyne, L. Dorfman, P. Gonzalez, and P. Mejia. 2011. *Sugary drinks FACTS: Evaluation sugary drink nutrition and marketing to youth.* New Haven, CT: Yale Rudd Center for Food Policy and Obesity.

Harrison, K., and A. L. Marske. 2005. Nutritional content of foods advertised during the television programs children watch most. *American Journal of Public Health* 95(9):1568-1574.

Hartline-Grafton, H., E. Vollinger, and J. Weill. 2011. *A review of strategies to bolster SNAP's role in improving nutrition as well as food security.* Washington, DC: Food Research and Action Center.

Henderson, V. R., and B. Kelly. 2005. Food advertising in the age of obesity: Content analysis of food advertising on general market and African American television. *Journal of Nutrition Education and Behavior* 37(4):191-196.

Higginson, C., T. R. Kirk, M. Rayner, and S. Draper. 2002. How do consumers use nutrition label information? *Nutrition and Food Science* 32(4):145-152.

Hoyer, W. D. 1984. An examination of consumer decision making for a common repeat purchase product. *Journal of Consumer Research* 11:822-829.

Huhman, M., L. D. Potter, F. L. Wong, S. W. Banspach, J. C. Duke, and C. D. Heitzler. 2005. Effects of a mass media campaign to increase physical activity among children: Year-1 results of the VERB campaign. *Pediatrics* 116(2):e277-e284.

Huhman, M., J. M. Berkowitz, F. L. Wong, E. Prosper, M. Gray, D. Prince, and J. Yuen. 2008. The VERB™ campaign's strategy for reaching African-American, Hispanic, Asian, and American Indian children and parents. *American Journal of Preventive Medicine* 34(6):S194-S209.

Huhman, M. E., L. D. Potter, M. J. Nolin, A. Piesse, D. R. Judkins, S. W. Banspach, and F. L. Wong. 2010. The influence of the VERB™ campaign on children's physical activity in 2002 to 2006. *American Journal of Public Health* 100(4):638-645.

Interagency Working Group on Food Marketed to Children. 2011. *Interagency Working Group on Food Marketed to Children preliminary proposed nutrition principles to guide industry self-regulatory efforts: Request for comments.* http://ftc.gov/os/2011/04/110428foodmarketproposedguide.pdf (accessed January 26, 2012).

IOM (Institute of Medicine). 2002. *The future of the public's health in the 21st century.* Washington, DC: National Academy Press.

IOM. 2005. *Preventing childhood obesity: Health in the balance*, edited by J. P. Koplan, C. T. Liverman, and V. A. Kraak. Washington, DC: The National Academies Press.

IOM. 2006. *Food marketing to children and youth: Threat or opportunity?*, edited by J. M. McGinnis, J. Gootman, and V. I. Kraak. Washington, DC: The National Academies Press.

IOM. 2009. *Local government actions to prevent childhood obesity*, edited by L. Parker, A. C. Burns, and E. Sanchez. Washington, DC: The National Academies Press.

IOM. 2010. *Front-of-package nutrition rating systems and symbols. Phase I report.* Washington, DC: The National Academies Press.

IOM. 2011a. *Examination of front-of-package nutrition rating systems and symbols: Promoting healthier choices.* Washington, DC: The National Academies Press.

IOM. 2011b. *Hunger and obesity: Understanding a food insecurity paradigm: Workshop summary.* Washington, DC: The National Academies Press.

Jensen, H. H. 2002. Food insecurity and the food stamp program. *American Journal of Agricultural Economics* 84(5):1215-1228.

Jilcott, S. B., E. D. Wall-Bassett, S. C. Burke, and J. B. Moore. 2011. Associations between food insecurity, Supplemental Nutrition Assistance Program (SNAP) benefits, and body mass index among adult females. *Journal of the American Dietetic Association* 111(11):1741-1745.

Kelly, B., C. Hughes, K. Chapman, J. C. Louie, H. Dixon, J. Crawford, L. King, M. Daube, and T. Slevin. 2009. Consumer testing of the acceptability and effectiveness of front-of-pack food labelling systems for the Australian grocery market. *Health Promotion International* 24(2):120-129.

Keystone Forum. 2006. *The Keystone Forum on away-from home foods: Opportunities for preventing weight gain and obesity.* Washington, DC: The Keystone Center.

Kim, S. Y., R. M. Nayga, and O. Capps. 2001. Food label use, self-selectivity, and diet quality. *Journal of Consumer Affairs* 35(2):346-363.

Kolish, E. 2011. The children's food and beverage advertising initiative: Meeting IOM's recommendations. Presented at the Presentation to the Committee on Accelerating Progress in Obesity Prevention, January 13, Irvine, CA.

Kraak, V. I., M. Story, E. A. Wartella, and J. Ginter. 2011. Industry progress to market a healthful diet to American children and adolescents. *American Journal of Preventive Medicine* 41(3):322-333.

Kunkel, D., C. McKinley, and P. Wright. 2009. *The impact of industry self-regulation on the nutritional quality of foods advertised on television to children.* Oakland, CA: ChildrenNow.

Larson, N. I., M. T. Story, and M. C. Nelson. 2009. Neighborhood environments: Disparities in access to healthy foods in the US. *American Journal of Preventive Medicine* 36(1):74-81.

Larsson, I., L. Lissner, and L. Wilhelmsen. 1999. The "Green Keyhole" revisited: Nutritional knowledge may influence food selection. *European Journal of Clinical Nutrition* 53(10):776-780.

Lawrence, R. G. 2004. Framing obesity. The evolution of news discourse on a public health issue. *Press/Politics* 9(3):56-75.

Layton, L., and D. Eggen. 2011. Industries lobby against voluntary nutrition guidelines for food marketed to kids. *The Washington Post*, July 9.

Lee, V., L. Mikkelsen, J. Srikantharajah, and L. Cohen. 2008. *Strategies for enhancing the built environment to support healthy eating and active living environments.* Oakland, CA: Prevention Institute, Healthy Eating Active Living Convergence Partnership, and PolicyLink.

Leftin, J., A. Gothro, and E. Eslami. 2010. *Characteristics of Supplemental Nutrition Assistance Program households: Fiscal year 2009.* Alexandria, VA: USDA/FNS.

Lin, C. T., J. Y. Lee, and S. T. Yen. 2004. Do dietary intakes affect search for nutrient information on food labels? *Social Science and Medicine* 59(9):1955-1967.

Lobstein, T., and S. Davies. 2009. Defining and labelling "healthy" and "unhealthy" food. *Public Health Nutrition* 12(3):331-340.

Louie, J. C., V. Flood, A. Rangan, D. J. Hector, and T. Gill. 2008. A comparison of two nutrition signposting systems for use in Australia. *N S W Public Health Bull* 19(7-8):121-126.

Luna, B. 2009. The maturation of cognitive control and the adolescent brain. In *From attention to goal directed behavior: Neurodynamical, methodological, clinical trends*, edited by F. Aboitiz and D. Cosmelli. Berlin, Germany: Springer. Pp. 249-274.

McDonald's. 2011. *McDonald's announces commitments to offer improved nutrition choices.* http://www.aboutmcdonalds.com/mcd/media_center/recent_news/corporate/commitments_to_offer_improved_nutrition_choices.html (accessed August 10, 2011).

Monsivais, P., A. Aggarwal, and A. Drewnowski. 2010. Are socio-economic disparities in diet quality explained by diet cost? *Journal of Epidemiology and Community Health*. E-pub.

Moore, E. S., and V. J. Rideout. 2007. The online marketing of food to children: Is it just fun and games? *Journal of Public Policy & Marketing* 26(2):202-220.

Morestin, F., M. Hague, M. Jacques, and F. Benoit. 2011. *Public policies on nutrition and labeling: Effects and implementation issues.* Quebec, Canada: National Collaborating Center for Healthy Public Policy (Public Health Agency of Canada).

Morrison, R. M., L. Mancino, and J. N. Vairyam. 2011. Will calorie labeling in restaurants make a difference? *Amber Waves* 9(1):10-17.

National Food Administration. 2011. *The Keyhole symbol.* http://www.slv.se/en-gb/Group1/Food-and-Nutrition/Keyhole-symbol/ (accessed August 1, 2011).

Nayga, R. M. 2000. Nutrition knowledge, gender, and food label use. *Journal of Consumer Affairs* 34(1):97-112.

Neuhouser, M. L., A. R. Kristal, and R. E. Patterson. 1999. Use of food nutrition labels is associated with lower fat intake. *Journal of the American Dietetic Association* 99(1):45-53.

New York City Department of Health and Mental Hygiene. 2010. *Farmers' markets initiatives: Promoting fresh fruits and vegetables in underserved communities.* http://www.nyc.gov/html/doh/downloads/pdf/cdp/cdp-farmers-market-report.pdf (accessed January 4, 2012).

NHS. 2011. *Food labels.* http://www.nhs.uk/Livewell/Goodfood/Pages/food-labelling.aspx (accessed September 2, 2011).

NRA (National Restaurant Association). 2011. *Kids Live Well: About.* http://www.restaurant.org/foodhealthyliving/kidslivewell/about/ (accessed August 10, 2011).

Ogden, C. L., M. M. Lamb, M. D. Carroll, and K. M. Flegal. 2010a. Obesity and socio-economic status in adults: United States, 2005-2008. *NCHS Data Brief* (50):1-8.

Ogden, C. L., M. M. Lamb, M. D. Carroll, and K. M. Flegal. 2010b. Obesity and socioeconomic status in children and adolescents: United States, 2005-2008. *NCHS Data Brief* (51):1-8.

Ollberding, N. J., R. L. Wolf, and I. Contento. 2010. Food label use and its relation to dietary intake among US adults. *Journal of the American Dietetic Association* 110(8):1233-1237.

Olson, C. M. 1999. Nutrition and health outcomes associated with food insecurity and hunger. *Journal of Nutrition* 129(2):521.

Pechmann, C., L. Levine, S. Loughlin, and F. Leslie. 2005. Impulsive and self-conscious: adolescents' vulnerability to advertising and promotion. *Journal of Public Policy and Marketing* 24(2):202-221.

Peeler, C. L., E. Kolish, M. Enright, and C. Burke. 2010. *The Children's Food and Beverage Advertising Initiative in action. A report on compliance and implementation during 2009.* Washington, DC: Council of Better Business Bureaus.

Pew Research Center for the People and the Press. 2010. *Ideological news sources: Who watches and why. Americans spending more time following the news.* Washington, DC: Pew Research Center for the People and the Press.

Powell, L. M., S. Slater, D. Mirtcheva, Y. Bao, and F. J. Chaloupka. 2007a. Food store availability and neighborhood characteristics in the United States. *Preventive Medicine* 44(3):189-195.

Powell, L. M., G. Szczypka, and F. J. Chaloupka. 2007b. Adolescent exposure to food advertising on television. *American Journal of Preventive Medicine* 33(Suppl. 4):S251-S256.

Powell, L. M., R. M. Schermbeck, G. Szczypka, F. J. Chaloupka, and C. L. Braunschweig. 2011. Trends in the nutritional content of television food advertisements seen by children in the United States: Analyses by age, food categories, and companies. *Archives of Pediatrics and Adolescent Medicine* 165(12):1078-1086.

Randolph, W., and K. Viswanath. 2004. Lessons learned from public health mass media campaigns: Marketing health in a crowded media world. *Annual Review of Public Health* 25:419-437.

Rank, M. R., and T. A. Hirschl. 2003. *Estimating the probabilities and patterns of food stamp use across the life course.* Chicago, IL: Joint Center for Poverty Research, University of Chicago and Northwestern University.

Rideout, V., U. G. Foehr, and D. F. Roberts. 2010. *Generation M2: Media in the lives of 8-18 year-olds.* Washington, DC: Kaiser Family Foundation.

Rideout, V., A. Lauricella, and E. Wartella. 2011. *Children, media, and race: Media use among white, black, Hispanic, and Asian American children.* Evanston, IL: Center on Media and Human Development, Northwestern University.

Roberto, C. A., P. D. Larsen, H. Agnew, J. Baik, and K. D. Brownell. 2010. Evaluating the impact of menu labeling on food choices and intake. *American Journal of Public Health* 100(2):312.

Rogers, K. 2011. Accelerating progress in obesity prevention. Presented at the Farm and Food Policy: Relationship to Obesity Prevention, May 19, 2011, Washington, DC.

RWJF (Robert Wood Johnson Foundation). 2009. *Action strategies toolkit: A guide for local and state leaders working to create healthy communities and prevent childhood obesity.* Princeton, NJ: RWJF.

Sacks, G., J. L. Veerman, M. Moodie, and B. Swinburn. 2011. "Traffic-light" nutrition labelling and "junk-food" tax: A modelled comparison of cost-effectiveness for obesity prevention. *International Journal of Obesity* 35:1001-1009.

Satia, J. A., J. A. Galanko, and M. L. Neuhouser. 2005. Food nutrition label use is associated with demographic, behavioral, and psychosocial factors and dietary intake among African Americans in North Carolina. *Journal of the American Dietetic Association* 105(3):392-402; discussion 402-403.

Scott, V., and A. F. Worsley. 1997. Consumer views on nutrition labels in New Zealand. *Australian Journal of Nutrition and Dietetics* 54:6-13.

Shenkin, J. D., and M. F. Jacobson. 2010. Using the food stamp program and other methods to promote healthy diets for low-income consumers. *American Journal of Public Health* 100(9):1562-1564.

Stead, M., G. Hastings, and L. McDermott. 2007. The meaning, effectiveness and future of social marketing. *Obesity Reviews* 8(Suppl. 1):189-193.

Steinberg, L. 2010. A dual systems model of adolescent risk-taking. *Developmental Psychobiology* 52(3):216-224.

Sutherland, L. A., L. A. Kaley, and L. Fischer. 2010. Guiding stars: the effect of a nutrition navigation program on consumer purchases at the supermarket. *American Journal of Clinical Nutrition* 91(4):1090S-1094S.

The Food Project. 2011. *Boston bounty bucks.* http://thefoodproject.org/bountybucks (accessed January 4, 2012).

Tirodkar, M. A., and A. Jain. 2003. Food messages on African American television shows. *American Journal of Public Health* 93(3):439-441.

Townsend, M. S., J. Peerson, B. Love, C. Achterberg, and S. P. Murphy. 2001. Food insecurity is positively related to overweight in women. *Journal of Nutrition* 131(6):1738-1745.

USDA (U.S. Department of Agriculture). 2007. *Implications of restricting the use of food stamp benefits: Summary*. Washington, DC: USDA.

USDA. 2011a. *Letter from Jessica Shahin, Associate Administrator, Supplemental Nutrition Assistance Program, USDA, to Elizabeth Berlin, Executive Deputy Commissioner, New York State Office of Temporary and Disability Assistance. August 19, 2011*. http://www.foodpolitics.com/wp-content/uploads/SNAP-Waiver-Request-Decision.pdf (accessed December 28, 2011).

USDA. 2011b. *SNAP-Ed plan guidance: FY2012*. http://www.nal.usda.gov/fsn/Guidance/FY2012SNAP-EdGuidance.pdf (accessed July 6, 2011).

USDA. 2011c. *Supplemental Nutrition Assistance Program: Eligible food items*. http://www.fns.usda.gov/snap/retailers/eligible.htm (accessed December 7, 2011).

USDA. 2011d. *Supplemental Nutrition Assistance Program participation and costs*. http://www.fns.usda.gov/pd/SNAPsummary.htm (accessed October 31, 2011).

USDA/FNS (Food and Nutrition Service). 2011a. *Benefit redemption patterns in the Supplemental Nutrition Assistance Program*, edited by L. Castner, and J. Henke. Alexandria, VA: USDA/FNS.

USDA/FNS. 2011b. *SNAP community partner outreach toolkit*. http://www.fns.usda.gov/snap/outreach/pdfs/toolkit/2011/Community/Basics/basics.pdf (accessed December 27, 2011).

Ver Ploeg, M., and K. Ralston. 2008. *Food stamps and obesity: What we know and what it means*. Economic information bulletin no. 34. Washington, DC: Economic Research Service.

Ver Ploeg, M., L. Mancino, and B. Lin. 2007. *Food and nutrition assistance programs and obesity: 1976-2002*. Economic Research Report Number 48. Washington, DC: U.S. Department of Agriculture, Economic Research Service.

Wakefield, M., B. Flay, M. Nichter, and G. Giovino. 2003. Role of the media in influencing trajectories of youth smoking. *Addiction* 98:79-103.

Wakefield, M. A., B. Loken, and R. C. Hornik. 2010. Use of mass media campaigns to change health behaviour. *The Lancet* 376(9748):1261-1271.

Wallack, L., and L. Dorfman. 1996. Media advocacy: A strategy for advancing policy and promoting health. *Health Education Quarterly* 23(3):293-317.

Wallack, L., and L. Dorfman. 2000. Putting policy into health communication: The role of media advocacy. In *Public communication campaigns*, 3rd ed., edited by R. Rice and C. Atkin. Thousand Oaks, CA: Sage. Pp. 389-401.

Wallack, L., L. Dorfman, D. Jernigan, and M. Themba. 1993. *Media advocacy and public health: Power for prevention.* Thousand Oaks, CA: Sage.

Walmart. 2011. *Walmart launches major initiative to make food healthier and healthier food more affordable.* http://walmartstores.com/pressroom/news/10514.aspx (accessed August 3, 2011).

Watkins, C. 2008. North American vegetable oil use in flux. *Inform* 19(7):493.

White House Task Force on Childhood Obesity. 2010. *Solving the problem of childhood obesity within a generation: White House Task Force on Childhood Obesity report to the President.* Washington, DC: Executive Office of the President of the United States.

Wilde, P., and M. Nord. 2005. The effect of food stamps on food security: A panel data approach. *Applied Economic Perspectives and Policy* 27(3):425.

Wong, F., M. Huhman, L. Asbury, R. Bretthauer-Mueller, S. McCarthy, P. Londe, and C. Heitzler. 2004. VERB™—a social marketing campaign to increase physical activity among youth. *Preventing Chronic Disease* 1(3).

Woodruff, K., L. Dorfman, V. Berends, and P. Agron. 2003. Coverage of childhood nutrition policies in California newspapers. *Journal of Public Health Policy* 24(2):150-158.

Wootan, M. G. 2011. *Putting nutrition into nutrition standards for marketing to kids: How marketed foods measure up to the interagency working group's proposed nutrition principles for food marketed to children.* Washington, DC: Center for Science in the Public Interest.

Yancey, A. K., B. L. Cole, R. Brown, J. D. Williams, A. Hillier, R. S. Kline, M. Ashe, S. A. Grier, D. Backman, and W. J. McCarthy. 2009. A cross-sectional prevalance study of ethnically targeted and general audience outdoor obesity-related advertising. *Milbank Quarterly* 87(1):155-184.

Zimmerman, R. S., P. M. Palmgreen, S. M. Noar, M. L. A. Lustria, H. Y. Lu, and M. Lee Horosewski. 2007. Effects of a televised two-city safer sex mass media campaign targeting high-sensation-seeking and impulsive-decision-making young adults. *Health Education and Behavior* 34(5):810.

8

Health Care and Work Environments

Health Care and Work Environments:
Goal, Recommendation, Strategies, and Actions for
Implementation

Goal: Expand the role of health care providers, insurers,
and employers in obesity prevention.

Recommendation 4: Health care and health service providers, employers, and insurers should increase the support structure for achieving better population health and obesity prevention.

Strategy 4-1: Provide standardized care and advocate for healthy community environments. All health care providers should adopt standards of practice (evidence-based or consensus guidelines) for prevention, screening, diagnosis, and treatment of overweight and obesity to help children, adolescents, and adults achieve and maintain a healthy weight, avoid obesity-related complications, and reduce the psychosocial consequences of obesity. Health care providers also should advocate, on behalf of their patients, for improved physical activity and diet opportunities in their patients' communities.

Potential actions include

- health care providers' standards of practice including routine screening of body mass index (BMI), counseling, and behavioral interventions for children, adolescents, and adults to improve physical activity behaviors and dietary choices;

- medical schools, nursing schools, physician assistant schools, and other relevant health professional training programs (including continuing education programs), including instruction in prevention, screening, diagnosis, and treatment of overweight and obesity in children, adolescents, and adults; and

- health care providers serving as role models for their patients and providing leadership for obesity prevention efforts in their communities by advocating for institutional (e.g., child care, school, and worksite), community, and state-level strategies that can improve physical activity and nutrition resources for their patients and their communities.

Strategy 4-2: Ensure coverage of, access to, and incentives for routine obesity prevention, screening, diagnosis, and treatment. Insurers (both public and private) should ensure that health insurance coverage and access provisions address obesity prevention, screening, diagnosis, and treatment.

Potential actions include

- insurers, including self-insured organizations and employers, considering the inclusion of incentives in individual and family health plans for maintaining healthy lifestyles;

- insurers considering (1) benefit designs and programs that promote obesity screening and prevention and (2) innovative approaches to reimbursing for routine screening and obesity prevention services (including preconception counseling) in clinical practice and for monitoring the performance of these services in relation to obesity prevention; and

- insurers taking full advantage of obesity-related provisions in health care reform legislation.

Strategy 4-3: Encourage active living and healthy eating at work.
Worksites should create, or expand, healthy environments by establishing, implementing, and monitoring policy initiatives that support wellness.

Potential actions include

- public and private employers promoting healthy eating and active living in the worksite in their own institutional policies and practices by, for example, increasing opportunities for physical activity as part of a wellness/health promotion program, providing access to and promotion of healthful foods and beverages, and offering health benefits that provide employees and their dependents coverage for obesity-related services and programs; and

- health care organizations and providers serving as models for the incorporation of healthy eating and active living into worksite practices and programs.

Strategy 4-4: Encourage healthy weight gain during pregnancy and breastfeeding, and promote breastfeeding-friendly environments. Health service providers and employers should adopt, implement, and monitor policies that support healthy weight gain during pregnancy and the initiation and continuation of breastfeeding. Population disparities in breastfeeding should be specifically addressed at the federal, state, and local levels to remove barriers and promote targeted increases in breastfeeding initiation and continuation.

Potential actions include

- all those who provide health care or related services to women of childbearing age offering preconception counseling on the importance of conceiving at a healthy BMI;

- medical facilities, prenatal services, and community clinics adopting policies consistent with the Baby-Friendly Hospital Initiative;

- local health departments and community-based organizations, working with other segments of the health sector, providing information on breastfeeding and the availability of related classes to pregnant women and new mothers, connecting pregnant women and new mothers with breastfeeding support programs to help them make informed infant feeding decisions, and developing peer support programs that empower pregnant women and mothers to obtain the help and support they need from other mothers who have breastfed;

- workplaces instituting policies to support breastfeeding mothers, including ensuring both private space and adequate break time; and

- the federal government using Prevention Fund dollars to support implementation of the Baby-Friendly Hospital Initiative nationwide, and providing funding to support community-level collaborative efforts and peer counseling with the aim of increasing the duration of breastfeeding.

Millions of individuals have the opportunity to be influenced by health care and work environments daily:

- More than 140 million American civilians were employed as of November 2011 (Bureau of Labor Statistics, 2011).
- In 2008, it was estimated that there were more than 6.2 million professionals in health care occupations (including physicians, registered dietitians, nurses, and counselors) in the United States. The field is projected to increase by 22 percent by 2018 (Bureau of Labor Statistics, 2010).
- As of June 2011, among Americans under age 65, nearly 23 percent were covered by a public health insurance plan, and 61 percent had private health insurance coverage (Martinez and Cohen, 2011).
- For 2011, the total number of Medicare beneficiaries in the United States was 48 million (KFF, 2011).

It is clear that health systems, health care providers, employers, and insurers are in a position to influence the health of the population. By engaging in obesity prevention and treatment strategies, such as providing community-level resources (education, support, and opportunities) for individuals and their families, health care and work environments can help catalyze individual and, ultimately, population health improvement. For example, as seen with smoking, another public health concern, cessation initiatives by insurance and health care providers that supported and encouraged policy holders and patients to quit, as well as workplace interventions that included counseling or support, had a noticeable effect on quitting rates (Cahill et al., 2008; CDC, 2011c).

As health care continues to evolve and as new forms of health systems emerge (such as patient-centered medical homes, accountable care organizations, and other new systems of care), attention to obesity prevention, screening, diagnosis, and treatment must be considered.[1]

RECOMMENDATION 4

Health care and health service providers, employers, and insurers should increase the support structure for achieving better population health and obesity prevention.

As depicted in Figure 8-1, health care and work environments are interconnected with the other four areas of focus addressed in this report and are a necessary component of the committee's comprehensive approach to accelerating progress in obesity prevention.

The committee's recommendations for strategies and actions to expand the role of health care and health service providers, employers, and insurers in obesity prevention are detailed in the remainder of this chapter. Indicators for measuring progress toward the implementation of each strategy, organized according to the scheme presented in Chapter 3 (primary, process, foundational) are presented in a box following the discussion of that strategy.

STRATEGIES AND ACTIONS FOR IMPLEMENTATION

Strategy 4-1: Provide Standardized Care and Advocate for Healthy Community Environments

All health care providers should adopt standards of practice (evidence-based or consensus guidelines) for prevention, screening, diagnosis, and treatment of overweight and obesity to help children, adolescents, and adults achieve and maintain a healthy weight, avoid obesity-related complications, and reduce the

---

[1]Attention to overweight prevention, screening, diagnosis, and treatment is implicit within obesity prevention and treatment efforts.

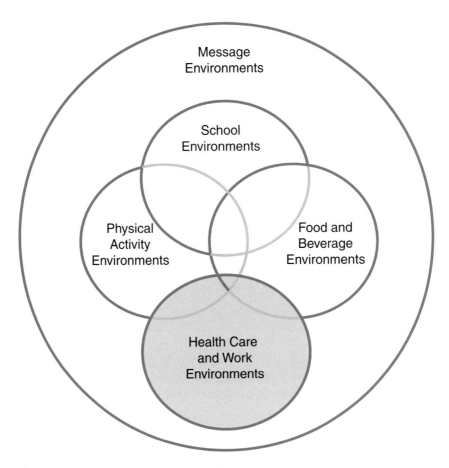

FIGURE 8-1 Five areas of focus of the Committee on Accelerating Progress in Obesity Prevention.
NOTE: The area addressed in this chapter is highlighted.

psychosocial consequences of obesity. Health care providers also should advocate, on behalf of their patients, for improved physical activity and diet opportunities in their patients' communities.

Potential actions include

- health care providers' standards of practice including routine screening of body mass index (BMI), counseling, and behavioral interventions for children, adolescents, and adults to improve physical activity behaviors and dietary choices;

- medical schools, nursing schools, physician assistant schools, and other relevant health professional training programs (including continuing education programs), including instruction in prevention, screening, diagnosis, and treatment of overweight and obesity in children, adolescents, and adults; and
- health care providers serving as role models for their patients and providing leadership for obesity prevention efforts in their communities by advocating for institutional (e.g., child care, school, and worksite), community, and state-level strategies that can improve physical activity and nutrition resources for their patients and their communities.

Context

Health care and health service providers have frequent opportunities to engage in screening for disease risk factors and to encourage their patients to engage in healthful lifestyles. The current health care system has an opportunity to incorporate obesity and lifestyle screening and prevention into routine practice as it has done with colon cancer, breast cancer, cervical cancer, and cardiovascular disease, for example. Health care professionals, both individually and through their professional organizations, can work to make obesity prevention part of routine preventive care.

To maximize the value of patient visits and help children, adolescents, and adults achieve and maintain a healthful lifestyle, health care providers should adopt standards of practice for the prevention, screening, diagnosis, and treatment of obesity that include screening of BMI, counseling, and behavioral interventions aimed at improving the physical activity and dietary behaviors of their patients.

Standards of practice, or clinical practice guidelines, are statements that include recommendations intended to optimize patient care that are informed by a systematic review of evidence and an assessment of the benefits and harms of alternative care options (IOM, 2011a). Such guidelines offer an evaluation of the quality of the relevant scientific literature and an assessment of the likely benefits and harms of particular interventions or treatments (IOM, 2011a). This information enables health care providers to proceed accordingly, selecting the best care for an individual patient based on his or her preferences. Health care providers have the opportunity to see children and adolescents, in particular, at regular and frequent intervals for well and acute care, and they are in a unique position to promote childhood obesity prevention in several ways.

Evidence

In 2000, the Centers for Disease Control and Prevention (CDC) recommended the use of age- and sex-adjusted BMI to screen for overweight children 2-19 years of age and developed revised standardized growth charts (Kuczmarski et al., 2002). In 2003, the American Academy of Pediatrics (AAP) recommended that health care providers calculate and plot BMI percentiles on a yearly basis for children and adolescents (Krebs and Jacobson, 2003). More recently, the Institute of Medicine (IOM) committee that produced the report *Early Childhood Obesity Prevention Policies* recommended that health care professionals consider a child's BMI, rate of weight gain, and parental weight as risk factors for obesity (IOM, 2011b).

If health care providers monitor the rate of weight gain using BMI, they are more likely to identify children who are at risk for overweight or obesity earlier than if they use traditional methods for plotting weight for age (Sesselberg et al., 2010; Wethington et al., 2011). Yet even though most health care providers report being familiar with BMI screening guidelines and have the tools to calculate patient BMIs, few providers report actually using BMI to assess overweight or obesity (Barlow et al., 2002; Hillman et al., 2009; Larsen et al., 2006; Wethington et al., 2011). Indeed, many health care providers are not properly diagnosing obesity (Dennison et al., 2009; Hamilton et al., 2003; Perrin et al., 2010). Some providers report not having enough time during patient visits for overweight screening (Boyle et al., 2009; Hopkins et al., 2011), and others report lack of reimbursement and inadequate resources (i.e., staff and/or access to nutrition specialists) as barriers to BMI screening, obesity diagnosis, and counseling on weight/health status (Barlow et al., 2002; Hopkins et al., 2011; Tsai et al., 2006). Clinicians who document overweight in the patient medical record are more likely to screen for BMI, provide counseling, and make referrals to specialists (Sesselberg et al., 2010; Wethington et al., 2011).

The United States is currently undergoing a transition to more universal and higher utilization of electronic health records (EHRs). This transition is the result of a recent government effort (through the Health Information Technology for Economic and Clinical Health [HITECH] Act) to support the adoption and "meaningful use" (meaning use intended to improve health and health care) of EHRs and health information technology (Blumenthal, 2011). Accelerated adoption of EHRs might facilitate the adoption of standards of practice that include BMI screening, assessment, and tracking, and would allow for the capture of quality improvement efforts and measures. Use of EHRs has been shown to significantly increase BMI assessment and documentation and treatment of obese adults among family physicians (Sesselberg et al., 2010).

Use of EHRs would allow BMI and BMI percentiles (which are important measures, particularly for children and pregnant women, because ideal weights vary by age) to be calculated automatically when patient vital signs are obtained. In addition, EHRs can incorporate decision-support tools that could provide prompts for brief motivational interviews, links to food and activity resources, or facilitated referrals to specialists. If EHR vendors included data fields to capture pediatric and adult BMI, document nutrition and activity counseling, and identify resources on healthy lifestyles for physicians and patients, they would facilitate the delivery of individual care, as well as allow for better population health management at the practice level and surveillance and monitoring of public health data at the community, local government, and state levels. Practice-level data could be fed into health information exchanges (HIEs), a system of aggregated health care information available electronically across organizations within a community, region, or hospital system. HIEs would allow for community-based, as well as clinically based, interventions by allowing public health and medical care providers to fully utilize decision support and resources.

Including BMI screening as part of routine visits would give health care providers a platform through which they could engage patients (and their families) on the health benefits of a healthy weight and lifestyle and the health consequences of overweight and obesity (including elevating parental concern about childhood obesity if a patient was at risk) (IOM, 2005). In addition to monitoring and tracking of BMI, other predictors of risk for obesity should be added to risk assessment, including birth weight and parental BMI (for pediatric patients) and maternal gestational weight gain, gestational diabetes, and smoking status (for adult patients) (Flegal et al., 1995; IOM, 2009b; Whitaker et al., 1997). If health care providers addressed risks for overweight and obesity, families would receive the full benefit of counseling and early intervention.

Although it is recommended that clinicians offer counseling and behavioral support to obese patients, however, studies have found that many health care providers do not feel prepared, competent, or comfortable in discussing weight with their patients and lack reliable models of treatment to guide their efforts (Appel et al., 2011; Hopkins et al., 2011). Few report offering specific guidance on physical activity, diet, or weight control, even though clinical preventive visits that include obesity-related discussions have been shown to increase levels of physical activity among sedentary patients (Calfas et al., 1996; Sesselberg et al., 2010; Smith et al.,

2011). Moreover, disparities are seen in which patients actually receive screening and counseling. A recent study of more than 9,000 adolescents, for example, found that overweight teens are receiving less screening and fewer preventive measures than normal-weight and obese patients during routine checkups (Jasik et al., 2011). This finding calls for accelerating educational and quality improvement efforts aimed at incorporating obesity care into practice.

In addition to BMI screening, the use of physical activity as a vital sign is considered a promising way to increase the frequency with which health care providers counsel patients about physical activity. It has been found to be a valid clinical screening tool (Greenwood et al., 2010), although more evidence is needed to determine whether it correlates with improved BMI and/or health status. To measure physical activity as a vital sign, health care providers could ask adult patients simple questions about days per week of physical activity and the intensity of that activity. Parents and their children also could be asked questions about how much time they spend in physical activity or physical education in school and how much time they spend outdoors. Because responses to such questions about typical behavior have been found to be highly correlated with BMI (Greenwood et al., 2010), they would provide an opportunity for health care providers to discuss physical activity with their patients.

Many health care providers are already focused on helping patients adopt healthy lifestyle behaviors, but a significant gap remains between current practice and universal and consistent lifestyle counseling (Huang et al., 2011). Increased education for health care providers, both during initial schooling/training and as part of continuing education, on how to incorporate BMI screening (measuring and assessment) and effective counseling and behavioral interventions into patient visits could lead to broader use of these practices (Klein et al., 2010). For example, training focused on human nutrition would allow a health care provider to counsel effectively on nutrition, while training in behavior change counseling could help a health care provider motivate a patient to make lifestyle changes. In fact, a recent study found that physician participation in a learning collaborative increased the number of primary care practices that provided anticipatory guidance on obesity prevention and that identified and treated overweight or obese children (Young et al., 2010).

By maintaining a healthy weight and lifestyle of their own, health care providers also have an opportunity to influence their patients. Studies suggest that providers' own weight, eating habits, and physical activity levels may influence how they approach these subjects with their patients (Hopkins et al., 2011).

Studies also have shown that physicians who engage in physical activity are more likely to counsel patients on the benefits of exercise (Abramson et al., 2000). Confidence scores from patients receiving health counseling from obese physicians are consistently lower than those from patients seeing normal-weight physicians (Hash et al., 2003).

Outside of their offices, health care providers can use their influence and authority to inform policy at the local, state, and national levels by advocating for health improvement and obesity prevention. Health care providers can be powerful advocates for obesity-preventing environmental and policy change in their communities. More than 90 percent of U.S. physicians surveyed supported physician participation in public roles defined as "community participation and individual and collective health advocacy" (Gruen et al., 2006, p. 2,473). Involvement in issues closely related to individual patients' health was rated as very important (Gruen et al., 2006). By engaging in advocacy, health care providers can play a pivotal role in incorporating knowledge of individual factors that promote or inhibit healthy lifestyle change into a wider community perspective.

Implementation

Recent surveys have found that approximately 44 percent of U.S. hospitals and nearly half of outpatient practices are employing EHRs (Classen and Bates, 2011). The challenge now is how to ensure meaningful use of EHRs for patient care, as data have suggested that simply using EHRs does not necessarily result in improved quality of care provided, even over time (Classen and Bates, 2011).

The U.S. Preventive Services Task Force recommends that children and adolescents be screened for obesity and that clinicians offer or make referrals for "comprehensive, intensive behavioral interventions to promote improvement in weight status" (USPSTF, 2010a, p. 362). These recommendations for children, adolescents, and adults also have been included in a list of preventive services to be provided with no copay under the federal health care reform legislation signed into law in March 2010 (USPSTF, 2010b). The American Academy of Family Physicians (AAFP) has stated that family physicians should offer assistance to patients who are obese or overweight or who request assistance in preventing obesity (Lyznicki et al., 2001). Health care professional organizations and provider groups support the adoption of practices that will contribute to obesity prevention. Recommendations, toolkits, resources, and guides currently are available to encourage and assist health care providers in adopting approaches to care that promote the prevention, screening, diagnosis, and treatment of overweight and obesity.

A number of initiatives designed to implement these recommendations have been undertaken. For example:

- Obesity prevention and treatment have been a strategic priority for the AAP for the past decade. The AAP also has a specific section on its website devoted to helping practitioners prevent and treat obesity, which includes practice tools, education and support, reimbursement information, and advocacy training (http://aap.org/obesity). In addition, Bright Futures, the AAP's national health promotion and disease prevention initiative, addresses children's health needs in the context of family and community (http://brightfutures.aap.org/). The AAP also has developed the Community Pediatrics Training Initiative program, which is "designed to improve residency training by supporting pediatricians in becoming leaders and advocates to create positive and lasting change on behalf of children's health" (AAP, 2011). Through this program, faculty and residents are provided with training, technical assistance and resources, and networking and funding opportunities.
- The Let's Move campaign (Let's Move, 2011), in partnership with the AAP, is working with the broader medical community to educate health care providers about obesity and ensure that they regularly monitor children's BMI, provide counseling on healthy eating early on, and even write prescriptions describing the simple things individuals and families can do to increase physical activity and healthy eating.
- The Texas Pediatric Society developed and distributed a toolkit to "aid pediatric practitioners in the prevention, early recognition, and clinical care of children and adolescents who are overweight or obese, with or without associated co-morbid conditions" (Texas Pediatric Society, 2008).
- The Blue Cross Blue Shield Association and the AAP developed a toolkit designed to help health care providers confront the obesity epidemic with their pediatric patients. It includes materials to help manage pediatric patients during office visits, guidelines that provide key assessment and diagnosis information, and tear-off patient chart sheets that can be used to track patient information (BCBSA, 2011).
- The American Medical Association's (AMA's) Healthier Life Steps program recently released the Physician's Guide to Personal Health Toolkit, which includes tools to support the personal efforts of providers to live a healthier lifestyle and serve as role models for their patients (AMA, 2010).

- The National Association of School Nurses (NASN) has developed a continuing education program, School Nurse Childhood Obesity Prevention Education (S.C.O.P.E.), designed specifically for school nurses, that "provides strategies for school nurses to assist students, families and the school community to address the challenges of obesity and overweight" (NASN, 2011).

Several health professional groups advocate, or encourage advocacy among their members, for obesity prevention by supporting programs and changes in policy and by working to promote awareness of the issues involved. For example:

- The AAP has recommended that physicians and health care professionals work with families and communities and advocate for the encouragement of physical activity and improved nutrition, especially through in-school programs (Krebs and Jacobson, 2003). In addition, the AAP has called for a ban on all junk food and fast-food ads during children's television shows as a means of slowing the rising tide of obesity. The statement also asks Congress, the Federal Trade Commission, and the Federal Communications Commission to eliminate junk food and fast-food ads on cell phones and other media, as well as to prohibit companies that make such products from paying to have their products featured in movies (Strasburger, 2011).
- The Academy of Nutrition and Dietetics, formerly known as the American Dietetic Association, has developed an integrated action plan for all of its registered dietitians and registered dietetic technicians, as well its organizational units, to work toward the prevention of childhood obesity. Included in this plan are strategies to expand the role of the registered dietitian from educator and counselor to advocate for community change and the promotion of healthy environments for children. The Commission on Dietetic Registration sponsors trainings for its members in its Childhood and Adolescent Weight Management program (Commission on Dietetic Registration, 2011). In addition, the Academy of Nutrition and Dietetics Foundation signature school-based nutrition education program, Energy Balance for Kids with Play (EB4K with Play), provides programming designed to result in behavior change in students through improvements in the school wellness environment and community and parental involvement, in addition to more traditional educational methods (Academy of Nutrition and Dietetics, 2011).

- The American Nurses Association (ANA), which represents 2.9 million registered nurses (the largest group of health care providers), publically supports the Let's Move campaign. It recognizes that "nurses have the capacity to touch the lives of parents and of children to help educate them on healthy choices," and has pledged to support programs that address childhood obesity and to develop and distribute educational materials (ANA, 2010).
- The AAFP's public health initiative Americans In Motion (AIM) is aimed at influencing the health of all Americans through "fitness" (physical activity, nutrition, and emotional well-being). AIM promotes family health care providers as fitness role models who serve as key resources for improving fitness among individuals, families, and communities. Additionally, the AAFP has stated that family health care providers should participate in local, state, and national efforts to prevent obesity and encourage physical activity for children, adolescents, and adults.

Together, these initiatives demonstrate institutional leadership in helping to train, support, and encourage health care providers to expand their role in current obesity prevention efforts.

Indicators for Assessing Progress in Obesity Prevention for Strategy 4-1

Process Indicators

- Increase in the proportion of primary care providers who regularly measure the body mass index of their patients.
  Source for measuring indicator: National Survey on Energy Balance-Related Care Among Primary Care Physicians

- Increase in the proportion of physician office visits by children, adolescents, and adult patients that include counseling and/or education related to physical activity and nutrition.
  Source for measuring indicator: NAMCS

NOTE: NAMCS = National Ambulatory Medical Care Survey.

Strategy 4-2: Ensure Coverage of, Access to, and Incentives for Routine Obesity Prevention, Screening, Diagnosis, and Treatment

Insurers (both public and private) should ensure that health insurance coverage and access provisions address obesity prevention, screening, diagnosis, and treatment.

Potential actions include

- insurers, including self-insured organizations and employers, considering the inclusion of incentives in individual and family health plans for maintaining healthy lifestyles;
- insurers considering (1) benefit designs and programs that promote obesity screening and prevention and (2) innovative approaches to reimbursing for routine screening and obesity prevention services (including preconception counseling) in clinical practice and for monitoring the performance of these services in relation to obesity prevention; and
- insurers taking full advantage of obesity-related provisions in health care reform legislation.

Context

The adverse health effects of obesity (Calle and Thun, 2004; Eckel and Krauss, 1998; Preis et al., 2009) drive up health care costs (Thorpe et al., 2004). As described in Chapter 2, the estimated cost of obesity-related illness based on restricted-use data from the Medical Expenditure Panel Survey for 2000-2005 is $190.2 billion annually (in 2005 dollars), representing nearly 21 percent of national health care spending in the United States (Cawley and Meyerhoefer, 2011). Additionally, the Robert Wood Johnson Foundation (RWJF) has estimated that $14 billion per year is spent on childhood obesity in direct health care costs (RWJF, 2007).

With more than 80 percent of Americans having health insurance coverage, private or public (DeNavas-Walt et al., 2011), health insurers should be interested in obesity prevention, diagnosis, screening, and treatment services as a way of reducing medical claims and associated costs. Obesity prevention and treatment services also should be a priority for federally qualified health centers, school-based wellness clinics, public health clinics, and other facilities affording the most vulnerable populations access to care.

Currently, some health plans and employers are addressing obesity for enrollees and employees, respectively, in the workplace (Simpson and Cooper, 2009), and some health plans have provided and should continue to provide financial resources to support school-based initiatives to reverse childhood obesity (Dietz et al., 2007; Simpson and Cooper, 2009). Yet insurers do not consistently pay for obesity prevention and treatment services unless there are comorbidities, such as diabetes, hypertension, or musculoskeletal issues. Obesity prevention should be considered a core service similar to cancer prevention screening and counseling.

Coverage of obesity prevention depends not only on health plans but also on employers. Two-thirds of insurance in the private market, while administered by health plans, is actually provided by self-insured employers, and a large number of businesses and organizations therefore have the ability to adjust benefits within their health plans (Heinen and Darling, 2009). In fact, health plans and businesses have embraced worker and workplace wellness programs that promote a healthier workforce and presumably reduce medical care costs (Heinen and Darling, 2009).

Health care insurers can address obesity by giving employers health plan options that include promising and innovative evidence-based strategies for encouraging policyholders and their families to maintain a healthy weight, increase physical activity, and improve the quality of their diet (IOM, 2005). Further, providing coverage for obesity treatment, prevention, screening, and diagnosis would give health care providers the opportunity and the means to provide the necessary care for each of their patients (whether diet and nutrition counseling, preconception counseling, or routine BMI screening).

Evidence

Although relatively little effort has been devoted to studying scientifically the specific impacts of various reimbursement and incentive approaches, evidence suggests that when one accounts for the high costs associated with obesity (see Chapter 2) over the long term, incentives for maintaining a healthy lifestyle become cost-effective, and in essence pay for themselves. Studies have shown that when employers and insurers provide incentives for weight loss and health maintenance, participants are more likely to engage in health-promoting behaviors and are more likely to lose weight (Archer et al., 2011; Arterburn et al., 2008; Simpson and Cooper, 2009) (see also Strategy 4-3). However, most studies of incentive programs have included only adult participants, and the programs were provided at no cost (variables not yet studied include out-of-pocket cost, convenience, and time).

Data from the Diabetes Prevention Program reveal that weight loss (through physical activity and diet) was effective in lowering the incidence of diabetes in individuals with prediabetes (NDIC, 2008). Additionally, emerging evidence suggests that obesity prevention efforts are especially important because, as a result of genetic and biological factors, people who become obese find it much more challenging to maintain any weight loss they may achieve (Sumithran et al., 2011). Moreover, while these physiologic compensatory mechanisms would be advantageous for a lean person in a food-scarce environment, energy-dense food is abundant and physical activity is largely unnecessary in most environments today, so relapse after weight loss is not surprising (Sumithran et al., 2011).

With respect to care delivery, health care providers often cite lack of reimbursement for obesity-related services as a barrier to providing such services (Cook et al., 2004). A survey of pediatricians found that for most, despite their knowledge of the problem and desire to address obesity prevention, inadequate reimbursement and lack of time were among major barriers to providing BMI screening and counseling during visits that were reported (Sesselberg et al., 2010). Although more evidence is needed to determine the most effective approaches, it is becoming clear that adequate coverage and reimbursement for obesity-related services are essential to addressing obesity prevention (Simpson and Cooper, 2009).

In sum, it is reasonable to believe that changes in health plan practices and policies could have a major effect on obesity prevention by reducing barriers to providing related care and incentives for engaging in a healthy lifestyle.

Implementation

While coverage for obesity-related health care services is highly variable, there has been some movement, especially over the past 5 years, toward providing reimbursement for obesity treatment and prevention in response to provider complaints and reevaluation of health plans by employers (Simpson and Cooper, 2009). Many employers also have begun to offer incentives or institute wellness policies that provide penalties or rewards based on an employees' (and in some cases their dependents') health status; often these incentives are monetary in nature (Mello and Rosenthal, 2008). Of note, in 2007 the Department of Labor released a clarification of the *Health Insurance Portability and Accountability Act* (HIPAA) of 1996, ruling that employers can use financial incentives in wellness programs to motivate workers to get healthy (Mello and Rosenthal, 2008).

An example of a monetary incentive is a plan offered by United Healthcare, a national insurer, which for a typical family includes a $5,000 yearly deductible that can be reduced to $1,000 if an employee is not obese and does not smoke. Other examples of incentive programs are providing discounted insurance or rebates for participation in health screening or the completion of weight loss or health education programs. Supporting such an approach, evidence from smoking cessation programs shows that full coverage or reimbursement improves quitting rates (Curry et al., 1998; Kaper et al., 2006). Insurers also have provided incentives to health care providers as a way to encourage BMI screening during pediatric visits (Simpson and Cooper, 2009).

At the state level, reimbursement for obesity-related services through Medicaid is highly variable. Despite documentation that coverage for obesity prevention in pediatric practice is available, many states are not aware of or create barriers to the delivery of such care (Simpson and Cooper, 2009). On the other hand, some states are promoting healthy behaviors through incentives for Medicaid and State Children's Health Insurance Program (SCHIP) participants (for example, awarding movie tickets, coupons, or gift certificates to parents who adhere to scheduled well-child visits). The Department of Health and Human Services recently announced that it will provide guidance for states on the inclusion of obesity services in Early and Periodic Screening, Diagnosis, and Treatment (EPSDT) benefits. Provisions in federal health care reform legislation require health insurers and government health programs to provide more checkups, screenings, and health counseling with little or no copayment by the patient. In addition, the legislation includes preventive and wellness services as "essential benefits" and contains incentives intended to encourage employers to implement and sustain wellness programs. It also allows for employers or insurers to provide incentives, such as reduced premiums, for participation in qualifying wellness programs.

Indicators for Assessing Progress in Obesity Prevention for Strategy 4-2

Process Indicators

* Increase in the number of health plans that include incentives for maintaining healthy lifestyles.
  Sources for measuring indicator: National Survey of Energy Balance-Related Care Among Primary Care Physicians and NAMCS

- Increase in the number of health plans that promote obesity screening and prevention and use innovative reimbursement strategies for screening and obesity prevention services.
  Sources for measuring indicator: National Survey of Energy Balance-Related Care Among Primary Care Physicians and NAMCS

- Increase in the number of health plans reporting and achieving obesity prevention and screening metrics, including universal BMI assessment, weight assessment, and counseling on physical activity and nutrition for children, adolescents, and adults.
  Source for measuring indicator: HEDIS

NOTE: BMI = body mass index; HEDIS = Healthcare Effectiveness Data and Information Set; NAMCS = National Ambulatory Medical Care Survey.

Strategy 4-3: Encourage Active Living and Healthy Eating at Work

Worksites should create, or expand, healthy environments by establishing, implementing, and monitoring policy initiatives that support wellness.

Potential actions include

- public and private employers promoting healthy eating and active living in the worksite in their own institutional policies and practices by, for example, increasing opportunities for physical activity as part of a wellness/ health promotion program, providing access to and promotion of healthful foods and beverages, and offering health benefits that provide employees and their dependents coverage for obesity-related services and programs; and
- health care organizations and providers serving as models for the incorporation of healthy eating and active living into worksite practices and programs.

Context

Employed adults spend a quarter of their lives at the worksite (Goetzel et al., 2009), and worksites are potential settings for promoting healthy eating and active living among large numbers of adults of various socioeconomic levels and ethnic and cultural backgrounds (Quintiliani et al., 2007). Advances in technology and changes in the structure of many worksites have lead to an increase in sedentary, low-physical-activity occupations over the past several decades (Church et al., 2011). The resulting decrease in energy expended throughout the workday is associated with increases in BMI (Choi et al., 2010; Church et al., 2011). In addition, adverse work conditions, such as high-demand environments, low-control environments, and long hours, have been found to increase the risk of obesity (Schulte et al., 2007). The rising prevalence of obesity in the United States, particularly within the workforce, is increasing employer costs, economic and otherwise.

The costs and resource use associated with obesity in the workplace have been examined widely. Studies have found that overall, overweight or obese employees have higher sick leave use, absenteeism, use of disability benefits, workplace injuries, and health care costs and lower productivity and work attendance than normal-weight employees (Gates et al., 2008; Schmier et al., 2006; Trogdon et al., 2008) (an overview of the economic consequences of obesity is provided in Chapter 2 [Table 2-2]). These variables can total more than $600 per year for each obese employee compared with the costs associated with normal-weight employees. Overweight employees have been estimated to cost employers more than $200 per year compared with costs for those who are of normal weight (Goetzel et al., 2010).

The worksite is a key venue affecting employee wellness. Creating an emotionally and physically healthy workplace, supporting employees' community-based physical activity, and offering onsite purchase of fruits and vegetables to bring home are examples of the potential results of a business focus on employee wellness. Worksite health promotion programs are employer initiatives designed to improve the health and well-being of workers (and often their dependents) and thereby reduce the costs associated with obesity in the workplace. These programs aim to prevent the onset of disease and to maintain health through primary, secondary, and tertiary prevention efforts. Primary prevention efforts in the workplace are directed at employed populations that are generally healthy, secondary prevention efforts are directed at individuals already at high risk because of certain lifestyle practices (such as smoking and maintaining a sedentary lifestyle), and tertiary prevention efforts focus on disease management (Goetzel and Ozminkowski, 2008).

Evidence

Worksites of all sizes represent an important venue (Schulte et al., 2008) for reaching the majority of the adult population. Worksite initiatives to promote and support healthy lifestyles have been shown to benefit both employers and employees (see Box 8-1) (CDC, 2011b).

Successful worksite wellness/health promotion programs have included strategies for providing employees with a healthy work environment; opportuni-

---

BOX 8-1
Potential Benefits of Workplace Wellness Programs

Potential benefits to employers:

- Reduces costs associated with chronic diseases

- Decreases absenteeism

- Reduces employee turnover

- Improves worker satisfaction

- Demonstrates concern for employees

- Improves morale

Potential benefits to employees:

- Ensures greater productivity

- Reduces absenteeism

- Improves fitness and health

- Provides social opportunity and a source of support within the workplace

SOURCE: CDC, 2011b.

ties for physical activity and health education; screening for obesity and related comorbidities; financial or nonmonetary incentives for participation in weight loss and/or health promotion efforts; and health benefit packages that include support for physical activity and nutrition (with respect to the latter feature, lack of health care coverage is associated with individuals forgoing needed care, including preventive care) (Archer et al., 2011; CDC, 2010; Romney et al., 2011). Some employees are willing to pay higher premiums for access to such wellness programs (Gabel et al., 2009).

The 2009 IOM report *Local Government Actions to Prevent Childhood Obesity* recommends that worksites, specifically those with high percentages of youth employees and government-run and -regulated worksites, develop policies and practices that build physical activity into routines (for example, exercise breaks at certain times of the day and in meetings or walking meetings) (IOM, 2009a). A review of the effectiveness of worksite physical activity and nutrition programs in promoting healthy weight among employees found that such programs had achieved modest improvements in employee weight status at 6- to 12-month follow-up (most of the studies examined in this review combined informational and behavioral strategies to influence physical activity and diet; fewer studies involved modifying the work environment [e.g., cafeteria, exercise facilities] to promote healthy choices) (Anderson et al., 2009).

Worksites also should ensure that healthy eating initiatives/programs are properly supported. One way of doing this is to ensure that employees (as well as guests, visitors, and clients/patients), have access to healthy food and beverage options if dining facilities, staff pantries, or vending machines are available in the work environment. There is strong evidence for the effectiveness of worksite obesity prevention and control programs that include improving access to healthy foods in vending machines and cafeterias (the report of the Healthy Eating Active Living Convergence Partnership provides several citations [Prevention Institute, 2008]) (see also Backman et al., 2011; Raulio et al., 2010).

Health promotion programs in the workplace are associated with reduced absenteeism, higher-quality performance and productivity, and lower health care costs (Aldana, 2001; Chapman, 2005; Goetzel and Ozminkowski, 2008; Heinen and Darling, 2009; Merrill et al., 2011; Pelletier, 2005). Therefore, such programs can be well worth the ongoing costs of their implementation (HHS, 2010) and can produce a direct financial return on investment (CDC, 2011b).

In sum, employers, while bearing both the direct medical and indirect productivity costs of obesity, have an opportunity to help increase and promote physical activity, healthy eating, and overall well-being among a large proportion of the adult population.

Implementation

Movement toward employer-based wellness programs is already occurring. As of 2008, the Bureau of Labor Statistics reported that 28 percent of full-time workers in the private sector and 54 percent of full-time workers in the public sector had access to worksite wellness programs, compared with 19 and 35 percent, respectively, a decade earlier (Stoltzfus, 2009). Additionally, in Washington State, for example, businesses, government agencies, and organizations came together to create the Access to Healthy Foods Coalition. Access to healthier options in the workplace is a goal of this coalition. In addition, making healthy foods and beverages available is part of a number of workplace wellness policies at large companies (examples include Power Group Companies, a Fortune 500 consulting firm, and Heinz, a global food company based in the United States). Health care reform legislation also may provide incentives for companies that offer workplace wellness solutions. Employers also could take advantage of existing stand-alone wellness, weight loss, physical activity, or incentive programs by providing access to or subsidizing membership fees for such programs during the work day or at the worksite. In the health care sector, several hospitals and health care organizations are already promoting active living and healthy eating. Examples include Health Care without Harm, a coalition that promotes a health care sector that does no harm and promotes the health of people and the environment; Kaiser Permanente's comprehensive food policy to promote individual and environmental health (the Healthy Picks program); and the growing number of hospital farmers' markets and gardens.

To aid employers in the development of worksite wellness programs, CDC developed LEAN Works, a free web-based resource that provides interactive tools and evidence-based resources to help employers design effective worksite obesity prevention and control programs (CDC, 2011b). In addition, employers can use CDC's obesity cost calculator to estimate the cost of obesity to their business, as well as the amount of money that could be saved by implementing various workplace interventions (CDC, 2011b).

Strategy 4-4: Encourage Healthy Weight Gain During Pregnancy and Breastfeeding, and Promote Breastfeeding-Friendly Environments

Health service providers and employers should adopt, implement, and monitor policies that support healthy weight gain during pregnancy and the initiation and continuation of breastfeeding. Population disparities in breastfeeding should be specifically addressed at the federal, state, and local levels to remove barriers and promote targeted increases in breastfeeding initiation and continuation.

Potential actions include

- all those who provide health care or related services to women of child-bearing age offering preconception counseling on the importance of conceiving at a healthy BMI;
- medical facilities, prenatal services, and community clinics adopting policies consistent with the Baby-Friendly Hospital Initiative;
- local health departments and community-based organizations, working with other segments of the health sector, providing information on breastfeeding and the availability of related classes to pregnant women and new mothers, connecting pregnant women and new mothers with breastfeeding support programs to help them make informed infant feeding decisions, and developing peer support programs that empower pregnant women and mothers to obtain the help and support they need from other mothers who have breastfed;
- workplaces instituting policies to support breastfeeding mothers, including ensuring both private space and adequate break time; and
- the federal government using Prevention Fund dollars to support implementation of the Baby-Friendly Hospital Initiative nationwide, and providing funding to support community-level collaborative efforts and peer counseling with the aim of increasing the duration of breastfeeding.

Context

Primary prevention of obesity begins before birth. Women of childbearing age today are heavier, a greater percentage are entering pregnancy overweight or obese, and many are gaining too much weight during pregnancy (IOM, 2009b). One of the most important modifiers of weight gain in pregnancy and its impact on maternal and child health is a woman's weight at the start of pregnancy (higher pregnancy weight gain has been associated with prepregnancy BMI) (IOM, 2009b). Addressing obesity prevention, intervention, and treatment in childhood and adolescence would result in young women entering their reproductive years at healthier weights. This is an example of taking a life-course approach to a healthy pregnancy and is important to reversing the transgenerational increase in obesity risk (Cnattingius et al., 2011).

Maternal gestational weight gain has been linked to obesity in childhood, as well as poorer maternal and infant outcomes (IOM, 2009a; Oken et al., 2007). Guidelines for maternal gestational weight gain have been released by the IOM (2009a), but focused attention is necessary to ensure their widespread implementation.

In its reexamination of pregnancy weight guidelines IOM (2009a) recognizes that preconception counseling and support will be needed to assist mothers to enter pregnancy at a healthy weight, and in turn, have healthier pregnancies and healthier infants. After birth, support for breastfeeding as a primary strategy for obesity prevention requires a joint effort of hospital and outpatient services and community-based support through the engagement of employers and local health care providers. Helping mothers continue breastfeeding in the early postpartum period through 6 months requires a supportive environment at home, in the community, and in the workplace. Strategies to increase breastfeeding duration in the workplace have been successful, as has providing peer support. The current federal Special Supplemental Nutrition Program for Women, Infants, and Children (WIC) regulations contain provisions that encourage women to breastfeed and provide appropriate nutritional support for breastfeeding participants (USDA/FNS, 2011). Strategies aimed at increasing breastfeeding initiation and maintenance are crucial to increasing the impact of breastfeeding on obesity prevention. Specific attention to the associations of breastfeeding with age and race/ethnicity would accelerate obesity prevention among the most vulnerable populations.

Evidence

Evidence suggests that preconceptional counseling improves women's knowledge about pregnancy-related risk factors, including excessive weight gain, as well as their behaviors to mitigate those risks (Elsinga et al., 2008). Pre- and inter-conceptional counseling also improves attitudes and behavior with respect to physical activity and nutrition in response to behavioral interventions (Hillemeier et al., 2008). Pregnancy weight gain has been associated with several short- and long-term effects for mother and child. In particular, observational data are accumulating that link maternal weight gain and later childhood adiposity. There is also a strong association between high pregnancy weight gain and postpartum weight retention in mothers (IOM, 2009a).

After birth, breastfeeding has been shown to be associated with a reduced risk of obesity in the child (Ip et al., 2007, 2009), a protective effect that can persist into adulthood (Owen et al., 2005). Evidence suggests that initiation, longer duration, and exclusivity of breastfeeding provide a protective effect and lower odds of becoming overweight or obese in childhood and adolescence (Harder et al., 2005). A review of 22 systematic reviews on early-life determinants of overweight and obesity found that breastfeeding may be a protective factor for later overweight and obesity (Monasta et al., 2010). A study of the association between breast-feeding and adiposity at age 3 years involving 884 children found that between birth and 6 months of age, infant weight change mediates associations of breast-feeding with BMI, but only partially mediates associations with indicators of child adiposity (van Rossem et al., 2011). And a study of another recent cohort of 5,047 children and their mothers in the Netherlands found that between 3 and 6 months of age, shorter breastfeeding duration and exclusivity during the first 6 months were associated with increased rates of growth, including weight and BMI (Durmus et al., 2011).

Additionally, a number of systematic reviews on the relationship between breastfeeding and childhood obesity have concluded that, as reported by the IOM (2011b), there is an association between breastfeeding and a reduction in obesity risk in childhood, although the nature of the study designs makes it difficult to infer causality. Several biologic mechanisms have been proposed to explain the effect of breastfeeding on obesity prevention, including that breastfeeding supports self-regulation of energy intake (Li et al., 2008, 2010; Mihrshahi et al., 2011; van Rossem et al., 2011).

Relative to breastfed infants, formula-fed infants exhibit higher and more pro-longed insulin responses to feedings (Lucas et al., 1981; Manco et al., 2011), and this effect may persist into childhood. In obese children, formula feeding has been associated with reduced insulin sensitivity and increased insulin secretion relative to breastfed children with the same BMI (Manco et al., 2011). Moreover, factors present in breast milk but not in formula, such as leptin, a cytokine that controls satiety and energy balance, may confer an obesity protective effect (Singhal et al., 2002).

Breastfeeding has been endorsed as a strategy for obesity prevention by the IOM (2009b), CDC (2011c), the AAP (Gartner et al., 2005), the American College of Obstetricians and Gynecologists (ACOG, 2007), and the Endocrine Society (August et al., 2008). Significant gaps remain, however, in both breastfeeding initiation and maintenance. While Merewood and colleagues (2005) found that almost 82 percent of infants have ever breastfed, maintenance at 6 months dropped to 60 percent and exclusive breastfeeding at 6 months to 25 percent (CDC, 2011a). Breastfeeding initiation has been associated with having given birth in a Baby-Friendly Hospital (Merewood et al., 2005). Yet while many hospitals have made progress toward becoming Baby-Friendly (Figure 8-2) there were only two states as of 2009 in which more than 20 percent of births occurred at hospitals that had completed the 10 steps to certification as Baby-Friendly.

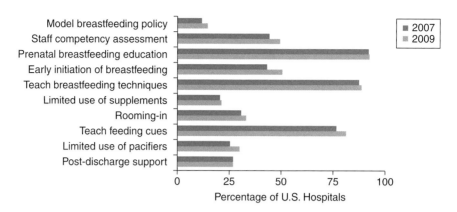

FIGURE 8-2 Percentage of U.S. hospitals with recommended policies and practices to support breastfeeding (2007 and 2009).
SOURCE: CDC, 2011d.

Implementation

The IOM has concluded that to improve maternal and child health outcomes, women not only should be within a normal BMI range when they conceive, but also should gain within the recommended guidelines (IOM, 2009b). To meet the recommendations for pregnancy weight gain, many women need preconception counseling, which may include plans for weight loss. Counseling is already an integral part of CDC's preconception recommendations (Johnson et al., 2006), which are designed to enable women to enter pregnancy in optimal health, avoid adverse health outcomes associated with childbearing, and reduce disparities in adverse pregnancy outcomes.

In 1991, the World Health Organization (WHO) and the United Nations Children's Fund (UNICEF) launched the Baby-Friendly Hospital Initiative to ensure that all hospitals and birthing centers would offer optimal breastfeeding support. In 1997, Baby-Friendly USA was established as the national authority for the Baby-Friendly Hospital Initiative in the United States. Promotion and support of breastfeeding at birth through the Baby-Friendly Hospital Initiative has resulted in significant increases in breastfeeding rates (Perez-Escamilla, 2007). There is also a dose-response relationship between the number of Baby-Friendly steps (see Box 8-2) in place and successful breastfeeding. In one study, mothers who experienced none of the Baby-Friendly steps were eight times less likely to continue breastfeeding to 6 weeks than mothers experiencing at least five steps (DiGirolamo et al., 2001). The Baby-Friendly Hospital Initiative has developed a guidance document for overcoming barriers to implementation (Baby-Friendly USA, 2004).

BOX 8-2
10 Steps to Successful Breastfeeding

1. Have a written breastfeeding policy that is routinely communicated to all health care staff.

2. Train all health care staff in skills necessary to implement this policy.

3. Inform all pregnant women about the benefits and management of breastfeeding.

4. Help mothers initiate breastfeeding within a half-hour of birth.

5. Show mothers how to breastfeed and how to maintain even if they should be separated from their infants.

6. Give newborn infants no food or drink other than breastmilk, unless medically indicated.

7. Practice rooming-in—allow mothers and infants to remain together—24 hours a day.

8. Encourage breastfeeding on demand.

9. Give no artificial teats or pacifiers (also called dummies or soothers) to breastfeeding infants.

10. Foster the establishment of breastfeeding support groups and refer mothers to them on discharge from the hospital or clinic.

SOURCE: WHO/UNICEF, 1989.

Texas is one state where the Baby-Friendly Hospital Initiative has received strong support. According to Shealy and colleagues (2005, p. 5), "The Texas Hospital Association and the Texas Department of Health have jointly developed the Texas Ten Step Hospital Program to recognize Texas hospitals that have achieved at least 85 percent adherence to the WHO/UNICEF Ten Steps.

Certification is entirely voluntary and based on the hospitals' reports; there are no external audits or site visits."

Support for breastfeeding maintenance as mothers return home to their communities and workplaces is crucial. A supportive worksite environment helps support breastfeeding continuation (Galtry, 1997), while lack of accommodation for breastfeeding mothers contributes to shorter breastfeeding duration (Corbett-Dick and Bezek, 1997). Convincing evidence supports the role of corporate lactation programs in increasing breastfeeding maintenance (see Box 8-3 for an example). Workplace lactation support programs also have resulted in improved work experiences for breastfeeding mothers; improved productivity and staff loyalty; enhanced public image of the employer; and decreased absenteeism, health care costs, and employee turnover (Bar-Yam, 1997; Cohen et al., 1995; Dodgson and Duckett, 1997).

Of note, 24 states, the District of Columbia, and Puerto Rico have laws regarding workplace lactation support. Provisions within the federal health care reform legislation specifically recommend that employers provide break time for employees to express breastmilk in a suitable space other than a bathroom for 1 year after their child's birth.[2] However, employers are not required to compensate employees for break time, and employers with fewer than 50 employees are exempt if the recommendations cause a hardship (U.S. Department of Labor, 2011). In addition, both the Surgeon General (HHS, 2011) and the report of the White House Obesity Task Force encourage workplace lactation support (White House Task Force on Childhood Obesity, 2010).

Studies of breastfeeding support have emphasized the "importance of person-centered communication skills and of relationships in supporting a woman to breastfeed" (Schmied et al., 2011, p. 58). Peer support programs are effective both independently and in combination with multifaceted interventions in increasing breastfeeding initiation and duration (Britton et al., 2007; Fairbank et al., 2000; Shealy et al., 2005). Home-visiting programs, which involve periodic visits by family health nurses or other health care providers, also have been found to be effective models for delivery of support for parents and their children, particularly for vulnerable populations, and have been found to be feasible options for addressing risk factors for childhood obesity (Hodnett and Roberts, 2000; Wen et al., 2009). Home-visiting programs are a method of care included within the federal health

---

[2] See http://www.usbreastfeeding.org/Portals/0/Workplace/HR3590-Sec4207-Nursing-Mothers.pdf (accessed November 4, 2011).

BOX 8-3
Example of a Worksite Breastfeeding Initiative:
California Public Health Foundation Special
Supplemental Nutrition Program for Women, Infants,
and Children

According to Shealy and colleagues (2005, p. 10):

> The California Public Health Foundation WIC (Special Supplemental Nutrition Program for Women, Infants, and Children) agencies provide a breastfeeding support program for their employees, most of whom are paraprofessionals. The program includes encouraging and recognizing breastfeeding milestones and providing training on breastfeeding, monthly prenatal classes, postpartum support groups, and a supportive work site environment. The work site environment includes pumping facilities, flexible break times, and access to a breast pump. A program hallmark is access to an experienced colleague known as a Trained Lactation Coach, or TLC, who breastfed her own children after returning to work. An evaluation of the California program revealed that more than 99 percent of employees returning to work after giving birth initiated breastfeeding, and 69 percent of those employees breastfed at least 12 months. Access to breast pumps and support groups were significantly associated with the high breastfeeding duration rates (Whaley et al., 2002).

care reform legislation. An example of a comprehensive community breastfeeding support program is provided in Box 8-4.

Key factors in successful peer support groups include the following (Britton et al., 2007; Shealy et al., 2005; USDA/FNS, 2004)

- peer mothers of similar sociocultural background;
- paid counselors (who may be more effective than volunteers with respect to retention and ability to sustain the program);
- training of peer counselors in breastfeeding management, nutrition, infant growth and development, counseling techniques, and criteria for making referrals;

- in both individual and group settings, peer counselors who are trained and are generally clinically monitored or overseen by a professional in lactation management support, such as an International Board Certified Lactation Consultant (IBCLC), nurse, nutritionist, or physician with specific training in skilled lactation care;
- leadership and support from management, staff access to IBCLCs, and community partnerships for making and receiving referrals; and
- integration of peer support within the overall health system, which appears to contribute to the ongoing maintenance of a program.

Indicators for Assessing Progress in Obesity Prevention for Strategy 4-4

Process Indicators

- Increase in the prevalence of initiation of any breastfeeding among new mothers.
  Source for measuring indicator: CDC breastfeeding report card

- Increase in the prevalence and duration of exclusive breastfeeding among new mothers.
  Source for measuring indicator: CDC breastfeeding report card

- Increase in the number of infants exclusively breastfed for 6 months.
  Source for measuring indicator: CDC breastfeeding report card

- Increase in the percentage of U.S. hospitals with recommended policies and practices to support breastfeeding.
  Source for measuring indicator: mPINC

- Increase in the percentage of U.S. workplaces with policies and practices that support breastfeeding.
  Source for measuring indicator: IFPS-II (in development)

Foundational Indicator

- Elimination of disparities in breastfeeding initiation and maintenance.
  Source for measuring indicator: NIS

NOTE: CDC = Centers for Disease Control and Prevention; IFPS-II = Infant Feeding Practices Survey II; mPINC = National Survey of Maternity Practices in Infant Nutrition and Care; NIS = National Immunization Survey.

INTEGRATION OF STRATEGIES FOR ACCELERATING PROGRESS IN OBESITY PREVENTION

The creation of systems to support healthy decision making at the community level is a necessary step linking individual health behavior change and choice to improvements in the physical and nutritional environments. Health care providers, employers, and insurers are all components of a system of support and service that enables individuals to access obesity prevention and treatment. However, these three components have tended to work independently. For example, individuals may hear messages in the workplace about healthy lifestyle change but have no access to additional visits with their health care provider or community resources because of a lack of health insurance coverage; conversely, individuals may see their health care provider for obesity treatment but lack healthy physical activity and nutrition choices at the worksite. Insurers may cover nutrition services but not physical activity. Integration of these interdependent entities can provide a system of community-level care with synergistic effects. Moreover, pregnant women and infants need to be surrounded by a system of broad-based support, with insurance coverage for all the services necessary to provide for a healthy pregnancy and early infancy. Health care providers and employers need to pay special attention to the support mothers and infants require to maintain healthy early infancy nutrition.

REFERENCES

AAP (American Academy of Pediatrics). 2011. *Community pediatrics training initiative*. http://www.aap.org/commpeds/cpti/about.htm (accessed December 2, 2011).

Abramson, S., J. Stein, M. Schaufele, E. Frates, and S. Rogan. 2000. Personal exercise habits and counseling practices of primary care physicians: A national survey. *Clinical Journal of Sport Medicine* 10(1):40-48.

Academy of Nutrition and Dietetics. 2011. *Energy balance 4 kids (EB4K) with play*. http://www.eatright.org/Media/content.aspx?id=6442465058 (accessed November 22, 2011).

ACOG (American Congress of Obstetricians and Gynecologists). 2007. ACOG committee opinion no. 361: Breastfeeding: Maternal and infant aspects. *Obstetrics and Gynecology* 109(2 Pt. 1):479-480.

Aldana, S. G. 2001. Financial impact of health promotion programs: A comprehensive review of the literature. *American Journal of Health Promotion* 15(5):296-320.

AMA (American Medical Association). 2010. *AMA healthier life steps: A physician's guide to personal health program*. http://www.ama-assn.org/ama/pub/physician-resources/public-health/promoting-healthy-lifestyles/healthier-life-steps-program/physicians-personal-health.page? (accessed August 15, 2011).

ANA (American Nurses Association). 2010. *News release: American Nurses Association supports nation's First Lady in combating childhood obesity.* http://www.nursingworld.org/FunctionalMenuCategories/MediaResources/PressReleases/2010-PR/Efforts-against-Childhood-Obesity.pdf (accessed November 11, 2011).

Anderson, L. M., T. A. Quinn, K. Glanz, G. Ramirez, L. C. Kahwati, D. B. Johnson, L. R. Buchanan, W. R. Archer, S. Chattopadhyay, G. P. Kalra, and D. L. Katz. 2009. The effectiveness of worksite nutrition and physical activity interventions for controlling employee overweight and obesity: A systematic review. *American Journal of Preventive Medicine* 37(4):340-357.

Appel, L. J., J. M. Clark, H.-C. Yeh, N.-Y. Wang, J. W. Coughlin, G. Daumit, E. R. Miller, A. Dalcin, G. J. Jerome, S. Geller, G. Noronha, T. Pozefsky, J. Charleston, J. B. Reynolds, N. Durkin, R. R. Rubin, T. A. Louis, and F. L. Brancati. 2011. Comparative effectiveness of weight-loss interventions in clinical practice. *New England Journal of Medicine* 365(21):1959-1968.

Archer, W. R., M. C. Batan, L. R. Buchanan, R. E. Soler, D. C. Ramsey, A. Kirchhofer, and M. Reyes. 2011. Promising practices for the prevention and control of obesity in the worksite. *American Journal of Health Promotion* 25(3):e12-e26.

Arterburn, D., E. O. Westbrook, C. J. Wiese, E. J. Ludman, D. C. Grossman, P. A. Fishman, E. A. Finkelstein, R. W. Jeffery, and A. Drewnowski. 2008. Insurance coverage and incentives for weight loss among adults with metabolic syndrome. *Obesity (Silver Spring)* 16(1):70-76.

August, G. P., S. Caprio, I. Fennoy, M. Freemark, F. R. Kaufman, R. H. Lustig, J. H. Silverstein, P. W. Speiser, D. M. Styne, and V. M. Montori. 2008. Prevention and treatment of pediatric obesity: An endocrine society clinical practice guideline based on expert opinion. *Journal of Clinical Endocrinology and Metabolism* 93(12):4576-4599.

Baby-Friendly USA. 2004. *Overcoming barriers to implementing the ten steps to successful breastfeeding.* http://www.babyfriendlyusa.org/eng/docs/BFUSAreport_complete.pdf (accessed July 3, 2011).

Backman, D., G. Gonzaga, S. Sugerman, D. Francis, and S. Cook. 2011. Effect of fresh fruit availability at worksites on the fruit and vegetable consumption of low-wage employees. *Journal of Nutrition Education and Behavior* 43(4 Suppl. 2):S113-S121.

Barlow, S. E., W. H. Dietz, W. J. Klish, and F. L. Trowbridge. 2002. Medical evaluation of overweight children and adolescents: Reports from pediatricians, pediatric nurse practitioners, and registered dietitians. *Pediatrics* 110(1 Pt. 2):222-228.

Bar-Yam, N. 1997. *Nursing mothers at work: An analysis of corporate and maternal strategies to support lactation in the workplace* [dissertation]. Waltham, MA: Heller School, Brandeis University.

BCBSA (Blue Cross Blue Shield Association). 2011. *Child obesity toolkit.* http://www.bcbsnm.com/provider/clinical/childhood_obesity.html (accessed September 19, 2011).

Blumenthal, D. 2011. Wiring the health system—origins and provisions of a new federal program. *New England Journal of Medicine* 365(24):2323-2329.

Boyle, M., S. Lawrence, L. Schwarte, S. Samuels, and W. J. McCarthy. 2009. Health care providers' perceived role in changing environments to promote healthy eating and physical activity: Baseline findings from health care providers participating in the healthy eating, active communities program. *Pediatrics* 123(Suppl. 5):S293-S300.

Britton, C., F. M. McCormick, M. J. Renfrew, A. Wade, and S. E. King. 2007. Support for breastfeeding mothers. *Cochrane Database of Systematic Reviews* (1):CD001141.

Bureau of Labor Statistics. 2010. *Career guide to industries, 2010-11 edition, healthcare.* http://www.bls.gov/oco/cg/cgs035.htm (accessed December 12, 2011).

Bureau of Labor Statistics. 2011. *The employment situation—November 2011.* http://www.bls.gov/news.release/pdf/empsit.pdf (accessed December 16, 2011).

Cahill, K., M. Moher, and T. Lancaster. 2008. Workplace interventions for smoking cessation. *Cochrane Database System Reviews* (4):CD003440.

Calfas, K. J., B. J. Long, J. F. Sallis, W. J. Wooten, M. Pratt, and K. Patrick. 1996. A controlled trial of physician counseling to promote the adoption of physical activity. *Preventive Medicine* 25(3):225-233.

Calle, E. E., and M. J. Thun. 2004. Obesity and cancer. *Oncogene* 23(38):6365-6378.

Cawley, J., and C. Meyerhoefer. 2011. The medical care costs of obesity: An instrumental variables approach. *Journal of Health Economics.* In press.

CDC (Centers for Disease Control and Prevention). 2010. Vital signs: Health insurance coverage and health care utilization—United States, 2006-2009 and January-March 2010. *Morbidity and Mortality Weekly Report* 59(44):1448-1454.

CDC. 2011a. *Breastfeeding report card—United States, 2011.* http://www.cdc.gov/breastfeeding/data/reportcard.htm (accessed August 3, 2011).

CDC. 2011b. *CDC's LEAN Works! A workplace obesity prevention program.* http://www.cdc.gov/LEANWorks/ (accessed August 15, 2011).

CDC. 2011c. Quitting smoking among adults—United States, 2001-2010. *Morbidity and Mortality Weekly Report* 60:1513-1519.

CDC. 2011d. *Vital signs: Hospital support for breastfeeding.* http://www.cdc.gov/VitalSigns/BreastFeeding/ (accessed August 3, 2011).

Chapman, L. S. 2005. Meta-evaluation of worksite health promotion economic return studies: 2005 update. *American Journal of Health Promotion* 19(6):1-11.

Choi, B., P. L. Schnall, H. Yang, M. Dobson, P. Landsbergis, L. Israel, R. Karasek, and D. Baker. 2010. Sedentary work, low physical job demand, and obesity in US workers. *American Journal of Industrial Medicine* 53(11):1088-1101.

Church, T. S., D. M. Thomas, C. Tudor-Locke, P. T. Katzmarzyk, C. P. Earnest, R. Q. Rodarte, C. K. Martin, S. N. Blair, and C. Bouchard. 2011. Trends over 5 decades in U.S. occupation-related physical activity and their associations with obesity. *PLoS ONE* 6(5):e19657.

Classen, D. C., and D. W. Bates. 2011. Finding the meaning in meaningful use. *New England Journal of Medicine* 365(9):855-858.

Cnattingius, S., E. Villamor, Y. T. Lagerros, A. K. Wikstrom, and F. Granath. 2011. High birth weight and obesity—a vicious circle across generations. *International Journal of Obesity (London)*. December 13.

Cohen, R., M. B. Mrtek, and R. G. Mrtek. 1995. Comparison of maternal absenteeism and infant illness rates among breast-feeding and formula-feeding women in two corporations. *American Journal of Health Promotion* 10(2):148-153.

Commission on Dietetic Registration. 2011. *Childhood and adolescent weight management*. http://www.cdrnet.org/whatsnew/childhood_module.cfm (accessed November 22, 2011).

Cook, S., E. M. Perrin, K. B. Flower, A. S. Ammerman, C. Homer, M. Weitzman, M. S. Johnson, and J. D. Klein. 2004. *Screening for obesity in pediatric primary care: A review of the literature*. Paper presented at Improving Health Services to Prevent Obesity in Children, Washington, DC.

Corbett-Dick, P., and S. K. Bezek. 1997. Breastfeeding promotion for the employed mother. *Journal of Pediatric Health Care* 11(1):12-19.

Curry, S. J., L. C. Grothaus, T. McAfee, and C. Pabiniak. 1998. Use and cost effectiveness of smoking-cessation services under four insurance plans in a health maintenance organization. *New England Journal of Medicine* 339(10):673-679.

DeNavas-Walt, C., B. D. Proctor, J. C. Smith, and U.S. Census Bureau. 2011. *Current population reports, p60-239, income, poverty, and health insurance coverage in the United States: 2010*. Washington, DC: U.S. Government Printing Office.

Dennison, B. A., J. Nicholas, R. de Long, M. Prokorym, and I. Brissette. 2009. Randomized controlled trial of a mailed toolkit to increase use of body mass index percentiles to screen for childhood obesity. *Preventing Chronic Disease* 6(4):A122.

Dietz, W., J. Lee, H. Wechsler, S. Malepati, and B. Sherry. 2007. Health plans' role in preventing overweight in children and adolescents. *Health Affairs* 26(2):430-440.

DiGirolamo, A. M., L. M. Grummer-Strawn, and S. Fein. 2001. Maternity care practices: Implications for breastfeeding. *Birth* 28(2):94-100.

Dodgson, J. E., and L. Duckett. 1997. Breastfeeding in the workplace. Building a support program for nursing mothers. *Official Journal of the American Association of Occupational Health Nurses* 45(6):290-298.

Durmus, B., L. van Rossem, L. Duijts, L. R. Arends, H. Raat, H. A. Moll, A. Hofman, E. A. Steegers, and V. W. Jaddoe. 2011. Breast-feeding and growth in children until the age of 3 years: The Generation R Study. *British Journal of Nutrition* 105(11):1704-1711.

Eckel, R. H., and R. M. Krauss. 1998. American Heart Association call to action: Obesity as a major risk factor for coronary heart disease. AHA nutrition committee. *Circulation* 97(21):2099-2100.

Elsinga, J., L. C. de Jong-Potjer, K. M. van der Pal-de Bruin, S. le Cessie, W. J. Assendelft, and S. E. Buitendijk. 2008. The effect of preconception counselling on lifestyle and other behaviour before and during pregnancy. *Women's Health Issues* 18(Suppl. 6):S117-S125.

Fairbank, L., S. O'Meara, M. J. Renfrew, M. Woolridge, A. J. Sowden, and D. Lister-Sharp. 2000. A systematic review to evaluate the effectiveness of interventions to promote the initiation of breastfeeding. *Health Technology Assessment* 4(25):1-171.

Flegal, K. M., R. P. Troiano, E. R. Pamuk, R. J. Kuczmarski, and S. M. Campbell. 1995. The influence of smoking cessation on the prevalence of overweight in the United States. *New England Journal of Medicine* 333(18):1165-1170.

Gabel, J. R., H. Whitmore, J. Pickreign, C. C. Ferguson, A. Jain, K. C. Shova, and H. Scherer. 2009. Obesity and the workplace: Current programs and attitudes among employers and employees. *Health Affairs* 28(1):46-56.

Galtry, J. 1997. Lactation and the labor market: Breastfeeding, labor market changes, and public policy in the United States. *Health Care for Women International* 18(5):467-480.

Gartner, L., J. Morton, R. A. Lawrence, A. J. Naylor, D. O'Hare, R. J. Schanler, A. I. Eidelman, and American Academy of Pediatrics Section on Breastfeeding. 2005. Breastfeeding and the use of human milk. *Pediatrics* 115(2):496-506.

Gates, D. M., P. Succop, B. J. Brehm, G. L. Gillespie, and B. D. Sommers. 2008. Obesity and presenteeism: The impact of body mass index on workplace productivity. *Journal of Occupational and Environmental Medicine* 50(1):39-45.

Goetzel, R. Z., and R. J. Ozminkowski. 2008. The health and cost benefits of work site health-promotion programs. *Annual Review of Public Health* 29:303-323.

Goetzel, R. Z., K. M. Baker, M. E. Short, X. Pei, R. J. Ozminkowski, S. Wang, J. D. Bowen, E. C. Roemer, B. A. Craun, K. J. Tully, C. M. Baase, D. M. DeJoy, and M. G. Wilson. 2009. First-year results of an obesity prevention program at the Dow chemical company. *Journal of Occupational and Environmental Medicine* 51(2):125-138.

Goetzel, R. Z., T. B. Gibson, M. E. Short, B. C. Chu, J. Waddell, J. Bowen, S. C. Lemon, I. D. Fernandez, R. J. Ozminkowski, M. G. Wilson, and D. M. DeJoy. 2010. A multi-worksite analysis of the relationships among body mass index, medical utilization, and worker productivity. *Journal of Occupational and Environmental Medicine* 52(Suppl. 1):S52-S58.

Greenwood, J. L., E. A. Joy, and J. B. Stanford. 2010. The Physical Activity Vital Sign: A primary care tool to guide counseling for obesity. *Journal of Physical Activity and Health* 7(5):571-576.

Gruen, R. L., E. G. Campbell, and D. Blumenthal. 2006. Public roles of US physicians: Community participation, political involvement, and collective advocacy. *Journal of the American Medical Association* 296(20):2467-2475.

Accelerating Progress in Obesity Prevention

Hamilton, J. L., F. W. James, and M. Bazargan. 2003. Provider practice, overweight and associated risk variables among children from a multi-ethnic underserved community. *Journal of the National Medical Association* 95(6):441-448.

Harder, T., R. Bergmann, G. Kallischnigg, and A. Plagemann. 2005. Duration of breast-feeding and risk of overweight: A meta-analysis. *American Journal of Epidemiology* 162(5):397-403.

Hash, R. B., R. K. Munna, R. L. Vogel, and J. J. Bason. 2003. Does physician weight affect perception of health advice? *Preventive Medicine* 36(1):41-44.

Heinen, L., and H. Darling. 2009. Addressing obesity in the workplace: The role of employers. *Milbank Quarterly* 87(1):101-122.

HHS (U.S. Department of Health and Human Services). 2010. *The Surgeon General's vision for a healthy and fit nation.* Rockville, MD: Office of the Surgeon General.

HHS. 2011. *The Surgeon General's call to action to support breastfeeding.* Washington, DC: HHS, Office of the Surgeon General.

Hillemeier, M. M., D. S. Downs, M. E. Feinberg, C. S. Weisman, C. H. Chuang, R. Parrott, D. Velott, L. A. Francis, S. A. Baker, A. M. Dyer, and V. M. Chinchilli. 2008. Improving women's preconceptional health: Findings from a randomized trial of the strong healthy women intervention in the central Pennsylvania women's health study. *Women's Health Issues* 18(Suppl. 6):S87-S96.

Hillman, J. B., S. D. Corathers, and S. E. Wilson. 2009. Pediatricians and screening for obesity with body mass index: Does level of training matter? *Public Health Reports* 124(4):561-567.

Hodnett, E. D., and I. Roberts. 2000. Home-based social support for socially disadvantaged mothers. *Cochrane Database System Reviews* (2):CD000107.

Hopkins, K. F., C. Decristofaro, and L. Elliott. 2011. How can primary care providers manage pediatric obesity in the real world? *Journal of the American Academy of Nurse Practitioners* 23(6):278-288.

Huang, T. T., L. A. Borowski, B. Liu, D. A. Galuska, R. Ballard-Barbash, S. Z. Yanovski, D. H. Olster, A. A. Atienza, and A. W. Smith. 2011. Pediatricians' and family physicians' weight-related care of children in the United States. *American Journal of Preventive Medicine* 41(1):24-32.

IOM (Institute of Medicine). 2005. *Preventing childhood obesity: Health in the balance.* Washington, DC: The National Academies Press.

IOM. 2009a. *Local government actions to prevent childhood obesity.* Washington, DC: The National Academies Press.

IOM. 2009b. *Weight gain during pregnancy: Reexamining the guidelines.* Washington, DC: The National Academies Press.

IOM. 2011a. *Clinical practice guidelines we can trust.* Washington, DC: The National Academies Press.

IOM. 2011b. *Early childhood obesity prevention policies.* Washington, DC: The National Academies Press.

Ip, S., M. Chung, G. Raman, P. Chew, N. Magula, D. DeVine, T. Trikalinos, and J. Lau. 2007. Breastfeeding and maternal and infant health outcomes in developed countries. *Evidence Report/Technology Assessment (Full Report)* (153):1-186.

Ip, S., M. Chung, G. Raman, T. A. Trikalinos, and J. Lau. 2009. A summary of the agency for healthcare research and quality's evidence report on breastfeeding in developed countries. *Breastfeeding Medicine* 4(Suppl. 1):S17-S30.

Jasik, C. B., S. H. Adams, C. E. Irwin, Jr., and E. Ozer. 2011. The association of BMI status with adolescent preventive screening. *Pediatrics* 128(2):e317-e323.

Johnson, K., S. F. Posner, J. Biermann, J. F. Cordero, H. K. Atrash, C. S. Parker, S. Boulet, and M. G. Curtis. 2006. Recommendations to improve preconception health and health care—United States. A report of the CDC/ATSDR preconception care work group and the select panel on preconception care. *Morbidity and Mortality Weekly Report Recommendations and Reports* 55(RR-6):1-23.

Kaper, J., E. J. Wagena, C. P. van Schayck, and J. L. Severens. 2006. Encouraging smokers to quit: The cost effectiveness of reimbursing the costs of smoking cessation treatment. *Pharmacoeconomics* 24(5):453-464.

KFF (The Henry J. Kaiser Family Foundation). 2011. *Total number of Medicare beneficiaries, 2011.* http://www.statehealthfacts.org/comparemaptable.jsp?ind=290&cat=6 (accessed January 4, 2012).

Klein, J. D., T. S. Sesselberg, M. S. Johnson, K. G. O'Connor, S. Cook, M. Coon, C. Homer, N. Krebs, and R. Washington. 2010. Adoption of body mass index guidelines for screening and counseling in pediatric practice. *Pediatrics* 125(2):265-272.

Krebs, N. F., and M. S. Jacobson. 2003. Prevention of pediatric overweight and obesity. *Pediatrics* 112(2):424-430.

Kuczmarski, R. J., C. L. Ogden, S. S. Guo, L. M. Grummer-Strawn, K. M. Flegal, Z. Mei, R. Wei, L. R. Curtin, A. F. Roche, and C. L. Johnson. 2002. 2000 CDC growth charts for the United States: Methods and development. *Vital and Health Statistics. Series 11: Data from the National Health Survey* (246):1-190.

Larsen, L., B. Mandleco, M. Williams, and M. Tiedeman. 2006. Childhood obesity: Prevention practices of nurse practitioners. *Journal of the American Academy of Nurse Practitioners* 18(2):70-79.

Let's Move. 2011. *Take action healthcare providers.* http://www.letsmove.gov/health-care-providers (accessed September 19, 2011).

Li, R., S. B. Fein, and L. M. Grummer-Strawn. 2008. Association of breastfeeding intensity and bottle-emptying behaviors at early infancy with infants' risk for excess weight at late infancy. *Pediatrics* 122(Suppl. 2):S77-S84.

Li, R., S. B. Fein, and L. M. Grummer-Strawn. 2010. Do infants fed from bottles lack self-regulation of milk intake compared with directly breastfed infants? *Pediatrics* 125(6):e1386-e1393.

Lucas, A., S. Boyes, S. R. Bloom, and A. Aynsley-Green. 1981. Metabolic and endocrine responses to a milk feed in six-day-old term infants: Differences between breast and cow's milk formula feeding. *Acta Paediatrica Scandinavica* 70(2):195-200.

Lyznicki, J. M., D. C. Young, J. A. Riggs, and R. M. Davis. 2001. Obesity: Assessment and management in primary care. *American Family Physician* 63(11):2185-2196.

Manco, M., A. Alterio, E. Bugianesi, P. Ciampalini, P. Mariani, M. Finocchi, C. Agostoni, and V. Nobili. 2011. Insulin dynamics of breast- or formula-fed overweight and obese children. *Journal of the American College of Nutrition* 30(1):29-38.

Martinez, M. E., and R. A. Cohen. 2011. *Health insurance coverage: Early release of estimates from the national health interview survey, January-June 2011*. National Center for Health Statistics. http://www.cdc.gov/nchs/nhis/releases.htm (accessed December 16, 2011).

Mello, M. M., and M. B. Rosenthal. 2008. Wellness programs and lifestyle discrimination—the legal limits. *New England Journal of Medicine* 359(2):192-199.

Merewood, A., S. D. Mehta, L. B. Chamberlain, B. L. Philipp, and H. Bauchner. 2005. Breastfeeding rates in US baby-friendly hospitals: Results of a national survey. *Pediatrics* 116(3):628-634.

Merrill, R. M., S. G. Aldana, T. P. Vyhlidal, G. Howe, D. R. Anderson, and R. W. Whitmer. 2011. The impact of worksite wellness in a small business setting. *Journal of Occupational and Environmental Medicine* 53(2):127-131.

Mihrshahi, S., D. Battistutta, A. Magarey, and L. A. Daniels. 2011. Determinants of rapid weight gain during infancy: Baseline results from the NOURISH randomised controlled trial. *BMC Pediatrics* 11:99.

Monasta, L., G. D. Batty, A. Cattaneo, V. Lutje, L. Ronfani, F. J. Van Lenthe, and J. Brug. 2010. Early-life determinants of overweight and obesity: A review of systematic reviews. *Obesity Reviews* 11(10):695-708.

NASN (National Association of School Nurses). 2011. *S.C.O.P.E.—School Nurse Childhood Obesity Prevention Education*. http://www.nasn.org/continuingeducation/livecontinuingeducationprograms/scope (accessed November 11, 2011).

NDIC (National Diabetes Information Clearinghouse). 2008. *Diabetes prevention program*. http://diabetes.niddk.nih.gov/dm/pubs/preventionprogram/ (accessed January 4, 2012).

Oken, E., E. M. Taveras, K. P. Kleinman, J. W. Rich-Edwards, and M. W. Gillman. 2007. Gestational weight gain and child adiposity at age 3 years. *American Journal of Obstetrics and Gynecology* 196(4):e321-e328.

Owen, C. G., R. M. Martin, P. H. Whincup, G. D. Smith, and D. G. Cook. 2005. Effect of infant feeding on the risk of obesity across the life course: A quantitative review of published evidence. *Pediatrics* 115(5):1367-1377.

Pelletier, K. R. 2005. A review and analysis of the clinical and cost-effectiveness studies of comprehensive health promotion and disease management programs at the worksite: Update VI 2000-2004. *Journal of Occupational and Environmental Medicine* 47(10):1051-1058.

Perez-Escamilla, R. 2007. Evidence based breast-feeding promotion: The baby-friendly hospital initiative. *Journal of Nutrition* 137(2):484-487.

Perrin, E. M., J. C. Jacobson Vann, J. T. Benjamin, A. C. Skinner, S. Wegner, and A. S. Ammerman. 2010. Use of a pediatrician toolkit to address parental perception of children's weight status, nutrition, and activity behaviors. *Academic Pediatrics* 10(4):274-281.

Preis, S. R., M. J. Pencina, S. J. Hwang, R. B. D'Agostino, Sr., P. J. Savage, D. Levy, and C. S. Fox. 2009. Trends in cardiovascular disease risk factors in individuals with and without diabetes mellitus in the Framingham Heart Study. *Circulation* 120(3):212-220.

Prevention Institute. 2008. *Promising strategies for creating healthy eating and active living environments.* http://www.convergencepartnership.org/atf/cf/%7B245A9B44-6DED-4ABD-A392-AE583809E350%7D/CP_Promising%20Strategies_printed.pdf (accessed July 7, 2011).

Quintiliani, L., J. Sattelmair, and G. Sorensen. 2007. *The workplace as a setting for interventions to improve diet and promote physical activity: Background paper prepared for the WHO/WEF joint event on preventing noncommunicable diseases in the workplace.* Geneva, Switzerland: WHO.

Raulio, S., E. Roos and R. Prattala. 2010. School and workplace meals promote healthy food habits. *Public Health Nutrition* 13(6A):987-992.

Romney, M. C., E. Thomson, and K. Kash. 2011. Population-based worksite obesity management interventions: A qualitative case study. *Population Health Management* 14(3):127-132.

RWJF (Robert Wood Johnson Foundation). 2007. *Newsroom: Foundation makes major commitment to combat childhood obesity.* http://www.rwjf.org/newsroom/product.jsp?id=22117 (accessed August 15, 2011).

Schmied, V., S. Beake, A. Sheehan, C. McCourt, and F. Dykes. 2011. Women's perceptions and experiences of breastfeeding support: A metasynthesis. *Birth* 38(1):49-60.

Schmier, J. K., M. L. Jones, and M. T. Halpern. 2006. Cost of obesity in the workplace. *Scandinavian Journal of Work, Environment and Health* 32(1):5-11.

Schulte, P. A., G. R. Wagner, A. Ostry, L. A. Blanciforti, R. G. Cutlip, K. M. Krajnak, M. Luster, A. E. Munson, J. P. O'Callaghan, C. G. Parks, P. P. Simeonova, and

D. B. Miller. 2007. Work, obesity, and occupational safety and health. *American Journal of Public Health* 97(3):428-436.

Schulte, P. A., G. R. Wagner, A. Downes, and D. B. Miller. 2008. A framework for the concurrent consideration of occupational hazards and obesity. *Annals of Occupational Hygiene* 52(7):555-566.

Sesselberg, T. S., J. D. Klein, K. G. O'Connor, and M. S. Johnson. 2010. Screening and counseling for childhood obesity: Results from a national survey. *Journal of the American Board of Family Medicine* 23(3):334-342.

Shealy, K. R., R. Li, S. Benton-Davis, and L. Grummer-Strawn. 2005. *The CDC guide to breastfeeding interventions.* http://www.cdc.gov/breastfeeding/pdf/breastfeeding_interventions.pdf (accessed November 4, 2011).

Simpson, L. A., and J. Cooper. 2009. Paying for obesity: A changing landscape. *Pediatrics* 123(Suppl. 5):S301-S307.

Singhal, A., I. S. Farooqi, S. O'Rahilly, T. J. Cole, M. Fewtrell, and A. Lucas. 2002. Early nutrition and leptin concentrations in later life. *American Journal of Clinical Nutrition* 75(6):993-999.

Smith, A. W., L. A. Borowski, B. Liu, D. A. Galuska, C. Signore, C. Klabunde, T. T. Huang, S. M. Krebs-Smith, E. Frank, N. Pronk, and R. Ballard-Barbash. 2011. U.S. Primary care physicians' diet-, physical activity-, and weight-related care of adult patients. *American Journal of Preventive Medicine* 41(1):33-42.

Stoltzfus, E. R. 2009. *Access to wellness and employee assistance programs in the United States.* http://www.bls.gov/opub/cwc/cm20090416ar01p1.htm (accessed February 2, 2012).

Strasburger, V. C. 2011. Children, adolescents, obesity, and the media. *Pediatrics* 128(1):201-208.

Sumithran, P., L. A. Prendergast, E. Delbridge, K. Purcell, A. Shulkes, A. Kriketos, and J. Proietto. 2011. Long-term persistence of hormonal adaptations to weight loss. *New England Journal of Medicine* 365(17):1597-1604.

Texas Pediatric Society. 2008. *Texas Pediatric Society obesity toolkit.* http://txpeds.org/texas-pediatric-society-obesity-toolkit (accessed September 19, 2011).

Thorpe, K. E., C. S. Florence, D. H. Howard, and P. Joski. 2004. The impact of obesity on rising medical spending. *Health Affairs* Suppl. Web Exclusives W4-480-486.

Trogdon, J. G., E. A. Finkelstein, T. Hylands, P. S. Dellea, and S. J. Kamal-Bahl. 2008. Indirect costs of obesity: A review of the current literature. *Obesity Reviews* 9(5):489-500.

Tsai, A. G., D. A. Asch, and T. A. Wadden. 2006. Insurance coverage for obesity treatment. *Journal of the American Dietetic Association* 106(10):1651-1655.

U.S. Department of Labor. 2011. *Wage and hour division (WHD): Breaktime for nursing mothers.* http://www.dol.gov/whd/nursingmothers/ (accessed November 4, 2011).

USDA/FNS (U.S. Department of Agriculture/Food and Nutrition Service). 2004. *Using loving support to implement best practices in peer counseling.* Tampa, FL: Best Start Social Marketing, Inc.

USDA/FNS. 2011. *Benefits and services: Breastfeeding promotion in WIC, current federal requirements.* http://www.fns.usda.gov/wic/Breastfeeding/mainpage.HTM (accessed August 3, 2011).

USPSTF (U.S. Preventive Service Task Force). 2010a. Screening for obesity in children and adolescents: US Preventive Services Task Force recommendation statement. *Pediatrics* 125(2):361-367.

USPSTF. 2010b. *USPSTF a and b recommendations.* http://www.uspreventiveservices-taskforce.org/uspstf/uspsabrecs.htm (accessed November 2, 2011).

van Rossem, L., E. M. Taveras, M. W. Gillman, K. P. Kleinman, S. L. Rifas-Shiman, H. Raat, and E. Oken. 2011. Is the association of breastfeeding with child obesity explained by infant weight change? *International Journal of Pediatric Obesity* 6(2-2):e415-e422.

Wen, L. M., M. De Domenico, D. Elliott, J. Bindon, and C. Rissel. 2009. Evaluation of a feasibility study addressing risk factors for childhood obesity through home visits. *Journal of Paediatrics and Child Health* 45(10):577-581.

Wethington, H. R., B. Sherry, and B. Polhamus. 2011. Physician practices related to use of BMI-for-age and counseling for childhood obesity prevention: A cross-sectional study. *BMC Family Practice* 12:80.

Whaley, S. E., K. Meehan, L. Lange, W. Slusser, and E. Jenks. 2002. Predictors of breast-feeding duration for employees of the special supplemental nutrition program for women, infants, and children (WIC). *Journal of the American Dietetic Association* 102(9):1290-1293.

Whitaker, R. C., J. A. Wright, M. S. Pepe, K. D. Seidel, and W. H. Dietz. 1997. Predicting obesity in young adulthood from childhood and parental obesity. *New England Journal of Medicine* 337(13):869-873.

White House Task Force on Childhood Obesity. 2010. *Report to the President: Solving the problem of childhood obesity within a generation.* http://www.letsmove.gov/sites/letsmove.gov/files/TaskForce_on_Childhood_Obesity_May2010_FullReport.pdf (accessed October 26, 2011).

WHO/UNICEF (World Health Organization/United Nations Children's Fund). 1989. *Protecting, promoting and supporting breast-feeding: The special role of maternity services.* Geneva, Switzerland: WHO.

Young, P. C., S. DeBry, W. D. Jackson, J. Metos, E. Joy, M. Templeman, and C. Norlin. 2010. Improving the prevention, early recognition, and treatment of pediatric obesity by primary care physicians. *Clinical Pediatrics* 49(10):964-969.

9

School Environments

School Environments:
Goal, Recommendation, Strategies, and Actions for
Implementation

Goal: Make schools a national focal point for obesity
prevention.

Recommendation 5: Federal, state, and local government
and education authorities, with support from parents,
teachers, and the business community and the private
sector, should make schools a focal point for obesity
prevention.

Strategy 5-1: Require quality physical education and opportunities for
physical activity in schools. Through support from federal and state governments, state and local education agencies and local school districts should
ensure that all students in grades K-12 have adequate opportunities to engage
in 60 minutes of physical activity per school day. This 60-minute goal includes
access to and participation in quality physical education.

For **Congress**, potential actions include

*   strengthening the local wellness policy requirement in Section 204 of the
    Healthy, Hunger-Free Kids Act of 2010 (Public Law 111-296, 111th Cong.,

2d sess. [December 13, 2010] 124, 3183) or the *Elementary and Secondary Education Act* (Public Law 89-10, 89th Cong., 1st sess. [April 11, 1965] 27, 20) by including a requirement for local education agencies to develop and implement a K-12 quality physical education curriculum with proficiency assessments.

For **state legislatures and departments of education,** potential actions include

- enacting policies with appropriate funding to ensure the provision of daily quality physical education at school for all students in grades K-12; and

- developing, requiring, and financially supporting the implementation of K-12 curriculum standards for quality physical education that (1) are aligned with guidance from practice and/or professional associations and appropriate instructional practice guidelines, and (2) ensure that at least 50 percent of class time is spent in vigorous or moderate-intensity physical activity.

For **local education agencies,** potential actions include

- adopting requirements that include opportunities for daily physical activity outside of physical education, such as active transport to school programs, intramural sports and activity programs, active recess, classroom breaks, after-school physical activity programming, and integration of physical activity into curricula lesson plans.

For **local school districts,** potential actions include

- improving and maintaining an environment that is conducive to safe physical education and physical activity.

Strategy 5-2: Ensure strong nutritional standards for all foods and beverages sold or provided through schools. All government agencies (federal, state, local, and school district) providing foods and beverages to children and adolescents have a responsibility to provide those in their care with foods and beverages that promote health and learning. The Dietary Guidelines for Americans provide specific science-based recommendations for optimizing dietary intake to prevent disease and promote health. Implementation of these guidelines would shift children's and adolescents' dietary intake to prevent obesity and risk factors associated with chronic disease risk by increasing the amounts of fruits, vegetables, and high-fiber grains they consume; decreasing their consumption of sugar-sweetened beverages, dietary fat in general, solid fats, and added sugars; and ensuring age-appropriate portion sizes of meals and other foods and beverages. Federal, state, and local decision makers are responsible for ensuring that nutrition standards based on the Dietary Guidelines are adopted by schools; these decision makers, in partnership with regulatory agencies, parents, teachers, and food manufacturers, also are responsible for ensuring that these standards are implemented fully and that adherence is monitored so as to protect the health of the nation's children and adolescents.

For the **U.S. Department of Agriculture (USDA),** potential actions include

- adopting nutrition standards for all federal child nutrition programs (i.e., the School Breakfast, National School Lunch, Afterschool Snack, Summer Food Service, and Special Milk programs) that are aligned with guidance on optimal nutrition; and

- adopting nutrition standards for all snacks and beverages sold/served outside of federal child nutrition programs that are aligned with guidance on optimal nutrition.

For **state legislatures and departments of education,** potential actions include

- adopting nutrition standards for foods sold/served outside of federal child nutrition programs that are aligned with guidance on optimal nutrition.

For **school boards and state departments of education,** potential actions include

- developing school district policies (including wellness policies for districts participating in federal child nutrition programs) and related regulations that include nutrition standards for foods sold/served outside of the federal programs that are aligned with guidance on optimal nutrition.

Strategy 5-3: Ensure food literacy, including skill development, in schools. Through leadership and guidance from federal and state governments, state and local education agencies should ensure the implementation and monitoring of sequential food literacy and nutrition science education, spanning grades K-12, based on the food and nutrition recommendations in the Dietary Guidelines for Americans.

For the **federal government,** potential actions include

- USDA developing K-12 food and nutrition curriculum guides that can be used by states and updating information in these guides as appropriate with each periodic revision of the Dietary Guidelines for Americans; and

- as USDA develops regulations to implement Section 204 of the *Healthy, Hunger-Free Kids Act of 2010* (Public Law 111-296, December 13, 2010), including a requirement for local education agencies to adopt and implement a K-12 food and nutrition curriculum based on state and federal guidance.

For **states, state legislatures, and departments of education,** potential actions include

- state legislatures and departments of education adopting, requiring, and financially supporting K-12 standards for food and nutrition curriculum based on USDA guidance;

- state departments of education establishing requirements for training teachers in effectively incorporating nutrition education into their curricula;

- states requiring teacher training programs to include curriculum requirements for the study of nutrition;

- state legislatures and departments of education adopting and requiring proficiency assessments for core elements of their state food and nutrition curriculum standards in accordance with the Common Core State Standards Initiative, and local education agency wellness policies articulating ways in which results of food and nutrition education proficiency assessments can be used to inform program improvement; and

- state and local departments of education working with local education agency wellness policies to link changes in the meals provided through child nutrition services with the food literacy and nutrition education curriculum to the extent possible.

Schools are uniquely positioned to support physical activity and healthy eating and therefore can serve as a focal point for obesity prevention among children and adolescents. Schools can be leaders in reversing trends that have made a physically active lifestyle more difficult and high-calorie, nutrient-poor foods more accessible. Children spend up to half of their waking hours in school. In an increasingly sedentary world, schools therefore provide the best opportunity for a population-based approach to increasing physical activity among the nation's youth. Likewise, because children and adolescents consume up to one-third or even one-half of their daily calories in school, schools have a unique opportunity to influence the quality of their diets.

The mission of schools is broader than simply teaching academic skills. Schools have an acknowledged responsibility for supporting the health and well-being of their students, for example, by requiring immunizations, providing health screenings, and offering meal programs that support a healthy diet. Both physical activity and a nutritious diet are associated with improved cognitive function and academic performance. Physically active and well-nourished students are better able to learn and less likely to miss school for health reasons (Florence et al., 2008; Taras, 2005a; Trudeau and Shepherd, 2010). Improvements in school physical activity and nutrition also will address social inequities, enabling children and adolescents with the fewest resources to have improved opportunities to become productive citizens.

RECOMMENDATION 5

Federal, state, and local government and education authorities, with support from parents, teachers, and the business community and the private sector, should make schools a focal point for obesity prevention.

School environments are interrelated with the other areas of focus addressed in this report, such as the physical activity and food and beverage environments, discussed in earlier chapters (see Figure 9-1). For example, schools not only provide physical education and serve foods and beverages to students, but also serve as powerful role models, providing a culture that can support, rather than undermine, the efforts of children and adolescents and parents to promote healthful living. As powerful influences, school food-related policies have been shown to affect not only what students consume at school but also what they and their parents perceive to be healthy choices. Immigrant families in particular look to public institutions to learn about cultural norms and practices (Gordon-Larsen et al., 2003). As far back as 1946, a report of the House Committee on Agriculture during hearings for the *National School Lunch Act*[1] stated that "the educational features of a properly chosen diet served at school should not be under-emphasized. Not only is the child taught what a good diet consists of, but his parents and family likewise are indirectly instructed."

Structuring school environments to encourage and support physical activity and healthy living offers a unique opportunity to reach nearly all children and adolescents, promoting their health both today and in the future, as lifelong health habits are initiated early in life. Today, the role of the school is more important than ever as fewer families have a parent at home who is not participating in the paid labor force, and children and adolescents are spending more time in before- and after-school programs outside of the home.

The *Healthy, Hunger-Free Kids Act of 2010*[2] created an opportunity to improve nutrition for students in the school setting. Recent efforts to change school physical education and food policies have been well received, but they are neither widespread, integrated, nor strong enough to produce the needed reduc-

---

[1]Public Law 396, 79th Cong., 2d sess. (June 4, 1976), 60, 231.
[2]Public Law 111-296, 111th Cong., 2d sess. (December 13, 2010), 124, 3183.

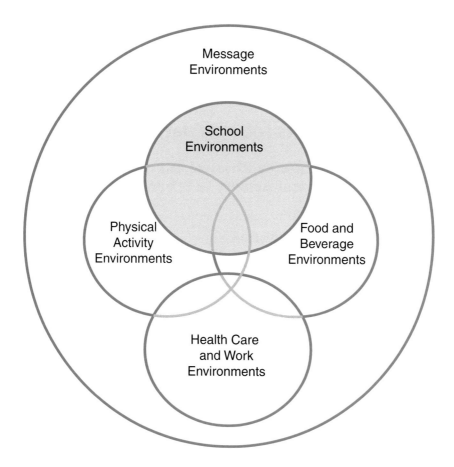

FIGURE 9-1 Five areas of focus of the Committee on Accelerating Progress in Obesity Prevention.
NOTE: The area addressed in this chapter is highlighted.

tion in childhood obesity rates. The committee recommends three strategies and associated actions to address these limitations. These strategies and actions are detailed in the remainder of this chapter. Indicators for measuring progress toward the implementation of each strategy, organized according to the scheme presented in Chapter 4 (primary, process, foundational), are presented in a box following the discussion of that strategy.

The strategies in this chapter are focused on school-aged children because of the broad reach of schools to children and adolescents. Early childhood education is not nationalized, nor is there sufficient evidence for all of the strategies presented in this chapter as applied to preschools to recommend all of them for younger children. The committee recognizes that the earlier years are critical times to promote children's health and has offered recommendations for physical activity in child care centers (Chapter 5, Strategy 1-3) and nutrition standards for government-owned and/or -operated child care centers (Chapter 6, Strategy 2-3).

STRATEGIES AND ACTIONS FOR IMPLEMENTATION

Strategy 5-1: Require Quality Physical Education and Opportunities for Physical Activity in Schools

Through support from federal and state governments, state and local education agencies and local school districts should ensure that all students in grades K-12 have adequate opportunities to engage in 60 minutes of physical activity per school day. This 60-minute goal includes access to and participation in quality physical education.

For **Congress,** potential actions include

- strengthening the local wellness policy requirement in Section 204 of the *Healthy, Hunger-Free Kids Act of 2010* (Public Law 111-296, December 13, 2010) or the *Elementary and Secondary Education Act* (Public Law 89-10, 89th Cong., 1st sess. [April 11, 1965] 27, 20) by including a requirement for local education agencies to develop and implement a K-12 quality physical education curriculum with proficiency assessments.

For **state legislatures and departments of education,** potential actions include

- enacting policies with appropriate funding to ensure the provision of daily quality physical education at school for all students in grades K-12; and
- developing, requiring, and financially supporting the implementation of K-12 curriculum standards for quality physical education that (1) are aligned with guidance from practice and/or professional associations and appropriate instructional practice guidelines, and (2) ensure that at least 50 percent of class time is spent in vigorous or moderate-intensity physical activity.

For **local education agencies,** potential actions include

- adopting requirements that include opportunities for daily physical activity outside of physical education, such as active transport to school programs, intramural sports and activity programs, active recess, classroom breaks, after-school physical activity programming, and integration of physical activity into curricula lesson plans.

For **local school districts,** potential actions include

- improving and maintaining an environment that is conducive to safe physical education and physical activity.

Context

Data from the 2006 School Health Policies and Programs Study (Lee et al., 2007) indicate that nationwide, 78 percent of schools require students to take some physical education as a requirement for graduation or promotion to the next grade or school level (69 percent of elementary schools, 84 percent of middle schools, and 95 percent of high schools). The frequency and length of activity breaks, opportunities for physical education, and adherence to expert guidance and assessment in implementing these requirements vary widely by school district, state, and grade level.

A small number of schools provide physical education opportunities at all grade levels every day or even a few days a week. In 2006, nearly 4 percent of all elementary schools (excluding kindergarten), 8 percent of all middle schools, and 2 percent of all high schools provided daily physical education or its equivalent for the entire school year for students in all grades. More schools provide physical education or its equivalent at least 3 days per week for the entire school year— almost 14 percent of elementary schools (excluding kindergarten), 15 percent of middle schools, and 3 percent of high schools (Lee et al., 2007).

Apart from physical education opportunities, the number and length of physical activity breaks required throughout the school day vary by state, district, and grade. Among all school districts, 39 percent require or recommend 30 minutes or more of recess per day, 23 percent require or recommend 20-29 minutes per day, and 16 percent require or recommend 10-19 minutes per day in elementary schools. Among all districts, 16 percent require and 25 percent recommend that elementary schools provide regular physical activity breaks; 10 percent of all districts require and 24 percent recommend that middle schools provide such breaks; and 4 percent of all districts require and 9 percent recommend that high schools provide such breaks (Lee et al., 2007). Among all states, 14 percent have a policy encouraging districts or schools to support or promote walking or biking to and from school, and nearly 18 percent of all districts have a policy that supports or promotes walking or biking to and from school.

Significant improvement has been seen in state and district policies to follow expert guidelines in implementing physical education policies. Between 2000 and 2006, the percentage of states that required or encouraged districts or schools to follow standards or guidelines based on the National Standards for Physical Education increased from 59 percent to 76 percent. In addition, the percentage of districts with a policy stating that schools must follow national, state, or district physical education standards or guidelines increased from 67 percent to 81 percent (Lee et al., 2007).

Finally, state assessment and graduation proficiency requirements for physical education are limited. The 2010 Shape of the Nation report (NASPE and AHA, 2010) found that 27 percent of states require that grades be given for physical education classes, but few include physical education in comprehensive assessment tests, if given. Of the 40 states that have an education "report card" for schools, only 5 include physical education in that report. Of the 45 states that require high school physical education, 75 percent specify the number of credits needed for graduation (12 states require 0.5 credit; 15 states require 1 credit; 3 states require 1.5 credits; 7 states requires 2 credits; and New Jersey requires 3.75 credits per year, the highest in the nation). In addition, 9 states require a health or wellness course to fulfill graduation requirements. Physical education is required only in grades K-12 in five states (Illinois, Iowa, Massachusetts, New Mexico, and Vermont) and is required in grades 1-12 in two states (New Jersey and Rhode Island).

The inconsistencies in frequency, duration, assessments, and requirements for physical education and opportunities for physical activity breaks throughout the day indicate that states and local education agencies can improve policies to help students achieve 60 minutes of physical activity per day.

Evidence

The 2005 Institute of Medicine (IOM) report *Preventing Childhood Obesity: Health in the Balance* recommends that children and adolescents participate in a minimum of 30 minutes of physical activity during the school day and that opportunities for physical activity and physical education be expanded. In addition, the report recommends that health curricula be enhanced to devote adequate attention to physical activity, reducing sedentary behaviors, nutrition, and energy balance, with a focus on behavioral skills (IOM, 2005). Many of these recommendations were based on a systematic review of the effectiveness of increasing the amount of time students spend in physical education, as well as large-scale school-based interventions that have been successful in increasing activity levels. Likewise, the Task Force on Community Preventive Services concluded that there is strong evidence that school-based physical education increases levels of physical activity, although evidence indicates minimal or inconsistent effects on body mass index (BMI) (Kahn et al., 2002). Another review found that two elementary school-based interventions—SPARK (Sports, Play, and Active Recreation for Kids) and CATCH (Coordinated Approach To Child Health)—and a small number of interventions involving older students were effective in increasing activity levels, with some interventions being associated with positive improvements in BMI (IOM, 2005). Reviews also have concluded that attending longer physical education classes did not affect academic performance (Kahn et al., 2002).

Schools' interest in physical activity begins with the brain (Trudeau and Shepherd, 2010). Movement and exercise increase breathing and heart rate so that more blood flows to the brain, thus enhancing energy production and waste removal. Physical activity oxygenates the brain, which is why taking a walk can help people "clear their head" and think better. Exercise has effects as well on higher mental executive functions involving memory, planning, organization, and the capability to juggle different intellectual tasks (Sibley and Etnier, 2003). Exercise also helps youth who have difficulty with impulse control (Kelder, 2010). A recent meta-analysis studying the impact of combinations of school-based interventions focused on increasing physical activity among children and adolescents aged 6-18 found "good evidence that school-based physical activity interventions have a positive impact on" duration of physical activity, television viewing, VO$_2$ max,[3] and blood cholesterol (Dobbins et al., 2009, p. 24). The authors also report that, in addition to the positive outcomes they studied, "the current evidence suggests that school-based physical activity interventions may be effective in the development of healthy lifestyle behaviors among children and adolescents, which will then translate into reduced risk for many chronic diseases and cancers in adulthood. The evidence also suggests that the best primary strategy for improving the long-term health of children and adolescents through exercise may be creating lifestyle patterns of regular physical activity that carry over to the adult years" (Dobbins et al., 2009, p. 2).

---

[3] Maximal oxygen uptake.

Mounting evidence shows a positive relationship between physical activity and academic performance. A systematic review of observational and longitudinal studies (Singh et al., 2012) suggests that there is a significant positive relationship between physical activity and academic performance, although just 2 of the 14 studies included in the review were judged as being of "high methodological quality." Nonetheless, this cautious conclusion was supported by two earlier reviews (Taras, 2005b; Trudeau and Shephard, 2008). A Centers for Disease Control and Prevention (CDC) synthesis of the literature on the association between school-based physical activity (including physical education, recess, classroom physical activity, and extracurricular physical activity) and academic performance (based on measures of academic achievement, academic behavior, and cognitive skills and attitudes) (CDC, 2010b) found 251 associations between the two. Of these, 50.5 percent were positive, 48 percent were not significant, and 1.5 percent were negative. In the context of school-based physical education, the available studies (n = 14) show that overall, increased time in physical education appears to have a positive or no relationship with academic achievement, and not a negative relationship. A review by Woodward-Lopez and colleagues (2010a) reports that physical activity is critical for optimal brain function and the ability to learn; positively influences academic performance; and can improve classroom behavior, attendance, and students' psychological well-being.

Implementation

It is important to encourage young people to participate in physical activities that are appropriate for their age, that are enjoyable, and that offer a wide variety of options. The focus at schools for decades has been on physical education and after-school extracurricular activities and sports. As described earlier, current district and state physical education policies and programs vary nationwide. At the national level, the *Healthy, Hunger-Free Kids Act of 2010*[4] requires, at a minimum, that goals for physical activity be included in all school wellness policies. The 1965 *Elementary and Secondary Education Act*,[5] which provides support for the development and improvement of physical education programs in schools, offers opportunities to encourage the development and adoption of consistent quality physical education at all grade levels across the country.

General physical education opportunities and after-school activities and sports usually are guided by a qualified instructor or coach. However, this is not always

---

[4]Public Law 111-296 (December 13, 2010).
[5]Public Law 89-10 (April 13, 1965).

the case. Noncurricular programs can contribute to increases in the frequency (daily), duration (60+ minutes), and intensity (vigorous or moderate or weight bearing) of activity (Kelder, 2010). A number of noncurricular physical activity strategies have been reviewed and are recommended as promising ways to increase physical activity throughout the school day (California Project LEAN, 2009; Jago and Baranowski, 2004; NASPE, undated). As reviewed by Kelder (2010, pp. 30-34), these evidence-based strategies include

- daily classroom physical activity breaks,
- organized physical activity during after-school programs,
- walking trails and active commuting (i.e., walking or biking) to/from school,
- access to the kind of equipment found in fitness clubs at school,
- walking programs or "open gym" in the morning before school begins,
- intramural sport teams for students not interested in competitive sports,
- evening events that provide a safe place for students to play, and
- annual campus or community events to heighten community awareness of physical activity and health.

Additionally, redesigned and renovated school playgrounds have been found to increase overall playground utilization and improve the physical activity levels of children and adults during school as well as after-school hours (Anthamatten et al., 2011; Brink et al., 2010; Colabianci et al., 2009; Ridgers et al., 2007). Combining quality physical education curriculum standards (i.e., guidelines of the National Standards for Physical Education) and proficiency assessments guided by professional experts with such additional noncurriculum opportunities for physical activity (before, during, and after school) will be necessary to help students achieve the recommended activity levels (i.e., 60 or more minutes of physical activity each day) and create a lifestyle pattern that will continue into their adult lives. Although these quality standards may pose a challenge given core curriculum requirements, combining physical education time with noncurricular physical activity strategies is a critical step in ensuring that children receive the recommended 60 minutes of daily physical activity and should be the goal for all schools.

Indicators for Assessing Progress in Obesity Prevention for Strategy 5-1

Primary Indicator

- Increase in the prevalence of children and adolescents meeting physical activity guidelines of 60 minutes per day of vigorous or moderate-intensity physical activity.*
  Sources for measuring indicator: YRBSS and NHANES (additional sources needed for measurement of indicator)

Process Indicators

- Increase in the proportion of school-aged children and adolescents enrolled in school physical education.
  Sources for measuring indicator: YRBSS and NYPANS (additional sources needed for measurement of indicator)

- Increase in the proportion of states with policies requiring that at least 50 percent of physical education time be spent in vigorous or moderate-intensity physical activity for each grade level.
  Sources for measuring indicator: CLASS (NCI), CDC's State School Health Profiles, CDC's School Health Policies and Programs Study

- Increase in the proportion of districts with policies requiring that at least 50 percent of physical education time be spent in vigorous or moderate-intensity physical activity for each grade level.
  Sources for measuring indicator: CDC's School Health Policy and Programs Study and Bridging the Gap District Wellness Policy Study

- Increase in the proportion of schools with policies requiring that at least 50 percent of physical education time be spent in vigorous or moderate-intensity physical activity for each grade level.
  Source for measuring indicator: CDC's School Health Policy and Programs Study

- Increase in the proportion of schools providing opportunities for school-based physical activity outside of physical education.
  Source for measuring indicator: CDC's School Health Policy and Programs Study

Foundational Indicators

- Increase in the frequency of CDC's School Health Policy and Programs Study to every 2 years.
  Source needed for measurement of indicator.

- Increase in the frequency of CDC's National Youth Physical Activity and Nutrition Survey to every 2 years.
  Source needed for measurement of indicator.

- Development of monitoring systems to capture objectively measured and context-specific data on participation in physical activity for all grade levels.
  Source needed for measurement of indicator.

NOTE: CDC = Centers for Disease Control and Prevention; CLASS = Classification of Laws Associated with School Students; NCI = National Cancer Institute; NHANES = National Health and Nutrition Examination Survey; NYPANS = National Youth Physical Activity and Nutrition Survey; YRBSS = Youth Risk Behavior Surveillance System.

---

*See Box B-1 in Appendix B.

Strategy 5-2: Ensure Strong Nutritional Standards for All Foods and Beverages Sold or Provided Through Schools

All government agencies (federal, state, local, and school district) providing foods and beverages to children and adolescents have a responsibility to provide those in their care with foods and beverages that promote health and learning. The Dietary Guidelines for Americans provide specific science-based recommendations for optimizing dietary intake to prevent disease and promote health. Implementation of these guidelines would shift children's and adolescents' dietary intake to prevent obesity and risk factors associated with chronic disease risk by increasing the amounts of fruits, vegetables, and high-fiber grains they consume; decreasing their consumption of sugar-sweetened beverages, dietary fat in general, solid fats, and added sugars; and ensuring age-appropriate portion sizes of meals and other foods and beverages. Federal, state, and local decision makers are responsible for ensuring that nutrition standards based on the Dietary Guidelines are adopted by schools; these decision makers, in partnership with regulatory agencies, parents, teachers, and food manufacturers, also are responsible for ensuring that these standards are implemented fully and that adherence is monitored so as to protect the health of the nation's children and adolescents.

For the **U.S. Department of Agriculture (USDA),** potential actions include

- adopting nutrition standards for all federal child nutrition programs (i.e., the School Breakfast, National School Lunch, Afterschool Snack, Summer Food Service, and Special Milk programs) that are aligned with guidance on optimal nutrition; and
- adopting nutrition standards for all snacks and beverages sold/served outside of federal child nutrition programs that are aligned with guidance on optimal nutrition.

For **state legislatures and departments of education,** potential actions include

- adopting nutrition standards for foods sold/served outside of federal child nutrition programs that are aligned with guidance on optimal nutrition.

For **school boards and state departments of education,** potential actions include

- developing school district policies (including wellness policies for districts participating in federal child nutrition programs) and related regulations that include nutrition standards for foods sold/served outside of the federal programs that are aligned with guidance on optimal nutrition.

Context

The relationship between access to healthy foods and dietary behaviors is well established (Larson et al., 2009; see also Chapter 6). Studies demonstrate that individuals with access to a greater abundance of healthy foods consume more fresh produce and other healthful items, and individuals with less access to these foods are less likely to eat a healthy diet (Treuhaft and Karpyn, 2010). Those institutions entrusted with caring for the nation's children and adolescents have an opportunity to provide food options for children and adolescents that will not promote obesity and compromise their health, but promote their health and learning.

Numerous government agencies at the federal, state, and local levels provide foods served to children and adolescents in schools. These agencies contribute financial and/or material resources to feed children and adolescents in schools, in after-school programs, and in summer feeding programs. Because of the scale of these programs, they are a critical partner in efforts to prevent obesity. The foods provided in school settings serve two purposes: nourishing children and adolescents, and educating them and their parents about healthy dietary patterns. "If a school's setting is intended to be a learning environment for children, the issue [of] healthful food choices needs to be a priority" (Pilant, 2006, p. 125). Currently, schools must offer meals consistent with the National School Lunch and Child Nutrition Act Amendments.[6] These regulations require that school meals provide a minimum percentage of the Recommended Dietary Allowances (RDAs) to protect against nutritional deficiencies that would impair children's growth and development.

Both the National School Lunch Program and the original national RDAs were created to foster the nutritional health of America's youth during the decade of World War II. Guidance on kinds and amounts of foods to be provided at each meal was institutionalized. In the decades that followed, less nutritious foods outside of the meal program began being sold at schools, providing additional revenues for school groups or food service departments. Although disputes about providing foods with little nutritional value to compete with school meals arose, these foods, termed competitive foods, remained. As the body of evidence about the dietary crisis among children and adolescents in the United States grew, so, too, did understanding of the association between the diets of children and adoles-

---

[6]Public Law 94-105, 94th Cong., 1st sess. (October 7, 1975). Amendments: Public Law 95-166, 95th Cong., 1st sess. (November 10, 1977); Public Law 97-35, 97th Cong., 1st sess. (August 13, 1981); Public Law 99-591, 99th Cong., 1st sess. (October 30, 1986).

cents and not only nutritional deficiencies, but also health problems (IOM, 2005, 2007, 2010; NRC, 1989). In recognition of the importance of providing foods to children and adolescents that will promote their health and reduce their risk of obesity, the *Healthy, Hunger-Free Kids Act of 2010*[7] gave USDA the mandate to develop regulations governing all foods sold and served on school campuses, including foods and beverages sold outside of school meal programs.

The guidance on school food for the *Healthy, Hunger-Free Kids Act* is found in two IOM reports. The first, *Nutrition Standards for Foods in Schools: Leading the Way Toward Healthier Youth* (IOM, 2007), recommends that competitive foods offered on school campuses contribute to rather than compete with an overall healthful eating environment. Based on the nutrition evidence in the Dietary Guidelines for Americans, the report outlines specific food and nutrition standards for all foods and beverages sold in schools outside of school meal programs. Soon afterward, the IOM Committee on School Meals was tasked with reviewing and assessing the food and nutrition needs of school-aged children and adolescents using the most recent Dietary Guidelines in order to recommend updates to the guidance regarding the foods and beverages served in the National School Lunch and School Breakfast Programs (IOM, 2010). The recommendations in both of these reports serve as the foundation for current school food strategies to accelerate progress toward preventing obesity.

Given that school breakfast and lunch programs may account for more than half of a child's daily calorie intake (IOM, 2010), their dietary impact can be substantial. Further, as noted above, the potential reach of school-based nutrition interventions is unparalleled, extending to nearly all children and adolescents in the United States, including the most difficult-to-reach, underserved populations (IOM, 2010).

Evidence

The 2010 Dietary Guidelines for Americans provide evidence-based dietary recommendations encompassing two concepts: helping individuals achieve and maintain a healthy weight and focus on consuming nutrient-dense foods and beverages. They include the following:

- Individuals should prepare, serve, and consume smaller portions at home, and eat smaller portions while eating out.
- Consumption of fruits and vegetables should be increased in childhood.

[7]Public Law 111-296 (December 13, 2010).

- Children should consume recommended levels of low-fat and fat-free dairy products.
- Children should consume more and a greater variety of high-fiber foods.
- Total fat should not exceed IOM-recommended ranges and should consist of primarily mono- and polyunsaturated fatty acids.
- Consumption of sugar-sweetened beverages should be discouraged.
- The intake of surplus energy in the form of empty calories from added sugars and solid fats should be controlled.

The guidance provided in the two above-cited IOM reports addresses each of these recommendations. It identifies the amount of each food group (fruits, vegetables, whole grains, milk, meat and other protein foods, and oils) needed by children and adolescents in each age category, and recommends that competitive foods contribute to meeting these specific food requirements as well. Appendix 7 in the 2010 Dietary Guidelines for Americans shows recommended average daily intake amounts for each food group or subgroup at all calorie levels. The last three recommendations listed above are addressed in the 2005 Dietary Guidelines as discretionary calories (calories from any source that can be used flexibly after nutrient needs have been fulfilled) and in the 2010 Dietary Guidelines as solid fats and added sugars. The 2005 and 2010 Dietary Guidelines (HHS, 2005, 2010) recommend specific daily limits on the amounts of solid fats and added sugars in the diets of children and adolescents in accordance with health standards (see 2010 Dietary Guidelines, Appendix 7). Assuming that children and adolescents eat at least one-third of their calories during the school day, the limit on calories from added solid fats and added sugars obtained during the school day ranges from 40 calories for the 1,600-calorie/day plan, to 86 calories for the 2,000-calorie/day plan, to 110 calories for the 2,400-calorie/day plan. An understanding of the trade-off between snack foods and whole foods, including fruits, vegetables, whole grains, and protein foods, informs the standards for competitive foods. Snack foods and beverages sold in schools have been displacing the foods needed for a healthy diet. Both of the above-cited IOM reports (2007, 2010) are grounded in evidence demonstrating that school meals influence children's overall daily dietary intake (USDA, 2007).

There is evidence that nutrition standards for foods sold in schools can be implemented by schools, garner positive responses from students, and reduce students' intake of less healthy foods, and may be associated with reductions in children's BMI increases. Recent studies examining state and local implementation of nutrition standards have demonstrated that schools are able to comply with new food and beverage standards (Cullen and Watson, 2009; Long et al., 2010; Phillips et al., 2010; Woodward-Lopez et al., 2010b) and that students respond favorably to the provision of more healthy foods in school (Gosliner et al., 2011). Limiting access to the least healthy foods and beverages in schools has been shown to lead to a reduction in students' overall consumption of these items (Schwartz et al., 2009; Woodward-Lopez et al., 2010b). In addition to changes in the school food environment that impact children's dietary intake (CDC, 2010a; Cullen et al., 2008; Mendoza et al., 2010), there is evidence of an association, although not necessarily causal, between policies limiting competitive foods and beverages and a reduction in child BMI increases over the past 10 years (Sanchez-Vaznaugh et al., 2010).

There may be concern that reduced revenues from competitive foods (including those sold in vending machines) will adversely affect a school's financial status. Woodward-Lopez and colleagues (2010b) assessed the impact of legislation in California that instituted nutrition standards for competitive foods and beverages. They report a decrease in competitive food and beverage sales from vending machines, snack bars and stores, and school fundraisers. Although food service à la carte sales decreased by 60 percent, increases in meal sales increased enough to compensate for the reduction in à la carte sales and lead to an increase in total school food revenues. Overall, the school food service bottom line deteriorated because food service expenditures outpaced revenue increases during the time period under study, but the food service directors who were interviewed for the study did not believe the increased costs were attributable to their wellness efforts (Woodward-Lopez et al., 2010b). In Seattle, recent anecdotal evidence shows that revenues from vending machine sales sharply decreased when healthier items replaced other foods in response to a school policy, leaving high school-associated student body governments with less funding than before. School officials are considering new vending machine offerings that still meet the nutrition standards, but are expected to garner increased sales (Wood, 2011).

Implementation

Implementation of this strategy and associated actions will have to occur at the federal, state, and local (district) levels. Box 9-1 details additional actions that can be taken to implement this strategy.

Federal level With the adoption of the *Child Nutrition and WIC Reauthorization Act of 2004*,[8] USDA was given the mandate to propose new meal patterns and nutrition standards for foods served in the National School Lunch Program and School Breakfast Program to align them with the Dietary Guidelines for Americans. The *Healthy, Hunger-Free Kids Act of 2010*[9] specified that schools would receive an additional reimbursement of 6 cents for each meal served that adheres to the new standards. USDA issued proposed revisions (USDA/FNS, 2011) in line with the IOM recommendations for school meals (IOM, 2008, 2010), which generated approximately 130,000 comments. In January 2012, USDA issued a final rule for the nutrition standards (USDA/FNS, 2012).

Also with the adoption of the *Healthy, Hunger-Free Kids Act of 2010*,[10] USDA was given the mandate to regulate competitive foods and beverages sold in schools, which would include foods sold in à la carte lines in the cafeteria, vending machines, in snack bars and stores, and for fundraisers. At the time that this report went to press, USDA was gathering evidence on this issue and developing a proposed rule for public comment. The act does not preempt stronger standards at the state or district level, so the federal standards are expected to provide a floor rather than a ceiling.

State level The federal government can create broad policies designed to encourage schools to provide healthier foods, but it is up to state and local governments to implement those policies in ways that promote healthful eating. Currently, most states have standards for competitive foods and beverages, but they vary greatly and tend to be weak overall. Most state standards focus specifically on foods and beverages sold outside of school meal programs (i.e., competitive foods and beverages) and do not address foods/beverages sold or served during summer months or in before- and after-school settings. Implementation studies in states with relatively strong standards—Arkansas, California, and Texas, in particular—have shown positive impacts of these standards on food/beverage availability and consumption and net energy intake.

After Arkansas Act 1220 was implemented, annual surveys of principals and superintendents showed that schools were more likely to require healthy food options at student parties and concession stands and to offer skim milk in the cafeteria, and less likely to make vending machines available during lunch periods

---

[8]Public Law 108-265, 108th Cong., 2d sess. (June 30, 2004), 118, 729.
[9]Public Law 111-296 (December 13, 2010).
[10]Public Law 111-296 (December 13, 2010).

Additional Potential Actions for Implementing School Nutritional Standards Based on the Dietary Guidelines for Americans

Guideline 1: Increase the contribution of fruits, vegetables, whole grains, low-fat and fat-free milk and milk products, and protein foods to the diets of children and adolescents aged 2 and older.

For Congress:

- Support full implementation of the *Healthy, Hunger-Free Kids Act of 2010* (Public Law 11-296, December 13, 2010).

- Upwardly adjust meal reimbursement rates as necessary for full implementation of nutrition requirements.

For the U.S. Department of Agriculture (USDA) and other federal agencies:

- Implement school meal standards consistent with Institute of Medicine (IOM) recommendations.

- Adopt the strictest IOM recommendations for all foods and beverages sold/ provided outside of school meal programs to allow only foods that contribute to meeting the nutritional requirements of children and adolescents (fruits, vegetables, whole grains, low-fat and fat-free dairy products, and other protein foods) to ensure that less healthy foods and beverages do not compete with those foods.

- Require programs to monitor compliance with nutrition standards.

- Amend local wellness policies to include strategies that support the implementation of nutrition standards in school meal and competitive food venues.

For state legislatures and departments of education:

- Evaluate programs aimed at improving students' intake of the above foods to highlight innovations and barriers to implementation.

- Support federal standards for school meals and competitive foods.

- Create professional development modules to help school nutrition professionals implement nutrition standards.

For local school districts and schools:

- Adopt supportive policies that encourage schools to adhere to updated federal nutrition standards.

- Develop and distribute a resource list to help school groups raise money without selling foods that fail to meet nutrition standards.

- Allocate adequate space and other necessary resources for the procurement, provision, and preparation of foods that meet nutrition standards.

- Encourage the participation of students and parents in menu development and product selection so that foods served are appealing to the student population.

- Maintain active wellness policy councils to support healthy food environments.

Guideline 2: Reduce the percentage of total energy in the diets of children and adolescents derived from added sugars and solid fats (fat intake should come primarily from mono- and polyunsaturated fatty acids).

For Congress:

- Support full implementation of the *Healthy, Hunger-Free Kids Act of 2010* (Public Law 11-296, December 13, 2010).

continued

BOX 9-1
Continued

For USDA and federal agencies:

- Adopt the strictest interpretation of the IOM school meal and competitive food standards.

- Provide guidance to schools and the food and beverage industry regarding the importance of the new standards and how to implement them to ensure that calories from sugars and solid fats are replaced with healthier calories.

- Require programs to monitor compliance with nutrition standards.

- Amend local wellness policies to include strategies that support the implementation of nutrition standards in school meal and competitive food venues.

For state legislatures and departments of education:

- Promote adequate school funding and suggestions for alternative school fundraisers to reduce the need for food sales to support school groups and programs.

- Develop monitoring systems to ensure that child care and recreation programs sponsored by the state but not participating in the National School Lunch Program comply with standards limiting foods and beverages with added sugars and solid fats.

For local school districts and schools:

- Work with students to develop a selection of appealing foods and beverages that do not include items high in added sugars and solid fats.

- Implement the strictest interpretation of the IOM school meal and competitive food standards.

- Create budgets that do not rely on snack food and beverage sales to support important school programs.

Guideline 3: Ensure that portion sizes as served are age-appropriate for children and adolescents.

For Congress:

- Support implementation of the *Healthy, Hunger-Free Kids Act of 2010* (Public Law 11-296, December 13, 2010).

For USDA and federal agencies:

- Develop guidance that establishes adequate but not excessive food portions for children and adolescents. Include maximum allowances for calories in school meals.

For state legislatures and departments of education:

- Develop portion size standards for foods and beverages served to children and adolescents in programs not within the reach of the National School Lunch, School Breakfast, and Summer Food Service programs.

For local school districts and schools:

- Ensure that food service staff are trained in and knowledgeable about appropriate portion sizes for children and adolescents of various ages.

- Develop strategies for monitoring portion sizes and ensuring that they are consistent with recommendations for children and adolescents of various ages. These may include relatively simple strategies such as offering smaller portions, using smaller dishware, or removing trays from the school lunchroom (Fischer et al., 2003; Just and Wansink, 2009; Rolls et al., 2004; Wansink, 2010).

or to include sodas in vending machines (Phillips et al., 2010). Woodward-Lopez and colleagues (2010b) observed in California an increase in standards-compliant items, a decrease in noncompliant items, and a reduction in at-school consumption of noncompliant items without an increase in home consumption of those items. They called the improvements modest, recognizing that many compliant items were fat- and sugar-modified products of low nutritional value. And an evaluation of the Texas School Nutrition Policy, an unfunded mandate, showed that post-policy changes included significant reductions in high-fat vegetable items served by school cafeterias and sales of large bags of chips at snack bars, and increases in sales of baked chips (Cullen and Watson, 2009).

A difference between adherence to nutrition standards for beverages and to nutrition standards for foods has been observed, and there are a number of possible reasons for this inconsistency. Samuels and colleagues (2009), Wood and colleagues (2010), and Woodward-Lopez and colleagues (2010b) explain that the way standards are written may make it easier to identify beverages that meet standards than foods that do so. A California policy specifies categories of compliant beverages (e.g., water, sports drinks, or milk with a certain fat percentage), but for foods, specifies nutrient limits instead of categories. Thus, determining whether a food is compliant requires multiple calculations to determine whether the amounts of calories, saturated fat, and other nutrients are compliant. Samuels and colleagues (2009) suggest that specifying compliant categories of foods would make policies easier for personnel to implement, but they acknowledge that establishing criteria for such categories would be a more complex task than it is for beverages. In addition, similar food products (for example, different flavors of similar products from the same brand) from the same manufacturer may vary in compliance because of slightly different nutrient compositions, causing confusion among personnel responsible for implementing the standards.

District level Beginning with the 2006-2007 school year, all local education agencies (i.e., school districts) participating in the federal child nutrition programs were required to adopt and implement a school wellness policy. As of school year 2009-2010, nearly all districts nationwide had such a policy, but they were fairly vague. The standards for competitive foods and beverages were one of the weakest elements, particularly in policies focused at the middle and high school levels (Chriqui et al., 2010). Box 9-1 provides additional suggested action steps for implementing this strategy.

Indicators for Assessing Progress in Obesity Prevention for Strategy 5-2

Primary Indicators

- Increase in the percentage of energy intake in schools attributable to the consumption of foods and beverages recommended by the Dietary Guidelines for Americans for children and adolescents aged 2 and older.*
  Sources for measuring indicator: NHANES, NYPANS, and YRBSS

- Reduction in the percentage of total energy in the diets of children and adolescents consumed at school derived from added sugars and solid fats (fat intake should come primarily from mono- and polyunsaturated fatty acids).
  Sources for measuring indicator: NHANES, NYPANS, and YRBSS

Process Indicators

- Adoption of regulations by the USDA that require all foods and beverages sold/served in schools to be aligned with the Dietary Guidelines for Americans recommendations.*
  Sources for measuring indicator: CLASS (NCI), CDC State School Health Profiles, and SHPPS

- Increase in the proportion of states with laws and regulations requiring that all foods sold/served in schools be aligned with the Dietary Guidelines for Americans recommendations.*
  Sources for measuring indicator: CLASS (NCI), CDC State School Health Profiles, and SHPPS

- Increase in the proportion of school districts with policies requiring that all foods sold/served in schools be aligned with the Dietary Guidelines for Americans recommendations.*
  Sources for measuring indicator: SHPPS and Bridging the Gap District Wellness Policy Study

- Increase in the percentage of public and private schools that adhere to the IOM's (2007) Tier 1 and Tier 2 food standards.
  Sources for measuring indicator: SNDA, USDA program monitoring/reporting, and SHPPS

Foundational Indicators

- Increase in the frequency of CDC's School Health Policy and Programs Study to every 2 years.
  Source needed for measurement of indicator.

- Increase in the frequency of CDC's National Youth Physical Activity and Nutrition Survey to every 2 years.
  Source needed for measurement of indicator.

- Addition of dietary questions to CDC's Middle School Youth Risk Behavior Surveillance System, particularly questions related to sugar-sweetened beverages and access to such beverages in schools.
  Source needed for measurement of indicator.

- Conduct of USDA's School Nutrition Dietary Assessment Study every 5 years.
  Source needed for measurement of indicator.

- Inclusion of population-representative subgroups of children and adolescents aged 2-5, 6-12, and 13-18 in CDC's NHANES.
  Source needed for measurement of indicator.

NOTE: CDC = Centers for Disease Control and Prevention; CLASS = Classification of Laws Associated with School Students; IOM = Institute of Medicine; NCI = National Cancer Institute; NHANES = National Health and Nutrition Examination Survey; NYPANS = National Youth Physical Activity and Nutrition Survey; SHPPS = School Health Policies and Practices Study; SNDA = School Nutrition Dietary Assessment Survey; USDA = U.S. Department of Agriculture; YRBSS = Youth Risk Behavior Surveillance System.

---

*See Box B-1 in Appendix B.

Strategy 5-3: Ensure Food Literacy, Including Skill Development, in Schools

Through leadership and guidance from federal and state governments, state and local education agencies should ensure the implementation and monitoring of sequential food literacy and nutrition science education, spanning grades K-12, based on the food and nutrition recommendations in the Dietary Guidelines for Americans.

For the **federal government,** potential actions include

- USDA developing K-12 food and nutrition curriculum guides that can be used by states and updating information in these guides as appropriate with each periodic revision of the Dietary Guidelines for Americans; and
- as USDA develops regulations to implement Section 204 of the *Healthy, Hunger-Free Kids Act of 2010* (Public Law 111-296, December 13, 2010), including a requirement for local education agencies to adopt and implement a K-12 food and nutrition curriculum based on state and federal guidance.

For **states, state legislatures, and departments of education,** potential actions include

- state legislatures and departments of education adopting, requiring, and financially supporting K-12 standards for food and nutrition curriculum based on USDA guidance;
- state departments of education establishing requirements for training teachers in effectively incorporating nutrition education into their curricula;
- states requiring teacher training programs to include curriculum requirements for the study of nutrition;
- state legislatures and departments of education adopting and requiring proficiency assessments for core elements of their state food and nutrition curriculum standards in accordance with the Common Core State Standards Initiative, and local education agency wellness policies articulating ways in which results of food and nutrition education proficiency assessments can be used to inform program improvement; and
- state and local departments of education, working with local education agency wellness policies, to link changes in the meals provided through child nutrition services with the food literacy and nutrition education curriculum to the extent possible.

Context

Current data on the efficacy of new programs designed to teach food and nutrition to children and adolescents in a school setting provide critical support for changes in the food environment to prevent obesity and promote health. The 2010 Dietary Guidelines for Americans recommend providing nutrition education programs in educational settings. The content of food and nutrition education should be based on the Dietary Guidelines, which provide the current evidence linking nutrition to the prevention of disease and promotion of health. During the last decade, however, despite an increased focus on efforts to prevent childhood obesity and evidence supporting the impact of nutrition education on dietary behaviors and weight outcomes, school programs providing nutrition education have remained inconsistent and underemphasized. Today, few schools offer the necessary intensity or quality of such education or a coordinated grade-level curricular approach. While 74 percent of elementary, 73 percent of middle, and 24 percent of high schools provided some nutrition content in every grade during the 2004-2005 school year (Briefel et al., 2009), data from CDC's School Health Policies and Practices Study illustrate the limitations of current practices. The median number of hours of required instruction that teachers provided on the topic of nutrition and dietary behavior during 2006 was 3.4 for elementary school students, 4.2 for middle school students, and 5.9 for high school students (Kann et al., 2007). Further, curriculum continuity often is absent from nutrition education—lessons taught in one grade are not coordinated/reinforced in subsequent school years as is the case for other subjects. A greater investment of educational time, as well as a K-12 curriculum based on the latest science on preventing disease and promoting nutritional health, would maximize opportunities for imparting the information needed to influence students' knowledge of nutrition and dietary behaviors.

The implementation of academic proficiency standards, including those of *No Child Left Behind Act* (Public Law 107-110, 107th Cong., 1st sess. [January 8, 2002], 115, 1425), has resulted in a narrowing of curriculum to fit specific standardized testing. Research suggests that teachers are limiting their curricula to content listed in curriculum frameworks and tested on examinations, while untested subjects such as social studies and science increasingly are excluded (Au, 2007; Grant, 2001; Kolbe, 2002; McNeil, 2000; Vogler and Virtue, 2007). Despite the widely recognized child obesity epidemic, nutrition education is among the subjects often omitted as a result of this narrowed focus. The committee recommends that proficiency standards for knowledge of food and nutrition parallel those for physical education and other core academic topics. These proficiency standards and associated measurements should be based on evidence of school nutrition education programs with demonstrated effectiveness in changing nutrition knowledge and behavioral outcomes among students.

Evidence

Although traditional education has not been solidly proven to change behavior, the type of nutrition education recommended by the committee is not the exclusively didactic nutrition education of the past, but is interactive and couples experiential education techniques with education on food systems, marketing, food literacy, and other elements integral to the development of healthful eating habits. This type of education has shown promise in impacting students' knowledge and behaviors.

Recently developed methods for teaching food and nutrition, in some cases using techniques based on experiential education (including food preparation, fruit and vegetable gardening, food tasting, and other hands-on approaches) can produce changes in knowledge without evidence of behavior change (Abood et al., 2008; DeVault et al., 2009; Gower et al., 2010; Katz et al., 2011; McGaffey et al., 2010; Moore et al., 2009, Morgan et al., 2010; Somerset and Markwell, 2009; Tuuri et al., 2009). Other studies have reported changes in students' dietary intake patterns as well (Contento et al., 2010; Day et al., 2008; Dunton et al., 2009; Fahlman et al., 2008; He et al., 2009; Heim et al., 2009; Kristjansdottir et al., 2010; Lo et al., 2008; Muth et al., 2008; Parmer et al., 2009; Wang et al., 2010) and in some cases, positive impacts on changes in their weight or BMI (Hatzis et al., 2010; Mihas et al., 2010; Plachta-Danielzik et al., 2011). Further, nutrition education when reinforced by the school food environment has been shown to lead to changes in behavior and/or weight status (Burgess-Champoux et al., 2008; Davis et al., 2009; Foster et al., 2008; Hollar et al., 2010a,b; Hoppu et al., 2010; Muckelbauer et al., 2009; Reinaerts et al., 2008; Taylor et al., 2008). These studies were conducted with students ranging from the kindergarten level through high school, with education doses varying by program. Those education interventions associated with demonstrated changes in student BMI were conducted with either elementary or middle school students and included variable numbers of classroom hours, from only a few during a 1-year period to up to 17 per year over a 6-year period.

In 2006, Knai and colleagues (2006) conducted a review of 15 nutrition education interventions (11 in primary schools and 4 in secondary schools) designed to increase fruit and vegetable intake in children and adolescents aged 5-18. To qualify for this review, a study had to measure fruit and vegetable intake at a follow-up of at least 3 months. Using a variety of methods to measure fruit and vegetable intake, 10 of the 15 interventions included in the review reported statistically significant positive change in consumption among intervention students compared with control students (Knai et al., 2006). Even using evidence drawn from an earlier period (1982-2004), the authors of the Academy of Nutrition and Dietetics position paper on individual-, family-, school-, and community-based interventions for pediatric overweight concluded: "There is fair evidence to support using nutrition education to change the type of food eaten, food preferences, or eating patterns as part of a school-based primary prevention program to effect changes in weight status/adiposity in elementary school and particularly in secondary school students" (Ritchie et al., 2006, p. 934).

The federal nutrition education programs that are administered to students in some selected grade levels and schools provide corroborating evidence for the efficacy of food and nutrition education in changing knowledge and behaviors. The Food Stamp Nutrition Education Program conducted a review of nationwide food and nutrition education programs in 2006. Fifty percent of implementing agencies (n = 22) believed that their outcome evaluations found positive behavior change among participants (Bell et al., 2006). Similarly, the National Institute of Food and Agriculture's 2010 annual report on the Expanded Food and Nutrition Education Program (EFNEP) shows that the majority of youth receiving nutrition education improved knowledge and skills in nutrition (USDA, 2010). And a USDA evaluation of a Team Nutrition pilot study for fourth graders in seven school districts around the country showed a significant positive impact on students' knowledge of the Food Guide Pyramid and healthy food choices (USDA, 1996). Multivariate analysis revealed that students exposed to more intervention components demonstrated the most significant changes in dietary behavior.

Implementation

The evidence is clear that nutrition education can positively influence children's food and nutrition knowledge and behaviors, but research indicates that more instructional time is needed. The total number of classroom hours for programs studied and found to be effective varied widely, but nearly always was more than the current average of 4-6 hours per year, which translates to just 1-2 minutes per day. This amount of instruction stands in contrast to physical activity, for which daily instructional time, opportunities, and positive messages are more likely to exist during the school day. Students are exposed to unhealthy foods virtually everywhere they go, and they must have the knowledge necessary to make informed choices. In the face of the extensive food marketing to which children and adolescents are exposed and must be able to interpret, a foundation of food and nutrition knowledge is important. It is difficult to imagine how children and adolescents can be expected to make healthy food choices in or out of school with so little instructional time spent on education about healthy foods and eating habits.

The amount of time schools should devote to nutrition education is not well defined. If quality nutrition education were a core subject area, it would receive 30 to 60 minutes per day, or 87 to 171 hours per year, of instructional time, similar to other academic subjects. It has been suggested that 50 hours/school year of instruction in nutrition is required to effect positive changes in eating behavior, but this number is not well substantiated and is based on best-practice estimates (Connell et al., 1985; Contento et al., 1995). The committee's recommendation is 20 to 50 hours per year. Fifty hours per year is approximately 15 minutes per day, which is considerably less time than is devoted to other subjects taught in schools, as well as physical education classes. It should be noted that, although nutrition education could be viewed as taking time away from core educational requirements, no evaluations of nutrition education have demonstrated a negative effect on academic performance. Furthermore, one nutrition education intervention showed a positive effect on academic test scores (Shilts et al., 2009).

Multicomponent school-based programs utilizing a variety of methods, such as nutrition education, changes in school food offerings, social marketing, school gardens, and parent involvement, have been shown to be effective in reducing the prevalence of obesity in at least some participants. Doak and colleagues (2006) reviewed the literature and assessed 25 school-based obesity prevention programs. They found that 68 percent of the programs (17 of the 25) were successful in reducing the BMI or skin-fold measurements of program participants. Gortmaker and colleagues (1999) evaluated a school-based health behavior intervention known as Planet Health, in which sessions were included within existing school curricula, among students in grades 6-8. The intervention reduced obesity (based on BMI and triceps skin fold) in girls in intervention schools compared with controls, but no differences were found among boys. One example of a multicomponent school health program that is accompanied by a large body of work is the CATCH program, which achieved positive results with respect to nutrition knowledge, intention, and food preferences and intake with approximately 12 to 20 hours of nutrition education per year (Edmundson et al., 1994; Luepker et al., 1996; Perry et al., 1990, 1997). The CATCH program provides compelling evidence of the multiple benefits of school-based food, nutrition, and physical education programs (Box 9-2).

BOX 9-2
The CATCH School-Based Food, Nutrition, and Physical Education Program

Background

The Coordinated Approach To Child Health (CATCH) program* was designed in the 1980s to improve physical activity and diet and to prevent the onset of tobacco use (Perry et al., 1990). In recent years, the CATCH program has aligned with the Centers for Disease Control and Prevention's coordinated school health model, in which eight components work interactively to educate young people about and provide support for a healthful lifestyle. The five main components of CATCH are (1) K-8 classroom curricula focusing on food, nutrition, and physical activity; (2) physical education activities; (3) child nutrition services; (4) family involvement; and (5) community involvement. An evidence base supports the program's efficacy in improving diet and increasing physical activity and preventing the onset of obesity in children.

Results and Evidence

- Results of long-term follow-up indicate that changes in diet and physical activity were maintained 3 years postintervention, until the children were in eighth grade (Nader et al., 1999).

- CATCH has been proven effective in promoting health among inner-city, border, rural, privileged, and underprivileged children. A school randomized replication study of CATCH in El Paso found significant effects in reducing the rate of increase of overweight and risk of overweight among a cohort of children in grades 3-5. By fifth grade, the rate of increase was 2 percent for girls and 1 per-

Accelerating Progress in Obesity Prevention

cent for boys in intervention schools, compared with 13 and 9 percent, respectively, in control schools (Coleman et al., 2005).

- PASS & CATCH, a version of CATCH making extensive use of classroom physical activities, has been shown to improve disadvantaged children's Stanford math and reading scores (Murray et al., under review).

- CATCH augments existing school health programming by inviting local community youth organizations to participate in the process of creating a healthier school environment. The effects of community support cannot be underestimated.

- An El Paso demonstration study of CATCH plus community support found a 7 percent reduction in child obesity prevalence (Hoelscher et al., 2010a).

- A recent Travis County demonstration study of CATCH showed an 8 percent reduction in overweight and obesity among fourth graders (Hoelscher et al., 2010b).

- According to a recent cost-effectiveness study of CATCH, the program's cost-effectiveness ratio was approximately $900 (representing the intervention cost per quality-adjusted life-year saved), and the net benefit was $68,125 (based on a comparison of the present value of averted future costs due to obesity with the cost of the CATCH intervention) (Brown et al., 2007).

---

*Formerly known as the Child and Adolescent Trial for Cardiovascular Health.

Indicators for Assessing Progress in Obesity Prevention for Strategy 5-3

Process Indicators

- Increase in the adoption of age-appropriate, sequential food and nutrition curriculum standards and performance measures for grades K-12 in all schools.
  Source for measuring indicator: SHPPS

- Increase in students' knowledge of nutrition, consistent with the Dietary Guidelines for Americans.*
  Source needed for measurement of indicator.

- Increase in the proportion of states with policies requiring a sequential food and nutrition curriculum for grades K-12.
  Sources for measuring indicator: CLASS (NCI) and SHPPS

- Increase in the proportion of states with nutrition education training requirements for teachers.
  Source needed for measurement of indicator.

Foundational Indicators

- Increase in the priority of advocacy efforts (among professional associations related to schools and nutrition) regarding the implementation of 20-50 hours of classroom nutrition education.
  Source needed for measurement of indicator.

NOTE: CLASS = Classification of Laws Associated with School Students; NCI = National Cancer Institute; SHPPS = School Health Policies and Practices Study.

---

*See Box B-1 in Appendix B.

INTEGRATION OF STRATEGIES FOR ACCELERATING PROGRESS IN OBESITY PREVENTION

Evidence outlined in this chapter points to opportunities to accelerate progress in preventing obesity among children and adolescents in three school-related areas: physical education, school foods, and food and nutrition education. During the past decade, states and municipal governments have implemented policies regarding competitive foods; many schools have made improvements in school meals and others in physical education programs. Some schools have added nutrition education programs in particular classrooms or grade levels. These programs and policies differ by class, grade, school, district and state.

Physical activity, school foods, and nutrition education generally have been treated separately within schools, and interdisciplinary obesity prevention efforts thus have rarely been realized. The breaking down of these silos began in many schools in fall 2006 when local education agencies sponsoring USDA-funded school meal programs were required to establish local wellness policies. A three-state USDA-funded Team Nutrition Local Wellness Demonstration Project reported that wellness committees brought together principals, food service directors, physical education teachers, school nurses, superintendents, parents, curriculum directors, school board members, and students (Wood et al., 2010). While none of the districts studied reported changes in all areas—including improvements in physical activity environments, implementation of physical education programs that meet state standards, increased opportunities for and participation by students and staff in physical activity, school food environments, and implementation of nutrition education in classes—most schools had made some improvements in some of these areas. Classroom nutrition instruction implemented concurrently with changes in meal program offerings was associated with improved healthy food choices (Wood et al., 2010). Thus school wellness policies can be a vehicle for change, suggesting comprehensive approaches to school wellness and providing consistent messages to school stakeholders. The report of the Wellness Demonstration Project goes on to say that local wellness policies have created a culture of change in schools that, coupled with the beginnings of an integrated approach to physical and food and nutrition and education, promises to provide momentum for the changes needed to accelerate progress toward obesity prevention in school environments (Wood et al., 2010).

The literature provides evidence of the benefits of multicomponent nutrition interventions, many specifically combining changes in the school food environment with food and nutrition education (Knai et al., 2006; Livingstone et al.,

2006; Peters et al., 2009). If well coordinated, a school lunch program can serve as an important adjunct to nutrition education. When multicomponent nutrition programs have been coupled with physical activity and physical education programs, even more dramatic changes have occurred, in some cases, changes in student adiposity (Brown and Summerbell, 2009; Coleman et al., 2005; Foster et al., 2008; Hollar et al., 2010a,b; Katz et al., 2008; Ritchie et al., 2006). In addition to achieving improvements in school meals and competitive foods, these programs often have included physical education and physical activity during the school day, strong nutrition education and promotion components, and family involvement, and some have included related community events.

Along with changes in the school environment and implementation of sequential food and nutrition education, it is important for teachers and other school staff to model healthy behaviors, and there is progress to be made in this area (Eaton et al., 2007; Hartline-Grafton et al., 2009). The Alliance for a Healthier Generation encourages school employee wellness programs in the belief that the conditions that affect the health of these employees influence the health and learning of students, and that protecting the health of school employees is essential to protecting student health and fostering students' academic success (Alliance for a Healthier Generation, 2011). Employee wellness programs are discussed further in Chapter 8 (Strategy 4-3) and have demonstrated positive outcomes in other settings. For example, a staff wellness intervention conducted in selected Special Supplemental Nutrition Program for Women, Infants, and Children (WIC) sites showed that intervention group staff were more likely than control group staff to report that the workplace environment supported their efforts to choose healthy foods and be physically active, and improved their counseling for WIC clients related to physical activity and weight (Crawford et al., 2004). In a staff wellness program in child care centers, employees in intervention sites reported providing more fresh fruits and vegetables to children and experiencing more positive changes in their comfort level with respect to discussing physical activity and nutrition with parents relative to employees in control sites (Gosliner et al., 2010). The committee believes that ensuring that school staff support the strategies set forth in this chapter—with words and actions—in the presence of students is likely critical for success.

The committee expects that changes in the school environment, implemented concurrently with this report's recommended changes in the rest of the system in which children live and play, will act synergistically to accelerate progress in obesity prevention (as illustrated by Figure 9-1, presented at the beginning of this chapter). Even if the effect of school-based interventions were to be relatively small, schools are an ideal setting in which to expose children and adolescents to knowledge and behaviors related to physical activity and nutrition. As shown in New York City (Berger et al., 2011) and by past interventions in CATCH schools (Box 9-2), changes in schools accompanied by changes in the community are associated with positive health outcomes. Furthermore, school-based interventions could have positive effects on children's behaviors outside of school, such as time spent viewing television (Robinson and Borzekowski, 2006) and consumption of healthy foods (IOM, 2010; Wang et al., 2010).

Objections to physical education and nutrition education programs coupled with changes in school foods will undoubtedly arise. The most serious objection is less likely to be lack of funding as it is to be concern about reduced time for academic subjects, with the potential result of lower test scores. With regard to reducing time spent on academic subjects, the committee acknowledges that integrating nutrition education with existing school curricula has shown limited success in reducing obesity (Austin et al., 2005; Gortmaker et al., 1999); however, this approach would need further testing at various grade levels before its use could be recommended in place of sequential nutrition education, in which knowledge and skills are reinforced and expanded each year as a stand-alone subject. The committee could find no evidence that such sequential programs lower academic test scores. To the contrary, some evidence indicates that school-based physical education (CDC, 2010b; Singh et al., 2012) and nutrition curriculum (Shilts et al., 2009) can positively influence academic achievement. Furthermore, well-nourished children are more able to learn and less likely to miss school for health reasons (Florence et al., 2008; Taras, 2005a). Studies have shown that students participating in school breakfast programs score higher on standardized tests and have better school attendance than similar children not participating in the program (Hoyland et al., 2009; Kleinman et al., 2002; Meyers et al., 1989; Powell et al., 1983, 1998). Assessments of recent interventions to improve school physical activity and nutrition environments have shown that these efforts can lead to an improvement in children's academic performance and to improved classroom behavior and attentiveness (Hollar, 2010a,b; Murphy et al., 1998; Nansel et al., 2010). As far back as 1904, Robert Hunter wrote about the need for students to have adequate physical activity and nutrition: "It is utter folly, from the point of view of learning, to have a compulsory school law which compels children, in that weak physical and mental state . . . to sit at their desks, day in and day out for several years, learning little or nothing . . . because hungry stomachs and languid bodies and thin blood are not able to feed the brain" (Hunter, 1965).

REFERENCES

Abood, D. A., D. R. Black, and D. C. Coster. 2008. Evaluation of a school-based teen obesity prevention minimal intervention. *Journal of Nutrition Education and Behavior* 40(3):168-174.

Alliance for a Healthier Generation. 2011. *School employee wellness.* http://www. healthiergeneration.org/schools.aspx?id=3393 (accessed December 28, 2011).

Anthamatten, P., L. Brink, S. Lampe, E. Greenwood, B. Kingston, and C. Nigg. 2011. An assessment of schoolyard renovation strategies to encourage children's physical activity. *International Journal of Behavior Nutrition and Physical Activity* 8:27.

Au, W. 2007. High-stakes testing and curricular control: A qualitative metasynthesis. *Educational Researcher* 36(5):258.

Austin, S. B., A. E. Field, J. Wiecha, K. E. Peterson, and S. L. Gortmaker. 2005. The impact of a school-based obesity prevention trial on disordered weight-control behaviors in early adolescent girls. *Archives of Pediatrics and Adolescent Medicine* 159(3):225-230.

Bell, L., F. Tao, J. Anthony, C. Logan, R. Ledsky, M. Ferreira, and A. Brown. 2006. *Food stamp nutrition education systems review: Final report.* Alexandria, VA: USDA/FNS, Office of Analysis, Nutrition, and Evaluation.

Berger, M., K. Konty, S. Day, L. D. Silver, C. Nonas, B. D. Kerker, C. Greene, T. Farley, and L. Harr. 2011. Obesity in K-8 students—New York City, 2006-2007 to 2010-2011 school years. *Morbidity and Mortality Weekly Report* 60(49):1673-1678.

Briefel, R. R., M. K. Crepinsek, C. Cabili, A. Wilson, and P. M. Gleason. 2009. School food environments and practices affect dietary behaviors of U.S. public school children. *Journal of the American Dietetic Association* 109(2):S91-S107.

Brink, L. A., C. R. Nigg, S. M. Lampe, B. A. Kingston, A. L. Mootz, and W. van Vliet. 2010. Influence of schoolyard renovations on children's physical activity: The Learning Landscapes Program. *American Journal of Public Health* 100(9):1672-1678.

Brown, H. S., A. Perez, Y.-P. Li, D. Hoelscher, S. Kelder, and R. Rivera. 2007. The cost-effectiveness of a school-based overweight program. *International Journal of Behavioral Nutrition and Physical Activity* 4(1):47.

Brown, T., and C. Summerbell. 2009. Systematic review of school-based interventions that focus on changing dietary intake and physical activity levels to prevent childhood obesity: An update to the obesity guidance produced by the National Institute for Health and Clinical Excellence. *Obesity Reviews* 10(1):110-141.

Burgess-Champoux, T. L., H. W. Chan, R. Rosen, L. Marquart, and M. Reicks. 2008. Healthy whole-grain choices for children and parents: A multi-component school-based pilot intervention. *Public Health Nutrition* 11(8):849-859.

Accelerating Progress in Obesity Prevention

California Project LEAN (Leaders Encouraging Activity and Nutrition). 2009. *Maximizing opportunities for physical activity during the school day.* Sacramento, CA: California Project LEAN.

CDC (Centers for Disease Control and Prevention). 2010a. Effects of switching from whole to low-fat/fat-free milk in public schools—New York City, 2004-2009. *Morbidity and Mortality Weekly Report* 59(3):70-73.

CDC. 2010b. *The association between school based physical activity, including physical education, and academic performance.* Atlanta, GA: HHS, CDC.

Chriqui, J. F., L. Schneider, F. J. Chaloupka, C. Gourdet, A. Bruursema, K. Ide, and O. Pugach. 2010. *School district wellness policies: Evaluating progress and potential for improving children's health three years after the federal mandate: School years 2006-07, 2007-08 and 2008-09, Volume 2.* Chicago, IL: Bridging the Gap Program, Health Policy Center, Institute for Health Research and Policy, University of Illinois.

Colabianchi, N., A. E. Kinsella, C. J. Coulton, and S. M. Moore. 2009. Utilization and physical activity levels at renovated and unrenovated school playgrounds. *Preventive Medicine* 48(2):140-143.

Coleman, K. J., C. L. Tiller, J. Sanchez, E. M. Heath, O. Sy, G. Milliken, and D. A. Dzewaltowski. 2005. Prevention of the epidemic increase in child risk of overweight in low-income schools: The El Paso coordinated approach to child health. *Archives of Pediatrics and Adolescent Medicine* 159(3):217-224.

Connell, D. B., R. R. Turner, and E. F. Mason. 1985. Summary of findings of the School Health Education Evaluation: Health promotion effectiveness, implementation, and costs. *Journal of School Health* 55(8):316-321.

Contento, I., G. I. Balch, Y. L. Bronner, D. M. Paige, S. M. Gross, and L. Bisignani. 1995. Nutrition education for school-aged children. *Journal of Nutrition Education* 27(6):298-311.

Contento, I. R., P. A. Koch, H. Lee, and A. Calabrese-Barton. 2010. Adolescents demonstrate improvement in obesity risk behaviors after completion of choice, control & change, a curriculum addressing personal agency and autonomous motivation. *Journal of the American Dietetic Association* 110(12):1830-1839.

Crawford, P. B., W. Gosliner, P. Strode, S. E. Samuels, C. Burnett, L. Craypo, and A. K. Yancey. 2004. Walking the talk: Fit WIC wellness programs improve self-efficacy in pediatric obesity prevention counseling. *American Journal of Public Health* 94(9):1480-1485.

Cullen, K. W., and K. B. Watson. 2009. The impact of the Texas public school nutrition policy on student food selection and sales in Texas. *American Journal of Public Health* 99(4):706-712.

Cullen, K. W., K. Watson, and I. Zakeri. 2008. Improvements in middle school student dietary intake after implementation of the Texas Public School Nutrition Policy. *American Journal of Public Health* 98(1):111-117.

Davis, E. M., K. W. Cullen, K. B. Watson, M. Konarik, and J. Radcliffe. 2009. A fresh fruit and vegetable program improves high school students' consumption of fresh produce. *Journal of the American Dietetic Association* 109(7):1227-1231.

Day, M. E., K. S. Strange, H. A. McKay, and P. J. Naylor. 2008. Action schools! BC—Healthy Eating: Effects of a whole-school model to modifying eating behaviours of elementary school children. *Canadian Journal of Public Health. Revue Canadienne de Sante Publique* 99(4):328-331.

DeVault, N., T. Kennedy, J. Hermann, M. Mwavita, P. Rask, and A. Jaworsky. 2009. It's all about kids: Preventing overweight in elementary school children in Tulsa, OK. *Journal of the American Dietetic Association* 109(4):680-687.

Doak, C. M., T. L. S. Visscher, C. M. Renders, and J. C. Seidell. 2006. The prevention of overweight and obesity in children and adolescents: A review of interventions and programmes. *Obesity Reviews* 7(1):111-136.

Dobbins, M., K. DeCorby, P. Robeson, H. Husson, and D. Tirilis. 2009. School-based physical activity programs for promoting physical activity and fitness in children and adolescents aged 6-18. *Cochrane Database of Systematic Reviews* (1).

Dunton, G. F., R. Lagloire, and T. Robertson. 2009. Using the RE-AIM framework to evaluate the statewide dissemination of a school-based physical activity and nutrition curriculum: "Exercise Your Options." *American Journal of Health Promotion* 23(4):229-232.

Eaton, D. K., E. Marx, and S. E. Bowie. 2007. Faculty and staff health promotion: Results from the school health policies and programs study 2006. *Journal of School Health* 77(8):557-566.

Edmundson, E. W., S. C. Luton, S. A. McGraw, S. H. Kelder, A. K. Layman, M. H. Smyth, K. J. Bachman, S. A. Pedersen, and E. J. Stone. 1994. CATCH: Classroom process evaluation in a multicenter trial. *Health Education Quarterly* (Suppl. 2):S27-S50.

Fahlman, M. M., J. A. Dake, N. McCaughtry, and J. Martin. 2008. A pilot study to examine the effects of a nutrition intervention on nutrition knowledge, behaviors, and efficacy expectations in middle school children. *Journal of School Health* 78(4):216-222.

Fisher, J. O., B. J. Rolls, and L. L. Birch. 2003. Children's bite size and intake of an entrée are greater with large portions than with age-appropriate or self-selected portions. *American Journal of Clinical Nutrition* 77(5):1164-1170.

Florence, M. D., M. Asbridge, and P. J. Veugelers. 2008. Diet quality and academic performance. *Journal of School Health* 78(4):209-215.

Foster, G. D., S. Sherman, K. E. Borradaile, K. M. Grundy, S. S. Vander Veur, J. Nachmani, A. Karpyn, S. Kumanyika, and J. Shults. 2008. A policy-based school intervention to prevent overweight and obesity. *Pediatrics* 121(4):e794-e802.

Gordon-Larsen, P., K. M. Harris, D. S. Ward, and B. M. Popkin. 2003. Acculturation and overweight-related behaviors among Hispanic immigrants to the US: The National Longitudinal Study of Adolescent Health. *Social Science and Medicine* 57(11):2023-2034.

Gortmaker, S. L., K. Peterson, J. Wiecha, A. M. Sobol, S. Dixit, M. K. Fox, and N. Laird. 1999. Reducing obesity via a school-based interdisciplinary intervention among youth: Planet health. *Archives of Pediatrics and Adolescent Medicine* 153(4):409-418.

Gosliner, W. A., P. James, A. K. Yancey, L. Ritchie, N. Studer, and P. B. Crawford. 2010. Impact of a worksite wellness program on the nutrition and physical activity environment of child care centers. *American Journal of Health Promotion* 24(3):186-189.

Gosliner, W., K. A. Madsen, G. Woodward-Lopez, and P. B. Crawford. 2011. Would students prefer to eat healthier foods at school? *Journal of School Health* 81(3):146-151.

Gower, J. R., L. J. Moyer-Mileur, R. D. Wilkinson, H. Slater, and K. C. Jordan. 2010. Validity and reliability of a nutrition knowledge survey for assessment in elementary school children. *Journal of the American Dietetic Association* 110(3):452-456.

Grant, S. G. 2001. An uncertain lever: Exploring the influence of state-level testing in New York state on teaching social studies. *Teachers College Record* 103(3):398-426.

Hartline-Grafton, H. L., D. Rose, C. C. Johnson, J. C. Rice, and L. S. Webber. 2009. Are school employees role models of healthful eating? Dietary intake results from the ACTION worksite wellness trial. *Journal of the American Dietetic Association* 109(9):1548-1556.

Hatzis, C. M., C. Papandreou, and A. G. Kafatos. 2010. School health education programs in Crete: Evaluation of behavioural and health indices a decade after initiation. *Preventive Medicine* 51(3-4):262-267.

He, M., C. Beynon, M. Sangster Bouck, R. St Onge, S. Stewart, L. Khoshaba, B. A. Horbul, and B. Chircoski. 2009. Impact evaluation of the northern fruit and vegetable pilot program: A cluster-randomised controlled trial. *Public Health Nutrition* 12(11):2199-2208.

Heim, S., J. Stang, and M. Ireland. 2009. A garden pilot project enhances fruit and vegetable consumption among children. *Journal of the American Dietetic Association* 109(7):1220-1226.

HHS/USDA (U.S. Department of Health and Human Services/U.S. Department of Agriculture). 2005. *Dietary guidelines for Americans.* Washington, DC: U.S. Government Printing Office.

HHS/USDA. 2010. *Dietary guidelines for Americans.* Washington, DC: U.S. Government Printing Office.

Hoelscher, D. M., S. H. Kelder, A. Perez, R. S. Day, J. S. Benoit, R. F. Frankowski, J. L. Walker, and E. S. Lee. 2010a. Changes in the regional prevalence of child obesity in 4th, 8th, and 11th grade students in Texas from 2000-2002 to 2004-2005. *Obesity* 18(7):1360-1368.

Hoelscher, D., A. Springer, N. Ranjit, S. Perry, A. Evans, M. Stigler, and S. Kelder. 2010b. Reductions in child obesity among disadvantaged school children with community involvement: The Travis County CATCH trial. *Obesity (Silver Spring)* 18(Suppl. 1):S36–S44.

Hollar, D., M. Lombardo, G. Lopez-Mitnik, T. L. Hollar, M. Almon, A. S. Agatston, and S. E. Messiah. 2010a. Effective multi-level, multi-sector, school-based obesity prevention programming improves weight, blood pressure, and academic performance, especially among low-income, minority children. *Journal of Health Care for the Poor and Underserved* 21(Suppl. 2):93-108.

Hollar, D., S. E. Messiah, G. Lopez-Mitnik, T. L. Hollar, M. Almon, and A. S. Agatston. 2010b. Effect of a two-year obesity prevention intervention on percentile changes in body mass index and academic performance in low-income elementary school children. *American Journal of Public Health* 100(4):646-653.

Hoppu, U., J. Lehtisalo, J. Kujala, T. Keso, S. Garam, H. Tapanainen, A. Uutela, T. Laatikainen, U. Rauramo, and P. Pietinen. 2010. The diet of adolescents can be improved by school intervention. *Public Health Nutrition* 13(6A):973-979.

Hoyland, A., L. Dye, and C. L. Lawton. 2009. A systematic review of the effect of breakfast on the cognitive performance of children and adolescents. *Nutrition Research Reviews* 22(02):220-243.

Hunter, R. 1965 (originally published in 1904). *Poverty, Harper Torchbooks edition.* New York: Harper & Row.

IOM (Institute of Medicine). 2005. *Preventing childhood obesity: Health in the balance,* edited by J. P. Koplan, C. T. Liverman, and V. A. Kraak. Washington, DC: The National Academies Press.

IOM. 2007. *Nutrition standards for foods in schools: Leading the way toward healthier youth.* Washington, DC: The National Academies Press.

IOM. 2008. *Nutrition standards and meal requirements for national school lunch and breakfast programs: Phase I. Proposed approach for recommending revisions.* Washington, DC: The National Academies Press.

IOM. 2010. *School meals: Building blocks for healthy children.* Washington, DC: The National Academies Press.

Jago, R., and T. Baranowski. 2004. Non-curricular approaches for increasing physical activity in youth: A review. *Preventive Medicine* 39(1):157-163.

Just, D. R., and B. Wansink. 2009. Smarter lunchrooms: Using behavioral economics to improve meal selection. *Choices* 24(3).

Kahn, E. B., L. T. Ramsey, R. C. Brownson, G. W. Heath, E. H. Howze, K. E. Powell, E. J. Stone, M. W. Rajab, and P. Corso. 2002. The effectiveness of interventions to increase physical activity. A systematic review. *American Journal of Preventive Medicine* 22(Suppl. 4):73-107.

Kann, L., S. K. Telljohann, and S. F. Wooley. 2007. Health education: Results from the School Health Policies and Programs Study 2006. *Journal of School Health* 77(8):408-434.

Katz, D. L., M. O'Connell, V. Y. Njike, M. C. Yeh, and H. Nawaz. 2008. Strategies for the prevention and control of obesity in the school setting: Systematic review and meta-analysis. *International Journal of Obesity (London)* 32(12):1780-1789.

Katz, D. L., C. S. Katz, J. A. Treu, J. Reynolds, V. Njike, J. Walker, E. Smith, and J. Michael. 2011. Teaching healthful food choices to elementary school students and their parents: The Nutrition Detectives program. *Journal of School Health* 81(1):21-28.

Kelder, S. 2010. *Stuck in the middle: The false choice between health and education in Texas middle schools.* Austin, TX: RGK Foundation.

Kleinman, R. E., S. Hall, H. Green, D. Korzec-Ramirez, K. Patton, M. E. Pagano, and J. M. Murphy. 2002. Diet, breakfast, and academic performance in children. *Annals of Nutrition and Metabolism* 46(Suppl. 1):24-30.

Knai, C., J. Pomerleau, K. Lock, and M. McKee. 2006. Getting children to eat more fruit and vegetables: A systematic review. *Preventive Medicine* 42(2):85-95.

Kolbe, L. J. 2002. Health and the goals of modern school health programs. *The State Education Standard* August:1-11.

Kristjansdottir, A. G., E. Johannsson, and I. Thorsdottir. 2010. Effects of a school-based intervention on adherence of 7-9-year-olds to food-based dietary guidelines and intake of nutrients. *Public Health Nutrition* 13(8):1151-1161.

Larson, N. I., M. T. Story, and M. C. Nelson. 2009. Neighborhood environments: Disparities in access to healthy foods in the U.S. *American Journal of Preventive Medicine* 36(1):74-81.

Lee, S. M., C. R. Burgeson, J. E. Fulton, and C. G. Spain. 2007. Physical education and physical activity: Results from the School Health Policies and Programs Study 2006. *Journal of School Health* 77(8):435-463.

Livingstone, M. B., T. A. McCaffrey, and K. L. Rennie. 2006. Childhood obesity prevention studies: lessons learned and to be learned. *Public Health Nutrition* 9(8A):1121-1129.

Lo, E., R. Coles, M. L. Humbert, J. Polowski, C. J. Henry, and S. J. Whiting. 2008. Beverage intake improvement by high school students in Saskatchewan, Canada. *Nutrition Research* 28(3):144-150.

Long, M. W., K. E. Henderson, and M. B. Schwartz. 2010. Evaluating the impact of a Connecticut program to reduce availability of unhealthy competitive food in schools. *Journal of School Health* 80(10):478-486.

Luepker, R. V., C. L. Perry, S. M. McKinlay, P. R. Nader, G. S. Parcel, E. J. Stone, L. S. Webber, J. P. Elder, H. A. Feldman, C. C. Johnson, S. H. Kelder, M. Wu, and CATCH Collaborative Group. 1996. Outcomes of a field trial to improve children's dietary patterns and physical activity. The Child and Adolescent Trial for Cardiovascular Health. CATCH Collaborative Group. *Journal of the American Medical Association* 275(10):768-776.

McGaffey, A., K. Hughes, S. K. Fidler, F. J. D'Amico, and M. N. Stalter. 2010. Can Elvis Pretzley and the Fitwits improve knowledge of obesity, nutrition, exercise, and portions in fifth graders? *International Journal of Obesity (London)* 34(7):1134-1142.

McNeil, L. M. 2000. *Contradictions of school reform: Educational costs of standardized testing.* New York: Routledge.

Mendoza, J. A., K. Watson, and K. W. Cullen. 2010. Change in dietary energy density after implementation of the Texas Public School Nutrition Policy. *Journal of the American Dietetic Association* 110(3):434-440.

Meyers, A. F., A. E. Sampson, M. Weitzman, B. L. Rogers, and H. Kayne. 1989. School breakfast program and school performance. *American Journal of Diseases of Children* 143(10):1234-1239.

Mihas, C., A. Mariolis, Y. Manios, A. Naska, A. Arapaki, T. Mariolis-Sapsakos, and Y. Tountas. 2010. Evaluation of a nutrition intervention in adolescents of an urban area in Greece: Short- and long-term effects of the VYRONAS study. *Public Health Nutrition* 13(5):712-719.

Moore, J. B., L. R. Pawloski, P. Goldberg, M. O. Kyeung, A. Stoehr, and H. Baghi. 2009. Childhood obesity study: A pilot study of the effect of the nutrition education program Color My Pyramid. *Journal of School Nursing* 25(3):230-239.

Morgan, P. J., J. M. Warren, D. R. Lubans, K. L. Saunders, G. I. Quick, and C. E. Collins. 2010. The impact of nutrition education with and without a school garden on knowledge, vegetable intake and preferences and quality of school life among primary-school students. *Public Health Nutrition* 13(11):1931-1940.

Muckelbauer, R., L. Libuda, K. Clausen, A. M. Toschke, T. Reinehr, and M. Kersting. 2009. Promotion and provision of drinking water in schools for overweight prevention: Randomized, controlled cluster trial. *Pediatrics* 123(4):e661-e667.

Murphy, J. M., M. E. Pagano, J. Nachmani, P. Sperling, S. Kane, and R. E. Kleinman. 1998. The relationship of school breakfast to psychosocial and academic functioning: Cross-sectional and longitudinal observations in an inner-city school sample. *Archives of Pediatrics and Adolescent Medicine* 152(9):899-907.

Murray, N. G., J. C. Garza, P. M. Diamond, M. Stigler, D. Hoelscher, S. Kelder, and J. Ward. under review. PASS & CATCH improves academic achievement. http://www.nemours.org/content/dam/nemours/www/filebox/service/preventive/nhps/pep/pass%2Bcatch.pdf (accessed December 12, 2011).

Muth, N. D., A. Chatterjee, D. Williams, A. Cross, and K. Flower. 2008. Making an IMPACT: Effect of a school-based pilot intervention. *North Carolina Medical Journal* 69(6):432-440.

Nader, P. R., E. J. Stone, L. A. Lytle, C. L. Perry, S. K. Osganian, S. Kelder, L. S. Webber, J. P. Elder, D. Montgomery, H. A. Feldman, M. Wu, C. Johnson, G. S. Parcel, and R. V. Luepker. 1999. Three-year maintenance of improved diet and physical activity: The CATCH cohort. *Archives of Pediatrics and Adolescent Medicine* 153(7):695-704.

Nansel, T. R., T. T. K. Huang, A. J. Rovner, and Y. Sanders-Butler. 2010. Association of school performance indicators with implementation of the healthy kids, smart kids programme: Case study. *Public Health Nutrition* 13(1):116-122.

NASPE (National Association for Sport and Physical Education). Undated. *Integrating physical activity into the complete school day*. Reston, VA: American Alliance for Health, Physical Education, Recreation and Dance.

NASPE and AHA (American Heart Association). 2010. *Shape of the nation report: Status of physical education in the USA*. Reston, VA: NASPE.

NRC (National Research Council, Committee on Diet and Health). 1989. *Diet and health: Implications for reducing chronic disease risk*. Washington, DC: National Academy Press.

Parmer, S. M., J. Salisbury-Glennon, D. Shannon, and B. Struempler. 2009. School gardens: An experiential learning approach for a nutrition education program to increase fruit and vegetable knowledge, preference, and consumption among second-grade students. *Journal of Nutrition Education and Behavior* 41(3):212-217.

Perry, C. L., E. J. Stone, G. S. Parcel, R. C. Ellison, P. R. Nader, L. S. Webber, and R. V. Luepker. 1990. School-based cardiovascular health promotion: The Child and Adolescent Trial for Cardiovascular Health (CATCH). *Journal of School Health* 60(8):406-413.

Perry, C. L., D. E. Sellers, C. Johnson, S. Pedersen, K. J. Bachman, G. S. Parcel, E. J. Stone, R. V. Luepker, M. Wu, P. R. Nader, and K. Cook. 1997. The Child and Adolescent Trial for Cardiovascular Health (CATCH): Intervention, implementation, and feasibility for elementary schools in the United States. *Health Education and Behavior* 24(6):716-735.

Peters, L. W., G. Kok, G. T. Ten Dam, G. J. Buijs, and T. G. Paulussen. 2009. Effective elements of school health promotion across behavioral domains: A systematic review of reviews. *BMC Public Health* 9:182.

Phillips, M. M., J. M. Raczynski, D. S. West, L. Pulley, Z. Bursac, C. H. Gauss, and J. F. Walker. 2010. Changes in school environments with implementation of Arkansas Act 1220 of 2003. *Obesity (Silver Spring)* 18(Suppl. 1):S54-S61.

Pilant, V. B. 2006. Position of the American Dietetic Association: Local support for nutrition integrity in schools. *Journal of the American Dietetic Association* 106(1):122-133.

Plachta-Danielzik, S., B. Landsberg, D. Lange, J. Seiberl, and M. J. Muller. 2011. Eight-year follow-up of school-based intervention on childhood overweight—the Kiel Obesity Prevention Study. *Obesity Facts* 4(1):35-43.

Powell, C., S. Grantham-McGregor, and M. Elston. 1983. An evaluation of giving the Jamaican government school meal to a class of children. *Human Nutrition. Clinical Nutrition* 37(5):381-388.

Powell, C. A., S. P. Walker, S. M. Chang, and S. M. Grantham-McGregor. 1998. Nutrition and education: A randomized trial of the effects of breakfast in rural primary school children. *American Journal of Clinical Nutrition* 68(4):873-879.

Reinaerts, E., R. Crutzen, M. Candel, N. K. De Vries, and J. De Nooijer. 2008. Increasing fruit and vegetable intake among children: Comparing long-term effects of a free distribution and a multicomponent program. *Health Education Research* 23(6):987-996.

Ridgers, N. D., G. Stratton, S. J. Fairclough, and J. W. Twisk. 2007. Children's physical activity levels during school recess: A quasi-experimental intervention study. *International Journal of Behavior, Nutrition, and Physical Activity* 4:19.

Ritchie, L. D., P. B. Crawford, D. M. Hoelscher, and M. S. Sothern. 2006. Position of the American Dietetic Association: Individual-, family-, school-, and community-based interventions for pediatric overweight. *Journal of the American Dietetic Association* 106(6):925-945.

Robinson, T. N., and D. L. G. Borzekowski. 2006. Effects of the SMART classroom curriculum to reduce child and family screen time. *Journal of Communication* 56(1):1-26.

Rolls, B. J., L. S. Roe, T. V. E. Kral, J. S. Meengs, and D. E. Wall. 2004. Increasing the portion size of a packaged snack increases energy intake in men and women. *Appetite* 42(1):63-69.

Samuels, S. E., S. Lawrence Bullock, G. Woodward-Lopez, S. E. Clark, J. Kao, L. Craypo, J. Barry, and P. B. Crawford. 2009. To what extent have high schools in California been able to implement state-mandated nutrition standards? *Journal of Adolescent Health* 45(Suppl. 3):S38-S44.

Sanchez-Vaznaugh, E. V., B. N. Sánchez, J. Baek, and P. B. Crawford. 2010. "Competitive" food and beverage policies: Are they influencing childhood overweight trends? *Health Affairs* 29(3):436-446.

Schwartz, M. B., S. A. Novak, and S. S. Fiore. 2009. The impact of removing snacks of low nutritional value from middle schools. *Health Education and Behavior* 36(6):999-1011.

Shilts, M. K., C. Lamp, M. Horowitz, and M. S. Townsend. 2009. Pilot study: EatFit impacts sixth graders' academic performance on achievement of mathematics and English education standards. *Journal of Nutrition Education and Behavior* 41(2):127-131.

Sibley, B. A., and J. L. Etnier. 2003. The relationship between physical activity and cognition in children: A meta-analysis. *Pediatric Exercise Science* 15:243-256.

Singh, A., L. Uijtdewilligen, J. W. R. Twisk, W. van Mechelen, and M. J. M. Chinapaw. 2012. Physical activity and performance at school: A systematic review of the literature including a methodological quality assessment. *Archives of Pediatrics and Adolescent Medicine* 166(1):49-55.

Somerset, S., and K. Markwell. 2009. Impact of a school-based food garden on attitudes and identification skills regarding vegetables and fruit: A 12-month intervention trial. *Public Health Nutrition* 12(2):214-221.

Taras, H. 2005a. Nutrition and student performance at school. *Journal of School Health* 75(6):199-213.

Taras, H. 2005b. Physical activity and student performance at school. *Journal of School Health* 75(6):214-218.

Taylor, R. W., K. A. McAuley, W. Barbezat, V. L. Farmer, S. M. Williams, and J. I. Mann. 2008. Two-year follow-up of an obesity prevention initiative in children: The APPLE project. *American Journal of Clinical Nutrition* 88(5):1371-1377.

Treuhaft, S., and A. Karpyn. 2010. *The grocery gap: Who has access to healthy food and why it matters.* Oakland, CA and Philadelphia, PA: PolicyLink and The Food Trust.

Trudeau, F., and R. J. Shephard. 2008. Physical education, school physical activity, school sports and academic performance. *International Journal of Behavioral Nutrition and Physical Activity* 5.

Trudeau, F., and R. J. Shephard. 2010. Relationships of physical activity to brain health and the academic performance of school children. *American Journal of Lifestyle Medicine* 4:138-150.

Tuuri, G., M. Zanovec, L. Silverman, J. Geaghan, M. Solmon, D. Holston, A. Guarino, H. Roy, and E. Murphy. 2009. "Smart Bodies" school wellness program increased children's knowledge of healthy nutrition practices and self-efficacy to consume fruit and vegetables. *Appetite* 52(2):445-451.

USDA (U.S. Department of Agriculture). 1996. *The story of team nutrition: Executive summary of the pilot study.* Alexandria, VA: USDA/FNS, Office of Evaluation, Nutrition, and Evaluation.

USDA. 2007. *School Nutrition Dietary Assessment Study—III: Volume I: School food service, school food environment, and meals offered and served.* Alexandria, VA: USDA.

USDA. 2010. *FY 2010: NIFA-national data: The Expanded Food and Nutrition Education Program.* Washington, DC: USDA.

USDA/FNS (Food and Nutrition Service). 2011. Nutrition standards in the National School Lunch and Breakfast Programs: Proposed rule. *Federal Register* 76(9):2494-2570.

USDA/FNS. 2012. Nutrition standards in the National School Lunch and School Breakfast Programs: Final rule. *Federal Register* 77(17):4088-4167.

Vogler, K. E., and D. Virtue. 2007. "Just the facts, ma'am": Teaching social studies in the era of standards and high-stakes testing. *Social Studies* 98(2):54-58.

Wang, M. C., S. Rauzon, N. Studer, A. C. Martin, L. Craig, C. Merlo, K. Fung, D. Kursunoglu, M. Shannguan, and P. Crawford. 2010. Exposure to a comprehensive school intervention increases vegetable consumption. *Journal of Adolescent Health* 47(1):74-82.

Wansink, B. 2010. From mindless eating to mindlessly eating better. *Physiology and Behavior* 100(5):454-463.

Wood, S. 2011. *Losing money, Seattle schools may ease ban on junk foods.* http://usnews.msnbc.msn.com/_news/2011/12/12/9394147-losing-money-seattle-schools-may-ease-ban-on-junk-foods (accessed December 12, 2011).

Wood, Y., M. M. Cody, and M. F. Nettles. 2010. *Team nutrition local wellness demonstration project report.* University, MS: National Food Service Management Institute.

Woodward-Lopez, G., H. Diaz, and L. Cox. 2010a. *Physical Education Research for Kids (PERK) report.* Orangevale, CA: The California Task Force on Youth and Workplace Wellness.

Woodward-Lopez, G., W. Gosliner, S. E. Samuels, L. Craypo, J. Kao, and P. B. Crawford. 2010b. Lessons learned from evaluations of California's statewide school nutrition standards. *American Journal of Public Health* 100(11):2137-2145.

10

Answering Questions About Leadership, Prioritization, and Assessment with a Systems Perspective

Key Messages

- Leadership, in the case of the committee's systems approach to accelerating obesity prevention, is a shared responsibility across sectors and levels, and one that may not follow typical hierarchical or individual sector-based approaches. It rests with all individuals, organizations, agencies, and sectors that can influence physical activity and food environments.

- The committee did not give priority to any one recommended action or set of actions above others. Rather, leaders are called on to identify priority actions over which they have control, using systems thinking in their implementation efforts.

- A greater awareness of the potential catastrophic consequences of the high rates of obesity, together with a common understanding that individuals and groups in every sector and at every level must play a critical role in prevention, will help catalyze the systemwide implementation of the committee's recommendations.

- Resources will be required to effectively monitor the full impact of the committee's recommendations and determine whether progress in obesity prevention is accelerating.

The unique perspective that a systems approach brings to the issue of obesity is highlighted at the end of the previous chapters presenting the committee's recommendations (Chapters 5-9). For example, Chapter 7, on message environments, points out some of the important intrasector and cross-sector insights that are gained by viewing these issues through a systems lens: "On their own, any one of these actions might help accelerate progress in obesity prevention, but together, their effect would be reinforced, amplified, and maximized. A social marketing campaign on its own, without a decrease in young people's exposure to food and beverage marketing, would be less effective. Likewise, a shift in food and beverage marketing would be more powerful when accompanied by a vigorous social marketing campaign." Likewise, Supplemental Nutrition Assistance Program (SNAP) Education (SNAP-Ed) would be much more effective if a sustained and targeted social marketing campaign were initiated and there were significant increases in food availability and affordability for SNAP recipients.

This unique perspective also influences the committee's views on how leadership, prioritization, and assessment should be handled. A theme that recurs throughout this report is that each of the committee's single recommendations, strategies, and potential actions has the potential to accelerate progress in obesity prevention, but that it is also important to view them as a whole system comprising the five critical areas depicted in Figure 10-1. As illustrated in the figure, this chapter addresses the important issues involved in the implementation of the committee's recommendations for accelerating progress in obesity prevention, using a simplified systems perspective, by answering three important questions: How should leadership be identified, defined, and exercised in response to the systems-oriented recommendations presented in this report? How can the systems thinking represented in this report guide the way a leader should approach implementation of the recommendations and the associated strategies and potential actions? What are the priorities on which leaders should act within and among the five interacting critical areas?

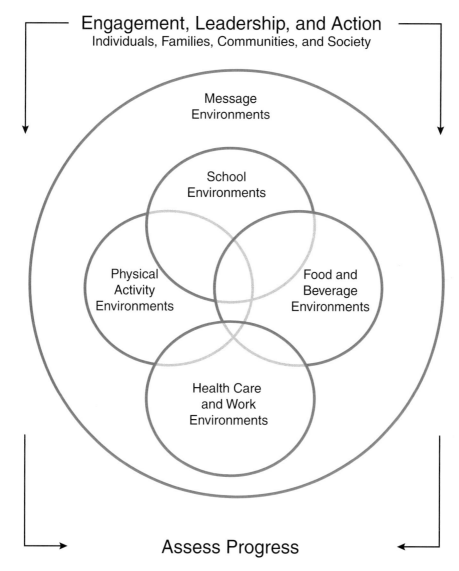

Engagement, Leadership, and Action
Individuals, Families, Communities, and Society

Message
Environments

School
Environments

Physical
Activity
Environments

Food and
Beverage
Environments

Health Care
and Work
Environments

Assess Progress

FIGURE 10-1 Comprehensive approach of the Committee on Accelerating Progress in Obesity Prevention.

This chapter also identifies a set of indicators—complementary to the more specific indicators in Chapters 5-9—that the committee recommends be used to assess progress in the implementation of its recommendations as a whole, an important step in effectively monitoring implementation and impact. The chapter concludes with suggestions for future systems research in obesity prevention.

DEFINING LEADERSHIP AND IDENTIFYING LEADERS

The issue of leadership is dealt with throughout this report. In Chapters 5-9, the potential and obvious leaders for each of the committee's recommendations are identified and called upon to take immediate action to accelerate progress in obesity prevention. These are typically the individuals, agencies, organizations, or sectors that are traditionally seen as having the knowledge, control, and responsibility for the particular environments, policies, and practices that must change. For example, the recommendations, strategies, and potential actions in Chapter 6 (on food and beverage environments) call on schools; the business community/private sector; non-governmental organizations; federal, state, and local governments; the food and beverage industry; and health care providers to take leadership on specific actions.

The report also introduces new ways to think about leadership. For example, Chapter 1 identifies and calls on another set of leaders—individuals, families, communities, and the larger society—for engagement, involvement, and action at multiple levels, pointing out that these levels are interdependent, and all are necessary to achieve impact. Their engagement can lead to, and is a prerequisite for, the exercise of leadership at these different levels. The initial discussion in Chapter 1 also highlights the importance of taking collaborative approaches, involving those affected by an issue in addressing the issues that affect them, and reducing disparities in racial/ethnic minority and low-income communities through "robust and long-term community engagement and civic participation among these disadvantaged populations." In addition, the chapter deals with the issue of responsibility, which is an important component of leadership, suggesting a new way to view personal responsibility—as a collective responsibility of the public and private sectors, and all those involved in each sector, to act to improve physical activity and nutrition environments. Chapter 3 includes some insights from systems thinking into new ways in which leaders can be identified or act, including the concepts of "facilitative leadership," which is "not necessarily located at any particular level or organization and is likely to encourage bottom-up solutions and activities"; "local creativity," which involves "mechanisms for local people to design locally relevant activities and solutions" and not "rigid requirements for activities imposed from outside the area"; and the possibility of "the visibility of obesity as an explicit policy goal or concern for nonhealth organizations. . . ."

A major premise that underlies all the points made above is that leadership in the case of the committee's systems approach to accelerating obesity prevention is a shared responsibility across sectors and levels, and one that may not follow typical hierarchical or individual sector-based approaches. In the committee's view, the problem of obesity is so complex and so embedded in Americans' everyday lives, culture, and physical environments that only integrated, systemic, cross-sector approaches to the problem will succeed. The committee's systems approach to accelerating progress in obesity prevention calls on all individuals, organizations, agencies, and sectors that do or can influence the environments that control physical activity and food consumption to assess and begin to act on their important roles as leaders in prevention. Some traditional leaders may turn away from their logical or designated roles in helping to solve this problem, but other organizations that have previously been concerned with obesity prevention may increase their efforts or broaden the scope of their activities, and many other less likely, unexpected, or less well-known candidates for leadership may step forward to address issues in sectors where they are stakeholders or have influence. For example, the broad articulation of the committee's system of recommendations will support ongoing organizational activity by groups such as county-level Cooperative Extension agencies that have nutrition expertise and strong community ties, while also encouraging many more leaders to identify themselves as important and willing actors, such as local banks that invest in community development or small businesses and faith-based organizations that provide services to their communities and congregations.

IMPLEMENTATION

Leaders who are identified and called upon by this report to act and who seek to carry out their designated roles, or leaders who self-identify—whether a group of mothers of young children concerned about the foods available in their community or an environmental specialist who sees the connections between her work on clean air and the importance of making physical activity a routine part of life—will share the moment of saying to themselves, "I can do something about this, and I want to play a role." From that point on, thinking about their role with a systems lens can guide their actions in new directions. They may consider various sectors, recommendations, strategies, and actions and find themselves on the systems "map" (as presented in Appendix B), figuratively or literally. However, they will act with new foresight—examining how what they plan to do will intersect with other actions that may be taken or are being taken already in various sectors.

They will examine actions by others, in their critical area or in the other four critical areas that are part of the whole system, that will help accelerate what they are attempting to accomplish. They may also see potential actions by others that, if taken, could advance them more rapidly toward their goals. This in turn may lead them not only to implement actions they have already identified, but also to encourage others, sometimes in different sectors, to act in new ways that support their own efforts.

In addition, these leaders may identify ongoing actions that work against what they are attempting to accomplish. This may lead them to change their strategies or work toward removal of the barriers in their or other sectors. They will also want to make sure that what they are planning to do does not have any obvious adverse consequences, and if there are additional positive consequences (side benefits) of what they are attempting, they will want to let others know about them in order to enlist additional support within or across sectors.

Finally, these leaders will want to examine their efforts over time with an eye to what others in their or other sectors are doing as it relates to their goals and how things may be changing overall. They also may want to communicate their actions, goals, and views to others who are working in their or other sectors to implement related changes. Examination of current or potential actions of others within the system and the development of creative, coordinated intra- or cross-sector relationships can lead to more effective efforts and greater opportunities for success. Some leaders, because of their roles, capacities, and broader influence, will choose to focus on an examination of what is happening in the whole system, within and across sectors and critical areas, and will act to understand and influence changes throughout the system.

PRIORITIES

Implicit in the preceding discussion of leadership and implementation is the assumption that individual leaders will determine which recommendations, strategies, and potential actions are their priorities or that those who choose to follow their lead will play a major role in determining these priorities. These leaders will likely start from where they have the most influence and likelihood of success, a decision that will result from a unique assessment of a range of variables. This follows naturally from the committee's systems perspective and definition and identification of leaders as described above, and from its approach to selecting recommendations, strategies, and potential actions as laid out in Chapter 4. The committee selected five major recommendations among hundreds of possibilities, with associated strategies and potential actions, for accelerating obesity prevention in the next decade. These are the committee's priorities for action. Beyond that prioritization, the committee did not go further, as it saw the implementation (or continuing implementation) of the entire system of recommendations, to the greatest extent possible, as the overarching priority. The committee did not give priority to any action or set of actions above any others, but rather envisioned leaders within sectors, and others, stepping up to implement different aspects of the system.

THE PUBLIC HEALTH CRISIS AS MOTIVATOR AND CATALYST FOR IMPLEMENTATION

This report describes the public health crisis of obesity in stark terms. It points out that almost one-third of children and two-thirds of adults in the United States are overweight or obese. In certain demographic groups, rates reach even higher levels. There are devastating health and social consequences for individuals—the great potential for illness, disability, and early death; social ostracism; discrimination in employment and income; depression; and an overall poor quality of life for many millions. Some estimate that one-third of all children born today (and one-half of Latino and black children) will develop type 2 diabetes in their lifetime, and that obesity may lead to a generation with a shorter life span than that of their parents.

As this report points out, the estimated cost of obesity-related illness based on data from the Medical Expenditure Panel Survey for 2000-2005 is $190.2 billion annually (in 2005 dollars), which represents 20.6 percent of annual health care spending in the United States (Cawley and Meyerhoefer, 2011). The U.S. economy already struggles today to cope with health care spending; this struggle will grow progressively more difficult as today's obese children mature.

Because of its views on leadership in accelerating obesity prevention, where that leadership resides, and how it is identified, the committee does not name or recommend one agent, leader, or "commission" to catalyze or lead the implementation of its system of recommendations for obesity prevention. Rather, it sees potential for many leaders across sectors and levels, from individuals working for improvements in physical activity at home and in their communities to federal agencies acting to prevent the negative effects of marketing on children's risk of obesity. The committee sees the primary catalyst for activation of its system of recommendations as a heightened awareness of the potential catastrophic consequences of the high rates of obesity in the United States for quality of life and the national budget, and a common understanding of the critical role that must be played by individuals in every sector and at every level.

The committee also sees the issue of funding the numerous changes that may be involved in implementing its recommendations as related to its concepts of motivator and catalyst and to the potential consequences for funding of taking a systems perspective. Experience in the politics of democracy shows that if an issue is truly understood as potentially catastrophic by citizens and their leaders, calls and support for change will emerge, and resources to engage in the battle will become more available. In addition, leaders will emerge at many levels, and their existing assets often will be brought into action or redeployed for new actions. Taking a systems perspective can help identify and open up new resources for funding from unexpected sources, and new assets that can support the cost of change can be discovered that would not otherwise be apparent. In addition, actions within a system can lead to alliances with individuals and sectors engaged in efforts that contribute significantly to obesity prevention but whose focus is related to another aspect of health or some other social outcome. The resources that can flow from these alliances have the potential to sustain obesity prevention efforts.

ASSESSMENT OF PROGRESS

Once implemented, the recommendations, strategies, and actions proposed in this report will be even more useful if they are evaluated to determine their individual and collective impact. While the recommendations included herein are based on the best evidence available to the committee as it prepared this report, new evidence will emerge and new evaluation research will be needed to fully examine the impact of the committee's individual and collective recommendations. However, such research will not happen without a sustained commitment on the part of decision makers to providing the resources necessary to support the work of monitoring the extent to which progress in obesity prevention is truly accelerating, as well as the impact of individual recommendations and the system of recommendations included in this report.

Using the framework developed in Chapter 4, the committee identified overarching (or system-level) indicators that focus on tracking progress toward reducing the incidence and prevalence of obesity and overweight in the United States. These indicators are intended for use in evaluating progress toward the adoption of the full system of strategies and actions described in Chapters 5 through 9. The committee also identified a foundational indicator focused on the broader dynamics of accelerating progress in obesity prevention, encompassing actions farther upstream from obesity prevention that are important for the successful implementation of all the recommended strategies and actions.

Notably, throughout the process of identifying indicators of progress, it became apparent to the committee that in many cases, national data sources do not yet exist for many of the proposed indicators. This is clearly an area of need going forward. More work is required to develop systems with which to monitor progress on the recommendations and strategies included in this report. Clearly not all of the systems for monitoring progress will be based on federally funded data sources. Rather, the committee envisions the need for a partnership among federal agencies, state agencies, foundation sources, and commercial sources, among others, to develop the systems necessary to monitor progress on the implementation of the committee's recommendations.

Indicators for Assessing Progress in Obesity Prevention with a Systems Perspective

Overarching Indicators

- Reduction in the proportion of adults who are obese.
  Source for measurement: NHANES

- Reduction in the proportion of adults who are overweight.
  Source for measurement: NHANES

- Reduction in the proportion of children and adolescents who are considered obese.
  Source for measurement: NHANES

- Reduction in the proportion of children and adolescents who are considered overweight.
  Source for measurement: NHANES

- Increase in the proportion of young children (aged 2-5) that are of normal weight status.
  Source for measurement: PNSS

- Increase in the proportion of adults who meet current federal physical activity guidelines.
  Source for measurement: NHIS

- Increase in the proportion of children and adolescents who meet current federal physical activity guidelines.
  Sources for measurement: YRBS, NYPAANS (for adolescents); source needed to measure proportion of children who meet current federal Physical Activity Guidelines

LOOKING TO THE FUTURE: MOVING TO THE NEXT LEVEL OF SYSTEMS ANALYSIS

As noted throughout the report and in Appendix B, a systems perspective consistently guided the committee's work, from the development of its vision to the formulation of recommendations, strategies, and actions with the greatest potential to accelerate progress in obesity prevention. However, a systems approach can provide additional opportunities for research and decision making. The committee's use of a systems perspective in viewing solutions to preventing obesity presents an important opportunity to create a research framework that takes this approach into account. This section offers a short discussion of quantitative systems-science methodologies that can be used to further test and refine the committee's system of recommendations and in turn improve future decision making on this dynamic, complex problem. As described in Chapter 4 (and presented in further detail in Appendix B), the committee's systems map serves many purposes, providing important information both to the committee and to readers of this report. In addition, it could in the future serve as a platform for the construction of more quantitative dynamic models. This type of dynamic systems model would enable the conduct of policy simulations exploring the impact over time of a system of recommended strategies and the impact of the five critical areas in which action is needed on each other and on key outcomes of interest. Systems mapping often is an important prerequisite for construction of such a quantitative model by researchers.

Complex problems, such as obesity, typically have been approached using correlation-based analytic methods (e.g., regression). These methods are useful for identifying linear relationships, but are limited because of their inability to establish and test a web of interrelated causal relationships. While correlation-based analytic methods can be valuable in providing detailed information about various aspects of a problem, used alone they can be insufficient for understanding problems that are driven by *interaction* among a large number of factors. Moreover, these conventional methods give limited insight into the mechanisms that underlie observed relationships (Auchincloss and Diez-Roux, 2008; NIH, 2011b).

Systems-science quantitative methodologies enable investigators to examine the dynamic interrelationships among variables at multiple levels of analysis (e.g., from individuals to society) simultaneously, often taking into account causal feedback processes among variables while also studying impacts on the behavior of the system as a whole over time (Midgely, 2003). Such models that utilize data (real or simulated) can incorporate knowledge about individual decision making and biological effects as well as broader flows of information or distributions of effect between factors to take into account the complex "real world" of interest (Hammond, 2009). Systems-science quantitative modeling can even yield policy and scientific insights when a randomized experiment is impractical, expensive, or unethical. Examples of systems-science methodologies and their uses are provided in Box 10-1.

Many systems modeling methods are not new and indeed are now used routinely in such fields as corporate management, economics, engineering, physics, energy, ecology, and biology precisely because these methods add value relative to alternative techniques or unaided decision making (NIH, 2011b). As appreciation for the complexity of many problems in the public health sphere has grown, there have recently been a number of calls to use systems science to examine public health problems (Homer and Hirsch, 2006; Leischow et al., 2008; Mabry et al., 2010; Madon et al., 2007; Milstein et al., 2007), including obesity in particular (Auchincloss and Diez-Roux, 2008; Hammond, 2009; Huang and Glass, 2008; NIH, 2011a).

BOX 10-1
Examples of Systems-Science Methodologies and Their Uses

Specific examples of systems-science methodologies include

- systems dynamics modeling (Homer and Hirsch, 2006; Sterman, 2006);

- agent-based modeling (Axelrod, 2006; Epstein, 2006; Miller and Page, 2007);

- discrete event simulation (Banks et al., 2010);

- network analysis (Scott, 2000; Wasserman and Faust, 1994);

- dynamic microsimulation modeling (Mitton et al., 2000); and

- Markov modeling (Sonnenberg and Beck, 1993).

These techniques, among others, are particularly well suited for

- understanding connections between a system's structure and its behavior over time;

- anticipating a range of plausible futures based on explicit scenarios for action or inaction in certain areas;

- identifying unintended or counterintuitive consequences of interventions;

- evaluating both the short- and long-term effects of policy options; and

- guiding investments in new research or data collection to address critical information needs.

REFERENCES

Auchincloss, A. H., and A. V. Diez-Roux. 2008. A new tool for epidemiology: The usefulness of dynamic-agent models in understanding place effects on health. *American Journal of Epidemiology* 168(1):1-8.

Axelrod, R. 2006. Agent-based modeling as a bridge between disciplines. In *Handbook of computational economics*. Vol. 2, edited by L. Tesfatsion and K. L. Judd. Amsterdam (NL): North-Holland. Pp. 1565-1584.

Banks, J., J. S. Carson II, B. L. Nelson, and D. M. Nicol. 2010. *Discrete-event system simulation*. 5th ed. Upper Saddle River, NJ: Pearson Prentice Hall.

Cawley, J., and C. Meyerhoefer. 2011. The medical care costs of obesity: An instrumental variables approach. *Journal of Health Economics* 31(1):219-230.

Epstein, J. M. 2006. Remarks on the foundations of agent-based generative social science. In *Handbook of computational economics*. Vol. 2, edited by L. Tesfatsion and K. L. Judd. Amsterdam (NL): North-Holland. Pp. 1585-1604.

Hammond, R. A. 2009. Complex systems modeling for obesity research. *Preventing Chronic Disease* 6(3):A97.

Homer, J. B., and G. B. Hirsch. 2006. System dynamics modeling for public health: Background and opportunities. *American Journal of Public Health* 96(3):452-458.

Huang, T. T., and T. A. Glass. 2008. Transforming research strategies for understanding and preventing obesity. *Journal of the American Medical Association* 300(15):1811-1813.

Leischow, S. J., A. Best, W. M. Trochim, P. I. Clark, R. S. Gallagher, S. E. Marcus, and E. Matthews. 2008. Systems thinking to improve the public's health. *American Journal of Preventive Medicine* 35(Suppl. 2):S196-S203.

Mabry, P. L., S. E. Marcus, P. I. Clark, S. J. Leischow, and D. Mendez. 2010. Systems science: A revolution in public health policy research. *American Journal of Public Health* 100(7):1161-1163.

Madon, T., K. J. Hofman, L. Kupfer, and R. I. Glass. 2007. Public health. Implementation science. *Science* 318(5857):1728-1729.

Midgely, G. 2003. *Systems thinking: Critical systems thinking and systemic perspectives on ethics, power and pluralism*. Vol. 4. Thousand Oaks, CA: Sage Publications.

Miller, J. H., and S. E. Page. 2007. *Complex adaptive systems: An introduction to computational models of social life*. Princeton, NJ: Princeton University Press.

Milstein, B., A. Jones, J. B. Homer, D. Murphy, J. Essien, and D. Seville. 2007. Charting plausible futures for diabetes prevalence in the United States: A role for system dynamics simulation modeling. *Preventing Chronic Disease* 4(3):A52.

Mitton, L., H. Sutherland, and M. J. Weeks. 2000. *Microsimulation modelling for policy analysis: Challenges and innovations*. New York: Cambridge University Press.

NIH (National Institutes of Health). 2011a. *Strategic plan for NIH obesity research: A report of the NIH Obesity Research Task Force*. NIH publication no. 11-5493. Washington, DC: U.S. Department of Health and Human Services.

NIH. 2011b. *Systems science*. http://obssr.od.nih.gov/scientific_areas/methodology/ systems_science/index.aspx (accessed November 18, 2011).

Scott, J. 2000. *Social network analysis: A handbook*. 2nd ed. London: Sage Publications.

Sonnenberg, F. A., and J. R. Beck. 1993. Markov models in medical decision making: A practical guide. *Medical Decision Making* 13(4):322-338.

Sterman, J. D. 2006. Learning from evidence in a complex world. *American Journal of Public Health* 96(3):505-514.

Wasserman, S., and K. Faust. 1994. *Social network analysis: Methods and applications* New York: Cambridge University Press.

A

Acronyms and Glossary

ACRONYMS

AAFP	American Academy of Family Physicians
AAP	American Academy of Pediatrics
ACA	*Patient Protection and Affordable Care Act of 2010*
ACOG	American College of Obstetricians and Gynecologists
AHA	American Heart Association
AIM	Americans In Motion
AMA	American Medical Association
ARRA	*American Recovery and Reinvestment Act*
BGCA	Boys & Girls Clubs of America
BMI	body mass index
BRFSS	Behavioral Risk Factor Surveillance System
CACFP	Child and Adult Care Food Program
CATCH	Coordinated Approach To Child Health (formerly Child and Adolescent Trial for Cardiovascular Health)
CDC	Centers for Disease Control and Prevention
CFBAI	Children's Food and Beverage Advertising Initiative
CSFII	Continuing Survey of Food Intakes by Individuals
CSPI	Center for Science in the Public Interest
DGAC	Dietary Guidelines Advisory Committee
DOE	U.S. Department of Education
DOT	U.S. Department of Transportation
EFNEP	Expanded Food and Nutrition Education Program

EHR	electronic health record
EPSDT	Early and Periodic Screening, Diagnosis, and Treatment
ERS	Economic Research Service
FDA	U.S. Food and Drug Administration
FTC	Federal Trade Commission
FY	fiscal year
GAO	Government Accountability Office (previously General Accounting Office)
HEDIS	Healthcare Effectiveness Data and Information Set
HHS	U.S. Department of Health and Human Services
HIE	health information exchange
HIPAA	*Health Insurance Portability and Accountability Act*
HITECH	Health Information Technology for Economic and Clinical Health
IBCLC	International Board Certified Lactation Consultant
IOM	Institute of Medicine
IWG	Interagency Working Group
L.E.A.D.	Locate Evidence, Evaluate Evidence, Assemble Evidence, Inform Decisions (framework)
MEPS	Medical Expenditure Panel Survey
MET	metabolic equivalent of task
mPINC	Maternity Practices in Infant Nutrition and Care
NASN	National Association of School Nurses
NASPE	National Association for Sport and Physical Education
NCCOR	National Collaborative on Childhood Obesity Research
NCHS	National Center for Health Statistics
NCI	National Cancer Institute
NHANES	National Health and Nutrition Examination Survey
NHIS	National Health Interview Survey
NHWS	National Health and Wellness Survey

NIH	National Institutes of Health
NRPA	National Recreation and Park Association
NSLP	National School Lunch Program
OECD	Organisation for Economic Co-operation and Development
PAG	Physical Activity Guidelines for Americans
PE	physical education
PSA	public service announcement
QALY	quality-adjusted life-year
RDA	Recommended Dietary Allowance
RWJF	The Robert Wood Johnson Foundation
SCHIP	State Children's Health Insurance Program
SHPPS	School Health Policies and Programs Study
SNAP	Supplemental Nutrition Assistance Program
SNAP-Ed	SNAP Education
SoFAS	solid fats and added sugars
SRTS	Safe Routes to School
SUS	Shape Up Somerville
UNICEF	United Nations Children's Fund
USDA	U.S. Department of Agriculture
USPSTF	U.S. Preventive Services Task Force
WHO	World Health Organization
WIC	Special Supplemental Nutrition Program for Women, Infants, and Children
YMCA	Young Men's Christian Association
YRBS	Youth Risk Behavior Survey
YRBSS	Youth Risk Behavior Surveillance System

GLOSSARY

Absenteeism   A persistent failure to appear for work, school, or other regular activities.

Active living   A way of life that integrates physical activity into daily routines. The two types of activities that make up active living are recreational or leisure, such as jogging, skateboarding, and playing basketball; and utilitarian or occupational, such as walking or biking to school, shopping, or running errands.

Adiposity   The state of an excess of body fat.

Advergame   A branded product that is built directly into an Internet-based game or video game, or game appearing in print materials.

Advertising   A paid public presentation and promotion of ideas, goods, or services by a sponsor that is intended to bring a product to the attention of consumers through a variety of media channels, such as broadcast and cable television, radio, print, billboards, the Internet, or personal contact.

Away-from-home foods   Foods categorized according to where they are obtained, such as restaurants and other places with wait service; fast-food establishments and self-service or carry-out eateries; schools, including day care, after-school programs, and summer camp; and other outlets, including vending machines, community feeding programs, and other people's homes.

Basal metabolism   The minimum amount of energy that an individual needs to maintain vital functions in a resting state.

BMI z-score   Number of standard deviations away from the population mean body mass index (BMI); in other words, the degree to which an individual's measurement deviates from what is expected for that individual.

Body mass index	An indirect measure of body fat, calculated as the ratio of a person's body weight in kilograms to the square of a person's height in meters.

$$\text{BMI (kg/m}^2) = \text{weight (kilograms)} \div \text{height (meters)}^2$$

$$\text{BMI (lb/in}^2) = \text{weight (pounds)} \div \text{height (inches)}^2 \times 703$$

In children and youth, BMI is interpreted using growth charts for age and gender and is referred to as BMI-for-age and sex, which is used to assess underweight, overweight, and obesity. According to the Centers for Disease Control and Prevention (CDC), a child with a BMI that is equal to or greater than the 95th percentile is considered to be obese. A child with a BMI that is equal to or between the 85th and 95th percentile is considered to be overweight.

Built environment The man-made elements of the physical environment; buildings, infrastructure, and other physical elements created or modified by people and the functional use, arrangement in space, and aesthetic qualities of these elements.

Calorie A calorie is defined as the amount of heat required to change the temperature of one gram of water from 14.5 degrees Celsius to 15.5 degrees Celsius. In this report, "calorie" is used synonymously with "kilocalorie," the unit of measure for energy obtained from food and beverages.

Calorie-dense food Foods and beverages that contribute few vitamins and minerals to the diet but contain substantial amounts of fat and/or sugar and are high in calories. Consumption of these foods, such as sugar-sweetened beverages, candy, and chips may contribute to excess caloric intake and unwanted weight gain in children.

Capacity building A multidimensional and dynamic process that improves the ability of individuals, groups, communities, organizations, and governments to meet their objectives or enhance performance to address population health. In public health, capacity building involves the ability to carry out essential functions, such as developing and sustaining partnerships, leveraging resources, conducting surveillance and monitoring, providing training and technical assistance, and conducting evaluations.

Community A social entity that can be spatial based on where people live in local neighborhoods, residential districts, or municipalities, or relational, as with people who have common ethnic or cultural characteristics or share similar interests.

Competitive foods Foods and beverages offered at schools other than meals and snacks served through the federally reimbursed school lunch, breakfast, and after-school snack programs. Competitive foods includes food and beverages items sold through à la carte lines, snack bars, student stores, vending machines, and school fundraisers.

Dietary Guidelines for Americans A federal summary of the latest dietary guidance for the public based on current scientific evidence and medical knowledge, issued by the Department of Health and Human Services and U.S. Department of Agriculture and revised every 5 years.

Disability A physical, intellectual, emotional, or functional impairment that limits a major activity, and may be a complete or partial impairment.

Disease An impairment, interruption, disorder, or cessation of the normal state of the living animal or plant body or of any of its components that interrupts or modifies the performance of the vital functions, being a response to environmental factors (e.g., malnutrition, industrial hazards, climate), to specific infective agents (e.g., worms, bacteria, or viruses), to inherent defects of the organism (e.g., various genetic anomalies), or to combinations of these factors; conceptually, a disease (which is usually tangible or measurable but may be symptom-free) is distinct from illness (i.e., the associated pain, suffering, or distress, which is highly individual and personal).

Disparities A term used to describe differences in quality of health and health care across racial, ethnic, and socioeconomic groups.

Energy balance A state in which energy intake is equivalent to energy expenditure, resulting in no net weight gain or weight loss. In this report, energy balance is used to indicate equality between energy intake and energy expenditure that supports normal growth without promoting excess weight gain.

Energy-dense foods Foods that are high in calories.

Energy density The amount of energy stored in a given food per unit volume or mass. Fat stores 9 kilocalories/gram (gm), alcohol stores 7 kilocalories/gm, carbohydrate and protein each store 4 kilocalories/gm, fiber stores 1.5 to 2.5 kilocalories/gm, and water has no calories. Foods that are almost entirely composed of fat with minimal water (e.g., butter) are more energy dense than foods that consist largely of water, fiber, and carbohydrates (e.g., fruits and vegetables).

Energy expenditure Calories used to support the body's basal metabolic functions plus those used for thermogenesis, growth, and physical activity.

Energy intake Calories ingested as food and beverages.

Environment The external influences on the life of an individual or community.

Epidemic A condition that is occurring more frequently and extensively among individuals in a community or population than is expected.

Exercise	Planned, structured, and repetitive body movements done to improve or maintain one or more components of physical fitness, such as muscle tone and strength.
Fast food	Foods designed for ready availability, use, or consumption and sold at eating establishments for quick availability or take-out.
Fat	The chemical storage form of fatty acids as glycerol esters, also known as triglycerides. Fat is stored primarily in adipose tissue located throughout the body, but mainly under the skin (subcutaneously) and around the internal organs (viscerally). Fat mass is the sum total of the fat in the body, while, correspondingly, the remaining, nonfat components of the body constitute the fat-free mass. Lean tissues such as muscle, bone, skin, blood, and the internal organs are the principal locations of the body's fat-free mass. In common practice, however, the terms "fat" and "adipose tissue" are often used interchangeably. Furthermore, "fat" is commonly used as a subjective or descriptive term that may have a pejorative meaning.
Fitness	A set of attributes, primarily respiratory and cardiovascular, relating to the ability to perform tasks requiring physical activity.
Food Guide Pyramid	An educational tool designed for the public that graphically illustrates recommendations from the Dietary Guidelines for Americans and nutrient standards such as the Dietary Reference Intakes and translates them into food-group-based advice that promotes a healthful diet.
Food insecurity	A household-level economic and social condition of limited or uncertain access to adequate food.
Food security	Consistent, dependable access to enough food for active, healthy living.

Food system	The interrelated functions that encompass food production, processing, and distribution; food access and utilization by individuals, households, communities, and populations; and food recycling, composting, and disposal.
Guidelines	In the present context, standardized information describing the best practices for addressing health problems commonly encountered in public health practice. The information is based on scientific evidence for the effectiveness and efficiency of the practices described. Where such evidence is lacking, guidelines are sometimes based on the consensus opinions of public health experts.
Health	A state of complete physical, mental, and social well-being, and not merely the absence of disease or infirmity.
Health promotion	The process of enabling people to increase control over and improve their health. To reach a state of complete physical, mental, and social well-being, an individual or group must be able to identify and to realize aspirations, to satisfy needs, and to change or cope with the environment. Health is a resource for everyday life, not the objective of living, and is a positive concept emphasizing social and personal resources, as well as physical capacities.
Healthy weight	In children and youth, a level of body fat at which comorbidities are not observed. In adults, a BMI at or between 18.5 and 24.9 kg/m^2.
Incidence	The frequency of new cases of a condition or disease within a defined time period. Incidence is commonly measured in terms of new cases per 1,000 (or 100,000) population at risk per year.
Indicator of progress	In the context of this report, an objective measure that can be used to assess the effect of, or association with, a given recommendation in accelerating progress toward obesity prevention.

Intervention	A policy, program, or action intended to bring about identifiable outcomes.
Marketing	An organizational function and a set of processes for creating, communicating, and delivering value to customers and for managing customer relationships in ways that benefit an organization and its stakeholders. Marketing encompasses a wide range of activities, including conducting market research; analyzing the competition; positioning a new product; pricing the product and services; and promoting products and services through advertising, consumer promotion, trade promotions, public relations, and sales.
Moderate-intensity physical activity	On an absolute scale, moderate-intensity physical activity is completed at 3.0 to 5.9 times the intensity of rest. On a scale that is relative to an individual's personal capacity, moderate-intensity physical activity is usually a 5 or 6 on a scale of 0 to 10.
Nutrient density	The amount of nutrients that a food contains per unit volume or mass. Nutrient density is independent of energy density although, in practice, the nutrient density of a food is often described in relationship to the food's energy density. Fruits and vegetables are nutrient dense but not energy dense. Compared with foods of high fat content, soda or soft drinks are not particularly energy dense because they are made up primarily of water and carbohydrate, but because they are otherwise low in nutrients, their energy density is high for their nutrient content.
Nutrition Facts panel	Standardized detailed nutritional information on the contents and serving sizes of nearly all packaged foods sold in the marketplace. The panel was designed to provide nutrition information to consumers and was mandated by the *Nutrition Labeling and Education Act* of 1994.

Obesity	An excess amount of subcutaneous body fat in proportion to lean body mass. In adults, a BMI of 30 or greater is considered obese. In this report, obesity in children and adolescents refers to age- and sex-specific BMIs that are equal to or greater than the 95th percentile of the CDC BMI growth charts. In most children, these values are known to indicate elevated body fat and to reflect the comorbidities associated with excessive body fatness.
Obesogenic	Environmental factors that may promote obesity and encourage the expression of a genetic predisposition to gain weight.
Overweight	In adults, a BMI between 25.0 and 29.9 is considered overweight. In this report, overweight in children and adolescents refers to age- and sex-specific BMIs at or above the 95th percentile of the CDC BMI growth charts.
Physical activity	Body movement produced by the contraction of skeletal muscles that results in energy expenditure above the basal level. Physical activity consists of athletic, recreational, housework, transport, or occupational activities that require physical skills and utilize strength, power, endurance, speed, flexibility, range of motion, or agility.
Physical education	Refers to a planned, sequential program of curricula and instruction that helps students develop the knowledge, attitudes, motor skills, self-management skills, and confidence needed to adopt and maintain physically active lifestyles.
Physical fitness	A set of attributes that people have or achieve that relates to the ability to perform physical activity. The ability to carry out daily tasks with vigor and alertness, without undue fatigue, and with ample energy to enjoy leisure-time pursuits and meet unforeseen emergencies.
Physical inactivity	Not meeting the type, duration, and frequency of recommended leisure time and occupational physical activities.

Policy	A written statement reflecting a plan or course of action of a government, business, community, or institution that is intended to influence and guide decision making. For a government, a policy may consist of a law, regulation, ordinance, executive order, or resolution.
Population health	The state of health of an entire community or population as opposed to that of an individual. It is concerned with the inter-related factors that affect the health of populations over the life course and the distribution of the patterns of health outcomes.
Presenteeism	The degree to which individuals attend regular activities such as work and school but are not fully functioning because of a medical or psychological condition.
Prevalence	The number of instances of a condition or disease in a population at a designated period of time, usually expressed as a percentage of the total population.
Prevention	With regard to obesity, *primary* prevention represents avoiding the occurrence of obesity in a population; *secondary* prevention represents early detection of disease through screening with the purpose of limiting its occurrence; and *tertiary* prevention involves preventing the sequelae of obesity in childhood and adulthood.
Price elasticity	The degree to which consumers change their purchasing and consumption behaviors in response to higher food/beverage prices.
Program	An integrated set of planned strategies and activities that support clearly stated goals and objectives designed to lead to desirable changes and improvements in the well-being of people, institutions, or environments or all of these.
Risk	The possibility or probability of loss, injury, disadvantage, or destruction.

Safety   The condition of being protected from or unlikely to cause danger, risk, or injury that may be either perceived or objectively defined.

School meals   Comprises the food service activities that take place within the school setting. The federal child nutrition programs include the National School Lunch Program, School Breakfast Program, Child and Adult Care Food Program, Summer Food Service Program, and Special Milk Program.

Sector   A distinct subset of a market, society, industry, or the economy in which the members share similar characteristics. Examples of the sectors discussed in this report include government or the public sector, communities, nonprofit and philanthropic organizations, health care, business/the private sector, schools, and households.

Sedentary   A way of living or lifestyle that requires minimal physical activity and that encourages inactivity through limited choices, disincentives, and/or structural or financial barriers.

Social marketing The application of commercial marketing principles to the analysis, planning, implementation, and evaluation of programs designed to influence voluntary behavioral changes in target audiences to improve their personal welfare and benefit society.

Solid fats   Fats with a high content of saturated and/or trans fatty acids, which are usually solid at room temperature. Common examples of solid fats include butter, beef fat, lard, shortening, coconut oil, palm oil, and milk fat, which is solid at room temperature but is suspended in fluid milk by homogenization.

Systematic review A review of a clearly formulated question that uses systematic and explicit methods to identify, select, and critically appraise relevant research and to collect and analyze data from the studies that are included in the review. Statistical methods (meta-analysis) may or may not be used to analyze and summarize the results of the included studies.

Systems approach   A paradigm or perspective involving a focus on the whole picture and not just a single element, awareness of the wider context, an appreciation for interactions among different components, and transdisciplinary thinking.

Systems thinking   An iterative learning process in which one takes a broad, holistic, long-term perspective on the world and examines the linkages and interactions among its elements.

Tween   A child in the middle of childhood and adolescence (between the ages of 9 and 13).

Unhealthy   Although there is no consensus on the definition of "unhealthy" foods/beverages, the term as used in this report refers to foods and beverages that are calorie-dense and low in naturally occurring nutrients. Such foods and beverages contribute little fiber and few essential nutrients and phytochemicals, but contain added fats, sweeteners, sodium, and other ingredients. Unhealthy foods and beverages displace the consumption of foods recommended in the Dietary Guidelines for Americans and may lead to the development of obesity.

Vigorous-intensity physical activity   On an absolute scale, vigorous-intensity physical activity is completed at 6.0 or more times the intensity of rest. On a scale relative to an individual's personal capacity, vigorous-intensity physical activity is usually a 7 or 8 on a scale of 0 to 10.

B

Methodology: Development of the Committee's Recommendations

To develop recommendations[1] for accelerating progress in obesity prevention, the committee undertook a series of steps. The process was informed primarily by the development of a set of guiding principles (detailed in Chapter 4). As described in Chapter 1, the committee was charged as a first step with reviewing obesity-related recommendations from previous Institute of Medicine (IOM) reports and other relevant sources. To this end, the committee identified recommendations to review, organized and grouped these recommendations, and developed a process for reviewing and filtering them. Complementary (and parallel) to the set of filtering criteria, an approach was used to help identify relationships and synergies among the recommendations with the most promise to accelerate progress in obesity prevention. Throughout the process, gaps were identified and considered in developing the final set of recommendations. From these efforts, a comprehensive approach to this study emerged that includes five critical areas, linked as an interrelated system. The committee's recommendations and strategies and potential actions for implementation are presented in Chapters 5-9 (and again in Appendix C). The following sections provide additional detail on how the committee developed its recommendations.

---

[1]As described in Box 4-1, the term "recommendations" as used in this report refers in general to a group of terms unless otherwise specified. Thus the committee's "recommendations" include the recommendations and their associated goals, strategies, and potential actions, and the review of prior "recommendations" includes what others have identified as recommendations, interventions, actions, and strategies.

IDENTIFICATION, ORGANIZATION, REVIEW, AND FILTERING OF PRIOR RECOMMENDATIONS

Identification and Organization

The committee began by compiling all previous obesity-related recommendations from the IOM and other relevant sources. It should be noted that the IOM and National Research Council (NRC) reports all were developed to fulfill a specific task that defines the scope of each report and consequently may limit the scope of its recommendations.

The general criterion used in deciding which recommendations to review was that they were relevant to population-based obesity prevention approaches; that is, they were intended to lower the mean body mass index (BMI) level and decrease the rate at which people enter the upper end of the BMI distribution. Although searches were not limited by the date of publication, the year 2005 marked the beginning of the National Academies' issuance of obesity prevention-related recommendations. The 2005 IOM report *Preventing Childhood Obesity: Health in the Balance* and the 2005 Transportation Research Board report *Does the Built Environment Influence Physical Activity?* demonstrated increasing recognition of the complex, multifaceted nature of the many factors that influence energy balance (IOM, 2005; TRB/IOM, 2005). This recognition led to the examination of obesity prevention strategies that moved beyond a biomedical model and an individual behavior change approach to encompass multilevel, multisector policy and environmental approaches. National Academies reports and reports outside of the National Academies that include recommendations emerging from this conceptualization were published mainly in 2005 and beyond (with some exceptions).

The criteria for including a report and consequently its recommendations in the committee's review were as follows:

- included only population-based obesity prevention strategies;
- used established procedures for making recommendations (e.g., evidence-based, transparency in decisions made);
- included only environmental and policy strategies (as opposed to strategies focused on individual behavior or biomedical approaches); and
- was derived from some type of expert task force or committee consensus.

The quest for relevant publications included an online search of several databases and publication lists of relevant organizations and a review of references in reports that were identified. Committee members, public workshop presenters and attendees, interested stakeholders, and the public also provided suggested sources for review (see the end of this appendix for a list of reports included in the review).

Approximately 800 obesity-prevention related recommendations were identified from these reports. To manage this large number of recommendations, the committee organized them into 10 broad topics (school foods; health care; food marketing; agriculture policy; physical activity, physical inactivity, transportation, and the built environment; pregnancy, early childhood, and child care; nutrition education and information; research, monitoring, and evaluation; food access and pricing; other). Within each broad topic, similar recommendations were grouped to help identify themes and continue to identify gaps.

Review and Filtering

Each recommendation that met the above inclusion criteria was reviewed and coded on several dimensions based on the committee's guiding principles (see Chapter 4) so the committee could assess its promise for accelerating progress in obesity prevention over the next decade. A textual description of each filter was provided to the coder to ensure consistency in judgments. The filters used were

- policy or funding dependent;
- reach/scope;
- potential magnitude of impact;
- evidence base;
- reduction of disparities;
- geographic implementation to date;
- degree to which recommendation is actionable;
- measurability;
- unintended consequences;
- timeline to implementation; and
- feasibility, practicality, and cost if known.

At least two coders were assigned to each recommendation or group of related recommendations. Each coder worked independently, and disagreements were resolved through discussion. If consensus was not readily obtained by the pair of coders, additional committee members were consulted. Once agreement had been reached, both coders' comments on the promise of the strategy were compiled, and a list of strategies based on the results of the coding exercise was developed. These recommendations were shared with the full committee, revised, updated, and consolidated as a result of further committee deliberations. The recommendations were judged against these filters using the information or evidence provided in the reports in which the recommendations were offered. Additionally, related information and evidence made available since the issuance of the original recommendations, as well as information on the progress of their implementation, was identified and considered to inform the coding process.

The search for and interpretation of relevant evidence for each recommendation was guided by a framework that was developed to inform decisions on obesity prevention, integrating research evidence into a broader policy context (IOM, 2010a). This framework with which to locate, evaluate, and assemble evidence to inform decisions on obesity prevention decision making (the L.E.A.D. framework) was used to identify, locate, and evaluate the type of evidence appropriate for the task of prioritizing the recommendations based on the best available scientific evidence. Being concerned with locating evidence to help in assessing the effects of the recommended interventions, the committee sought effectiveness studies, as well as studies examining the presumed mechanism of the intervention effects. Guided by the L.E.A.D. framework, the committee broadened its search to include empirical comparative studies and evaluations commonly referred to as impact assessments or outcome evaluations. Additionally, the committee considered implementation evidence to determine whether an intervention is still needed, whether it had the intended effects with the expected impact, and whether changes to the intervention might be necessary in the future. Finally, the committee took into consideration political and practical concerns such as the cost, feasibility, and practicality of implementing the interventions. To identify research related to an intervention's effectiveness, implementation, and relevance, the committee searched a wide variety of data sources, including the scientific literature; grey and unpublished literature; surveys, polls, and rankings; and government policies and programs. The committee focused its searches by first seeking and using literature syntheses and updates, and if no recent syntheses were found, searched for evidence on the particular recommendation of interest and also reached out to states, communities, and localities that have implemented an intervention for implementation-related research.

IDENTIFICATION OF LINKAGES AMONG FILTERED RECOMMENDATIONS

As described in Chapter 4 and recommended by the L.E.A.D. framework, mapping the determinants of a problem can elucidate potential mechanisms and dynamic pathways on which a more comprehensive approach should focus. Accordingly, the committee mapped the pathways through which the most promising recommendations (as identified through the above process) relate, thus taking a comprehensive systems approach that links the committee's recommendations.

As the committee gathered and reviewed prior recommendations, it became increasingly clear that to identify which recommendations were most likely to accelerate progress in obesity prevention, the committee needed to understand and map how the various recommendations would interact and reinforce or perhaps inhibit progress. To this end, it was necessary to understand that for each recommendation under consideration, there was a primary mechanism by which change would be effected and that each had a set of prerequisites, accelerants, and inhibitors that could potentially come into play during its implementation. The *primary mechanism* describes the pathway, or how and why a recommendation would help prevent obesity. *Prerequisites* are elements necessary for a recommendation to be implemented or to be successful. Examples include public acceptance and willingness and adherence to or enforcement of existing policies and regulations. *Accelerants* are factors that will speed up the effectiveness or leverage the impact of a recommendation. Examples include appropriate resources and well-organized coalitions and partnerships, as well as tools and templates to offer guidance. *Inhibitors* are elements that will slow the effectiveness of a recommendation or impede its implementation. Examples include existing legislation, regulations, or policies that prohibit action; a lack of guidance for implementation; a lack of pilot programs implementing the recommendation; and a lack of public, private, or political will and leadership.

The committee undertook a process of participatory model building to create a systems map that would illustrate how the recommendations were interrelated. As discussed in further detail in Chapters 2 and 3, the committee discussed the determinants of obesity and what changes have occurred in the United States over the past several decades as the obesity epidemic emerged. The committee analyzed how past decisions influenced the current landscape, and considered why so many private, public, individual, and societal decisions have been ineffective in achieving intended objectives. Deliberations and discussions led the committee to accept that answers to such questions might lie in the dynamic behavior of social, personal, environmental, political, and physical systems (Forrester, 1991), and that using system mapping as a tool (i.e., a systems map) would enable the committee to organize and make sense of the task at hand.

The result of these deliberations was the emergence of a comprehensive strategy to link actions in five critical areas that served as the basis for the committee's recommendations. The next section provides a detailed discussion of the map of the committee's recommendations as an interrelated system of interventions.

DEVELOPMENT OF THE SYSTEMS MAP

The systems map in this report is a visual tool designed to aid in identifying linkages among and between the committee's recommendations and implementing strategies. It allows visual communication of the latent potential effects of the recommendations and strategies both individually and synergistically, as well as how they fit within the broader societal context. This map makes it possible to identify strategies that may serve as prerequisites for other actions or may help reinforce their impact. It also allows the discovery of "long chain" effects of strategies that go beyond their immediate focus and impact. Finally, the map facilitated the design of a cohesive set of strategies that support each other as a system, increasing the effectiveness of the committee's recommendations by approaching them from multiple directions (see Figure B-1).

How to Read the Map

The map contains three shapes: squares, circles, and arrows. Squares are labeled with letters (A through E) and represent the committee's five recommendations, as listed in the accompanying legend. Circles are labeled with numbers (1 through 20) and represent the strategies suggested for implementing the recommendations. The coloring of the strategies reflects the sector(s) of action they represent: the business community/private sector, the public sector, citizens and civic/community organizations, health care, and worksites/employers. The recommendations and strategies shown on the map and listed on the legend are described in detail in Chapters 5 through 9.

An arrow indicates a connection between one strategy and another, between a strategy and a recommendation, or between two recommendations. The arrows are directional, indicating the flow of influence *from* one shape *to* another. An arrow pointing from a circle to a square can be read as "this strategy influences or affects this recommendation." Arrows may also be bidirectional, indicating *positive feedback* between the two shapes at its endpoints.

Construction of the Map

The systems map was constructed using an iterative process. Early in this process, the entire committee was given a background presentation on systems approaches and their use in other policy arenas. Working groups within the committee also participated in a thought exercise in which they were asked to identify key systems links between strategies and recommendations that met the inclusion criteria outlined above. Based on this exercise, discussions with the committee, and input and assistance from IOM staff, an initial systems map was developed and used to help frame the committee's discussion of strategies and recommendations. As the committee's deliberations proceeded, key systems connections were identified by committee members and staff. These connections, along with feedback on the map's design and a finalized set of recommendations and strategies, were used to generate the final systems map. It is also important to note that as individuals take a systems perspective when implementing these recommendations and strategies, additional connections may be identified.

Each connection (arrow), whether between two strategies (circles), two recommendations (squares), or one strategy and one recommendation, represents a carefully considered relationship of influence or impact identified by the committee and/or staff that is based on the best available evidence or conceptual support. In all cases, a clear mechanism for the flow of influence can be identified.

For example, Figure B-2 shows that the strategy of a nutrition labeling system (a circle labeled 3 in the upper lefthand portion of the map) impacts the strategy of food literacy in schools (a circle labeled 5 at the left and lower in the map) because a simplified nutrition labeling system makes it easier for students to act on the nutrition guidelines taught in schools. Thus an arrow points from circle 13 to circle 15 on the map.

Elsewhere on the map, the strategy of a social marketing program (a circle labeled 11 in the upper center of the map) both impacts and is impacted by the strategy of physical activity-related community programs (a circle labeled 2 nearby) (see Figure B-3). The two are mutually reinforcing. Thus arrows connect the two circles in both directions.

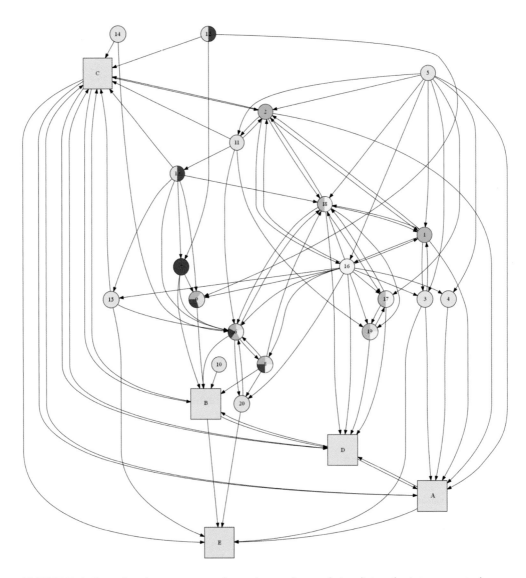

FIGURE B-1 Committee's systems map for understanding and visualizing the interconnectedness of its recommendations and strategies.

Legend for Figure B-1	
Strategies* (Circles)	*Recommendations** [Squares]
(1) Physical and built environment	[A] Prioritize promotion of physical activity by increasing access and opportunities for such activity.
(2) Physical activity-related community pro-grams	[B] Reduce unhealthy food and beverage options and increase healthier options.
(3) Physical education and physical activity in schools	[C] Transform the message environment.
(4) Physical activity in child care centers	[D] Increase the support provided by health care providers, insurers, and employers.
(5) Science and practice of physical activity	[E] Make schools a national focal point for obesity prevention.
(6) Sugar-sweetened beverages	
(7) Food and beverage options for children in restaurants	*Sector of action* (Color)
	• Business community/private sector (Red)
(8) Nutritional standards for all food and beverages	• Public sector (Blue)
	• Citizens and civic community organiza-tions (Green)
(9) Food and beverage retailing and distribu-tion policies	• Health care (Yellow)
	• Worksites/employers (Orange)
(10) U.S. agriculture policy and research	
(11) Social marketing program	
(12) Food and beverage marketing standards for children	
(13) Nutrition labeling system	
(14) Nutrition education policies	
(15) Food literacy in schools	
(16) Health care and advocacy	
(17) Coverage of and access to and incen-tives for obesity prevention, screening, diagnosis, and treatment	
(18) Healthy eating and active living at work	
(19) Weight gain and breastfeeding	
(20) School food and beverage standards	

*The strategies and recommendations as seen in the legend have been abbreviated. Appendix C provides the complete content of each strategy and recommendation.

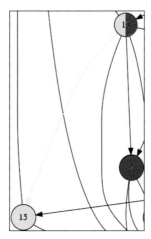

FIGURE B-2 A directional connection arrow on the map. A small section of the map is magnified here, and the arrow is highlighted in yellow.

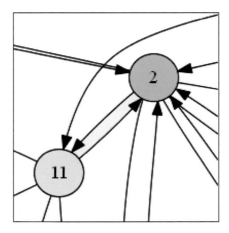

FIGURE B-3 A bidirectional connection on the map. A small section of the map is magnified here, and the two directional arrows are highlighted in yellow.

Use of the Map

The map represents a visual systems organization of the recommendations and strategies presented in the report. This systems view can be used to identify several kinds of patterns in the content of the report, many of which would be less evident in a linear or categorical textual organization of the concepts.

One important type of pattern is that of *synergy* between strategies that extends their influence to a greater number of recommendations. For example, strategy 14 (nutrition education policies) directly affects only recommendation C (transform the message environment). A categorical mapping of recommendations and strategies would show only this connection. However, the systems map also shows that through its connection to strategy 6 (sugar-sweetened beverages), strategy 14 also indirectly influences recommendation B (reduce unhealthy food and beverage options and increase healthier options) (Figure B-4). This type of

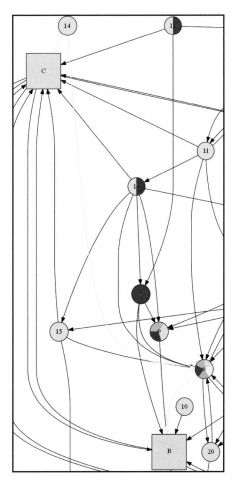

FIGURE B-4 An example of synergy. A subset of the map is magnified here. Direct influence of strategy 14 on recommendation C is shown, as well as indirect influence of strategy 14 via strategy 6 on recommendation B. Arrow tips of key connections are highlighted in yellow.

synergy between strategies helps define a systems approach to obesity prevention and demonstrates the potential for acceleration; the overall set of interventions may add up to more than simply the sum of its parts.

A related structural pattern is a *positive feedback* or "reinforcing" loop. A good example can be found in the center-right portion of the map, linking strategies 1 (physical and built environment), 16 (health care and advocacy), and 18 (healthy eating and active living at work). Bidirectional links connect strategies 18 and 1; another set of bidirectional links connects strategies 1 and 16; and strategy 16 connects back to strategy 18. Figure B-5 shows how these three strategies are mutually reinforcing and together may be more successful than any one on its own. The connections in this feedback cycle also link actions across three different sectors: citizens and civic/community organizations (strategy 1), health care (strategies 16/18), and worksites/employers (strategy 18). The positive feedback reinforcement between the three ultimately directly benefits recommendation D (increase the support provided by health care providers, insurers, and employers), as both strategy 16 and 18 flow into that recommendation.

A third type of pattern that can be identified using the map are "long chain" effects of strategies that go well beyond their immediate focus or impact. For example, strategy 15 (food literacy in schools) is linked directly only to recom-

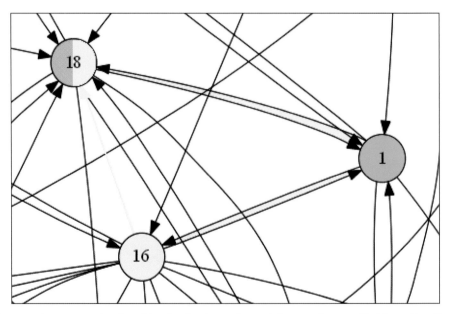

FIGURE B-5 An example of positive feedback. A subset of the map is magnified here. Key directional and bidirectional arrows are highlighted in yellow.

mendations C (transform the message environment) and E (make schools a national focal point for obesity prevention). Using the systems map, however, it can be seen that the impact of strategy 15 flows through to *all the other recommendations* (Figure B-6). It affects recommendation B via strategy 6 (sugarsweetened beverages), a two-step connection. It affects recommendation D by a slightly longer chain, from strategy 15→6→18 (healthy eating and active living at work). Finally, it reaches recommendation A by a long chain from strategy 15→6→18→1 (physical and built environment). Thus the systems map shows that

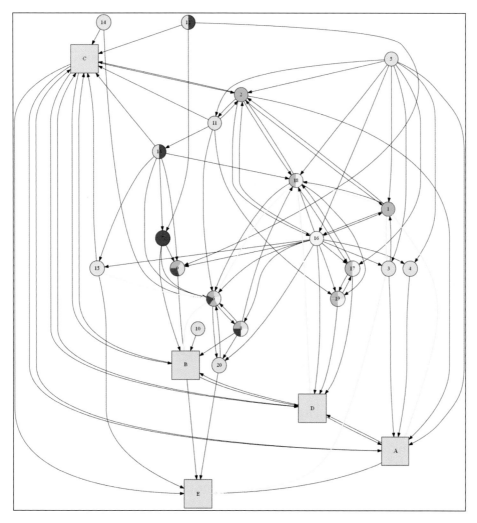

FIGURE B-6 An example of long-chain connections. Key directional arrows are highlighted in yellow.

nutrition education in schools can play a role directly or indirectly in *all* of the recommendations in the report and is a systemically important strategy.

The map also can be used to assess the package of recommendations and strategies in the report as a whole from a systems perspective and can serve as a national roadmap for action to accelerate progress in obesity prevention that is based on research evidence and the current level of progress in each area considered. The simultaneous implementation of the package of recommendations and strategies would create combined impacts that could further accelerate progress in preventing obesity. Indeed, a straightforward analysis of the map shows multiple connections and multiple pathways leading to each of the five recommendations—suggesting powerful overall systemic synergy as the strategies work together to achieve the recommendations. Similarly, relationship patterns such as those identified in the examples above are numerous, suggesting that the strategies themselves have important reinforcement potential. Finally, and also important from a systems perspective, the map shows many connections between strategies that focus on different recommendations or that involve different sectors of action. For example, strategies 13 and 15 (highlighted in Figure B-2) are connected to each other—even though strategy 13 feeds directly only to recommendation B and partially involves the business community/private sector, while strategy 15 feeds directly only to recommendation E and involves only the public sector. This coordination across sectors and recommendations is a key feature of the overall coordinated approach presented in this report.

Aside from the insight it provides into the system as a whole, the map is arranged to permit different audiences to quickly identify areas of individual interest. For example, the color coding of the strategies permits sectoral actors to identify those strategies in which they may be directly involved. Similarly, readers with an interest in a particular recommendation can quickly trace all of the strategies that feed directly or indirectly into that recommendation, as well as synergy with other recommendations (arrows between squares).

BASIS FOR PHYSICAL ACTIVITY AND DIETARY RECOMMENDATIONS

The committee looked to the 2008 Physical Activity Guidelines for Americans and the 2010 Dietary Guidelines for Americans to serve as the basis for defining adequate physical activity, healthy eating, and healthy foods (HHS/USDA, 2010; Physical Activity Guidelines Advisory Committee, 2008). In 2011, the release of MyPlate (http://www.choosemyplate.gov) provided additional guidance on healthy eating for the committee. These guidelines are based on the latest scientific evidence and provide information on achieving adequate activity levels, choosing a nutritious diet, and maintaining a healthy weight to reduce the risk of many adverse health outcomes. The key physical activity guidelines and overarching concepts of the dietary guidelines are outlined in Box B-1.

The Physical Activity and Dietary Guidelines for Americans support the prevention of overweight and obesity through the overarching concept of maintaining calorie balance over time to achieve and sustain a healthy weight. To maintain calorie balance, the guidelines highlight that individuals should improve physical activity and eating behaviors, increase physical activity and reduce sedentary behavior, control total calorie intake, and maintain appropriate calorie balance over the life span. More specifically, the guidelines provide information on key physical activity goals over the life span, as well as foods to avoid and foods with which to replace them.

REPORTS INCLUDED IN THE COMMITTEE'S REVIEW (as of September 2010)

Institute of Medicine and National Research Council (by year)

Does the built environment influence physical activity? (TRB/IOM, 2005)

Preventing childhood obesity: Health in the balance (IOM, 2005)

Food marketing to children and youth: Threat or opportunity? (IOM, 2006a)

WIC food packages: Time for a change (IOM, 2006b)

Nutrition standards for foods in schools: Leading the way toward healthier youth (IOM, 2007a)

Progress in preventing childhood obesity: How do we measure up? (IOM, 2007b)

Adolescent health services: Missing opportunities (NRC/IOM, 2009)

Local government actions to prevent childhood obesity (IOM, 2009a)

Weight gain during pregnancy: Reexamining the guidelines (IOM, 2009b)

Bridging the evidence gap in obesity prevention: A framework to inform decision making (IOM, 2010a)

Review of the nutrition guidelines for the Child and Adult Care Food Program (IOM, 2011b)

School meals: Building blocks for healthy children (IOM, 2010b)

Early childhood obesity prevention policies (IOM, 2011a)

BOX B-1
Physical Activity and Dietary Guidelines for Americans

The Physical Activity and Dietary Guidelines for Americans promote energy balance and support prevention of obesity. The Physical Activity Guidelines are for Americans 6 years of age and older, and the Dietary Guidelines are for Americans 2 years of age and older. These guidelines provide a strong evidence base on how proper physical activity levels and a healthy diet help individuals maintain a healthy body weight and contribute to progress in obesity prevention. Key Physical Activity Guidelines and overarching concepts in the Dietary Guidelines include the following:

1. Focus on increasing physical activity levels.[a]

   - Children and adolescents should participate in a minimum of 60 minutes of moderate-intensity physical activity each day.

   - Adults and older adults should participate each week in a minimum of 150 minutes of moderate-intensity physical activity, 75 minutes of vigorous physical activity, or an equivalent combination of both.

   - When older adults cannot engage in 150 minutes of moderate-intensity physical activity because of physical limitations, they should be as physically active as their abilities will allow.

Non-Academies Reports (by year)

Recommendations to increase physical activity in communities (Task Force on Community Preventive Services, 2002)

Public health strategies for preventing and controlling overweight and obesity in school and worksite settings: A report on recommendations of the Task Force on Community Preventive Services (Katz et al., 2005)

The Keystone Forum on away-from home foods: Opportunities for preventing weight gain and obesity (Keystone Forum, 2006)

2. Maintain calorie balance over time to achieve and sustain a healthy weight.[b]

   - Increase physical activity and reduce sedentary behavior, improve physical activity and eating behaviors, control total calorie intake, and maintain appropriate calorie balance during each stage of life.

3. Focus on consuming nutrient-dense foods and beverages[b]

   - Establish a healthy eating pattern by reducing intake of sodium and calories from solid fats, added sugars, and refined grains and replacing them with nutrient-dense foods and beverages, including fruits and vegetables, whole grains, fat-free or low-fat milk or milk products, seafood, lean meats and poultry, eggs, beans and peas, and nuts and seeds.

Individuals can visit http://www.ChooseMyPlate.gov and http://www.cdc.gov/physicalactivity/everyone/guidelines for advice on how to follow these guidelines.

---

[a]Physical Activity Guidelines for Americans (http://www.health.gov/paguidelines/).
[b]Dietary Guidelines for Americans (http://www.health.gov/dietaryguidelines/).

Expert committee recommendations on the assessment, prevention and treatment of child and adolescent overweight and obesity (Childhood Obesity Action Network, 2007)

Recommendations for prevention of childhood obesity (Davis et al., 2007)

Promising strategies for creating healthy eating and active living environments (Lee et al., 2008a)

Strategies for enhancing the built environment to support healthy eating and active living environments (Lee et al., 2008b)

Physical Activity Guidelines for Americans (HHS, 2008)

Recommended community strategies and measurements to prevent obesity in the United States (Khan et al., 2009)

Action strategies toolkit: A guide for local and state leaders working to create healthy communities and prevent childhood obesity (RWJF, 2009)

Shaping a healthier generation: Successful state strategies to prevent childhood obesity (Mulheron and Vonasek, 2009)

Legislative task force on diabetes and obesity: Report to the California legislature (Greenwood et al., 2009)

F as in fat: How obesity threatens America's future (Trust for America's Health, 2010)

Solving the problem of childhood obesity within a generation: White House Task Force on Childhood Obesity report to the President (White House Task Force on Childhood Obesity, 2010)

National physical activity plan for the United States (National Physical Activity Plan, 2010)

Statement of policy, comprehensive obesity prevention (NACCHO, 2010)

The Surgeon General's vision for a healthy and fit nation (HHS, 2010)

School-based obesity prevention strategies for state policymakers (CDC, date unknown)

REFERENCES

CDC (Centers for Disease Control and Prevention). Date unknown. *School-based obesity prevention strategies for state policymakers.* http://www.cdc.gov/healthyyouth/policy/pdf/obesity_prevention_strategies.pdf (accessed December 1, 2011).

Childhood Obesity Action Network. 2007. *Expert committee recommendations on the assessment, prevention and treatment of child and adolescent overweight and obesity.* Boston, MA: National Initiative for Children's Healthcare Quality.

Davis, M. M., B. Gance-Cleveland, S. Hassink, R. Johnson, G. Paradis, and K. Resnicow. 2007. Recommendations for prevention of childhood obesity. *Pediatrics* 120(Suppl. 4):S229-S253.

Forrester, J. W. 1991. System dynamics and the lessons of 35 years. In *The systemic basis of policy making in the 1990s,* edited by K. B. De Greene. Cambridge, MA: MIT Press.

Greenwood, M. R. C., P. B. Crawford, and R. M. Ortiz. 2009. *Legislative task force on diabetes and obesity: Report to the California legislature.* Santa Clara, CA: Offices of Santa Clara County Supervisors.

HHS (U.S. Department of Health and Human Services). 2008. *Physical activity guidelines for Americans.* Washington, DC: HHS.

HHS. 2010. *The Surgeon General's vision for a healthy and fit nation.* Rockville, MD: Office of the Surgeon General.

HHS/USDA (U.S. Department of Agriculture). 2010. *Dietary guidelines for Americans.* Washington, DC: U.S. Government Printing Office.

IOM (Institute of Medicine). 2005. *Preventing childhood obesity: Health in the balance.* Washington, DC: The National Academies Press.

IOM. 2006a. *Food marketing to children and youth: Threat or opportunity?* Edited by J. M. McGinnis, J. Gootman, and V. I. Kraak. Washington, DC: The National Academies Press.

IOM. 2006b. *WIC food packages: Time for a change.* Washington, DC: The National Academies Press.

IOM. 2007a. *Nutrition standards for foods in schools: Leading the way toward healthier youth.* Washington, DC: The National Academies Press.

IOM. 2007b. *Progress in preventing childhood obesity: How do we measure up?* Washington, DC: The National Academies Press.

IOM. 2009a. *Local government actions to prevent childhood obesity.* Washington, DC: The National Academies Press.

IOM. 2009b. *Weight gain during pregnancy: Reexamining the guidelines.* Washington, DC: The National Academies Press.

IOM. 2010a. *Bridging the evidence gap in obesity prevention: A framework to inform decision making.* Washington, DC: The National Academies Press.

IOM. 2010b. *School meals: Building blocks for healthy children.* Washington, DC: The National Academies Press.

IOM. 2011a. *Early childhood obesity prevention policies.* Washington, DC: The National Academies Press.

IOM. 2011b. *Review of the nutrition guidelines for the Child and Adult Care Food Program.* Washington, DC: The National Academies Press.

Katz, D. L., M. O'Connell, M. C. Yeh, H. Nawaz, V. Njike, L. M. Anderson, S. Cory, and W. Dietz. 2005. Public health strategies for preventing and controlling overweight and obesity in school and worksite settings: A report on recommendations of the Task Force on Community Preventive Services. *Morbidity and Mortality Weekly Report* 54(RR-10):1-12.

Keystone Forum. 2006. *The Keystone Forum on away-from home foods: Opportunities for preventing weight gain and obesity.* Washington, DC: The Keystone Center.

Khan, L. K., K. Sobush, D. Keener, K. Goodman, A. Lowry, J. Kakietek, and S. Zaro. 2009. Recommended community strategies and measurements to prevent obesity in the United States. *Morbidity and Mortality Weekly Report* 58(RR-7):1-26.

Lee, V., L. Mikkelsen, J. Srikantharajah, and L. Cohen. 2008a. *Promising strategies for creating healthy eating and active living environments.* Oakland, CA: Prevention Institute, Healthy Eating Active Living Convergence Partnership, and PolicyLink.

Lee, V., L. Mikkelsen, J. Srikantharajah, and L. Cohen. 2008b. *Strategies for enhancing the built environment to support healthy eating and active living environments.* Oakland, CA: Prevention Institute, Healthy Eating Active Living Convergence Partnership, and PolicyLink.

Mulheron, J., and K. Vonasek. 2009. *Shaping a healthier generation: Successful state strategies to prevent childhood obesity.* Washington, DC: National Governors Association, Center for Best Practices.

NACCHO (National Association of County and City Health Officials). 2010. *Statement of policy, comprehensive obesity prevention.* Washington, DC: NACCHO.

National Physical Activity Plan. 2010. *National physical activity plan for the United States.* http://www.physicalactivityplan.org/index.php (accessed December 1, 2011).

NRC (National Research Council)/IOM. 2009. *Adolescent health services: Missing opportunities.* Washington, DC: The National Academies Press.

Physical Activity Guidelines Advisory Committee. 2008. *Physical Activity Guidelines Advisory Committee report.* Washington, DC: HHS.

RWJF (Robert Wood Johnson Foundation). 2009. *Action strategies toolkit: A guide for local and state leaders working to create healthy communities and prevent childhood obesity.* Princeton, NJ: RWJF.

Task Force on Community Preventive Services. 2002. Recommendations to increase physical activity in communities. *American Journal of Preventive Medicine* 22(4, Suppl. 1):67-72.

TRB (Transportation Research Board)/IOM. 2005. *Does the built environment influence physical activity?* Washington, DC: The National Academies Press.

Trust for America's Health. 2010. *F as in fat: How obesity threatens America's future.* Washington, DC: Trust for America's Health.

White House Task Force on Childhood Obesity. 2010. *Solving the problem of childhood obesity within a generation: White House Task Force on Childhood Obesity report to the President.* Washington, DC: Executive Office of the President of the United States.

C

The Committee's Recommendations, Strategies, and Action Steps

The Committee on Accelerating Progress in Obesity Prevention offers the following recommendations and strategies and action steps for implementation (see Chapters 5 through 9 for individual research evidence and support). Each recommendation, strategy, and action step has positive acceleration potential, but the committee is recommending that the simultaneous implementation of these recommendations by key stakeholders and sectors will create combined impacts (or "synergies") that can further accelerate progress in preventing obesity.

GOAL 1: Make physical activity an integral and routine part of life.

RECOMMENDATION 1

Communities, transportation officials, community planners, health professionals, and governments should make promotion of physical activity a priority by substantially increasing access to places and opportunities for such activity.

Strategy 1-1: Enhance the Physical and Built Environment

Communities, organizations, community planners, and public health professionals should encourage physical activity by enhancing the physical and built environment, rethinking community design, and ensuring access to places for such activity.

Potential actions include

- communities, urban planners, architects, developers, and public health professionals developing and implementing sustainable strategies for improving
  the physical environment of communities that are as large as several square
  miles or more or as small as a few blocks in size in ways that encourage
  and support physical activity; and
- communities and organizations developing and maintaining sustainable
  strategies to create and/or enhance access to places and programs where
  people can be physically active in a safe and enjoyable way.

Strategy 1-2: Provide and Support Community Programs Designed to Increase Physical Activity

Communities and organizations should encourage physical activity by providing and supporting programs designed to increase such activity

Potential actions include

- developing and implementing ongoing physical activity promotion campaigns that involve high-visibility, multiple delivery channels and multiple
  sectors of influence;
- developing and implementing physical activity strategies that fit into
  people's daily routines—strategies that are most effective when tailored to
  specific interests and preferences; and
- developing and implementing strategies that build, strengthen, and maintain
  social networks to provide supportive relationships for behavior change
  with respect to physical activity.

Strategy 1-3: Adopt Physical Activity Requirements for Licensed Child Care Providers

State and local child care and early childhood education regulators should
establish requirements for each program to improve its current physical activity
standards.

Potential actions include

- requiring each licensed child care site to provide opportunities for physical activity, including free play, and outdoor play, at a rate of 15 minutes per hour of care; as a minimum, immediate first step, each site providing at least 30 minutes of physical activity per day for half-day programs, and 1 hour for full-day programs.

Strategy 1-4: Provide Support for the Science and Practice of Physical Activity

Federal, state, and local government agencies should make physical activity a national health priority through support for the translation of scientific evidence into best-practice applications.

For **federal-level government agencies,** potential actions include

- the Department of Health and Human Services (HHS) establishing processes for the regular and routine communication of scientific advances in understanding the health benefits of physical activity, particularly with respect to obesity prevention (these processes could include, but are not limited to, regularly scheduled updates of the Physical Activity Guidelines for Americans and reports of the U.S. Surgeon General); and
- all federal government agencies with relevant interests developing priority strategies to promote and support the National Physical Activity Plan, a trans-sector strategy for increasing physical activity among Americans.

For **state and local health departments,** potential actions include

- developing plans and strategies for making promotion of physical activity a health priority at the state and local levels.

GOAL 2: Create food and beverage environments that ensure that healthy food and beverage options are the routine, easy choice.

RECOMMENDATION 2

Governments and decision makers in the business community/private sector[1] should make a concerted effort to reduce unhealthy food and beverage options[2] and substantially increase healthier food and beverage options at affordable, competitive prices.

Strategy 2-1: Adopt Policies and Implement Practices to Reduce Overconsumption of Sugar-Sweetened Beverages

Decision makers in the business community/private sector, in nongovernmental organizations, and at all levels of government should adopt comprehensive strategies to reduce overconsumption of sugar-sweetened beverages.[3]

For **schools and other locations where children and adolescents are cared for,** potential actions include

- prohibiting access to sugar-sweetened beverages;
- providing a variety of beverage options that are competitively priced and are recommended by and included in the Dietary Guidelines for Americans; and
- making clean, potable water available.

For the **business community/private sector, nongovernmental organizations, and governments,** potential actions include

---

[1]The business community/private sector includes private employers and privately owned and/or operated locations frequented by the public, such as movie theaters, shopping centers, sporting and entertainment venues, bowling alleys, and other recreational/entertainment facilities.

[2]Although there is no consensus on the definition of "unhealthy" foods/beverages, the term refers in this report to foods and beverages that are calorie-dense and low in naturally occurring nutrients. Such foods and beverages contribute little fiber and few essential nutrients and phytochemicals, but contain added fats, sweeteners, sodium, and other ingredients. Unhealthy foods and beverages displace the consumption of foods recommended in the Dietary Guidelines for Americans and may lead to the development of obesity.

[3]Sugar-sweetened beverages are defined to include all beverages containing added caloric sweeteners, including, but not limited to, sugar- or otherwise calorically sweetened regular sodas, less than 100 percent fruit drinks, energy drinks, sports drinks, and ready-to-drink teas and coffees.

- making clean, potable water readily available in public places, worksites, and recreation areas;
- making a variety of beverage options that are competitively priced readily available in public places, worksites, and recreation areas;
- implementing fiscal policies aimed at reducing overconsumption of sugar-sweetened beverages through (1) pricing and other incentives to make healthier beverage options recommended by the Dietary Guidelines for Americans more affordable and, for governments, (2) substantial and specific excise taxes on sugar-sweetened beverages (e.g., cents per ounce of liquid, cents per teaspoon of added sugar), with the revenues being dedicated to obesity prevention programs;
- supporting the work of community groups and coalitions to educate the public about the risks associated with overconsumption of sugar-sweetened beverages; and
- developing social marketing campaigns aimed at reducing overconsumption of sugar-sweetened beverages.

For the **food and beverage industry,** potential actions include

- developing and promoting a variety of beverage options for consumers, including a range of healthy beverage options, beverages with reduced sugar content, and smaller portion sizes (e.g., 8-ounce containers).

For **health care providers** such as physicians, dentists, registered dietitians, and nurses, potential actions include

- performing routine screening regarding overconsumption of sugar-sweetened beverages and counseling on the health risks associated with consumption of these beverages.

Strategy 2-2: Increase the Availability of Lower-Calorie and Healthier Food and Beverage Options for Children in Restaurants

Chain and quick-service restaurants should substantially reduce the number of calories served to children and substantially expand the number of affordable and competitively priced healthier options available for parents to choose from in their facilities.

Potential actions include

- developing a joint effort (modeled after the Healthy Weight Commitment initiative) to set a specific goal for substantially reducing the total annual calories served to children in these facilities; and
- ensuring that at least half of all children's meals are consistent with the food and calorie guidelines of the Dietary Guidelines for Americans for moderately active 4- to 8-year-olds and are competitively priced.

Strategy 2-3: Utilize Strong Nutritional Standards for all Foods and Beverages Sold or Provided Through the Government, and Ensure That These Healthy Options Are Available in All Places Frequented by the Public

Government agencies (federal, state, local, and school district) should ensure that all foods and beverages sold or provided through the government are aligned with the age-specific recommendations in the Dietary Guidelines for Americans. The business community and the private sector operating venues frequented by the public should ensure that a variety of foods and beverages, including those recommended by the Dietary Guidelines for Americans, are sold or served at all times.

For **government agencies,** potential actions include

- the federal government expanding the healthy vending/concession guidelines to include all government-owned and/or -operated buildings, worksites, facilities,[4] and other locations where foods and beverages are sold/served; and
- all state and local government-owned and -operated buildings, worksites, facilities, and other locations where foods and beverages are sold/served (including through vending machines and concession stands) adopting and implementing a healthy food and beverage vending/concession policy.

---

[4]"Government-owned and -operated buildings, worksites, and facilities" is defined broadly to include not only places of work but also locations such as government-owned and/or -operated child care centers, hospitals, and other health care/assisted living facilities, military bases, correctional facilities, and educational institutions.

For the **business community/private sector,** potential actions include

- the business community and private-sector entities that operate places frequented by the public ensuring that a variety of food and beverage options are competitively priced and available for purchase and consumption in these places,[5] including food and beverages that are aligned with the recommendations of the Dietary Guidelines for Americans.

Strategy 2-4: Introduce, Modify, and Utilize Health-Promoting Food and Beverage Retailing and Distribution Policies

States and localities should utilize financial incentives such as flexible financing or tax credits, streamlined permitting processes, and zoning strategies, as well as cross-sectoral collaborations (e.g., among industry, philanthropic organizations, government, and the community) to enhance the quality of local food environments, particularly in low-income communities. These efforts should include encouraging or attracting retailers and distributors of healthy food (e.g., supermarkets) to locate in underserved areas and limiting the concentration of unhealthy food venues (e.g., fast-food restaurants, convenience stores). Incentives should be linked to public health goals in ways that give priority to stores that also commit to health-promoting retail strategies (e.g., through placement, promotion, and pricing).

Potential actions include

- states creating cross-agency teams to analyze and streamline regulatory processes and create tax incentives for retailing of healthy foods in underserved neighborhoods;
- states and localities creating cross-sectoral collaborations among the food and beverage industry, philanthropy, the finance and banking sector, the real estate sector, and the community to develop private funding to facilitate the development of healthy food retailing in underserved areas; and
- localities utilizing incentive tools to attract retailing of healthy foods (e.g., supermarkets and grocery stores) to underserved neighborhoods, such as through flexible financing or tax credits, streamlined permitting processes,

---

[5] "Places frequented by the public" includes, but is not limited to, privately owned and/or operated locations frequented by the public such as movie theaters, shopping centers, sporting and entertainment venues, bowling alleys, and other recreational/entertainment facilities.

zoning strategies, grant and loan programs, small business/economic development programs, and other economic incentives.

Strategy 2-5: Broaden the Examination and Development of U.S. Agriculture Policy and Research to Include Implications for the American Diet

Congress, the Administration, and federal agencies should examine the implications of U.S. agriculture policy for obesity, and should ensure that such policy includes understanding and implementing, as appropriate, an optimal mix of crops and farming methods for meeting the Dietary Guidelines for Americans.

Potential actions include

- the President appointing a Task Force on Agriculture Policy and Obesity Prevention to evaluate the evidence on the relationship between agriculture policies and the American diet, and to develop recommendations for policy options and future policy-related research, specifically on the impact of farm subsidies and the management of commodities on food prices, access, affordability, and consumption;
- Congress and the Administration establishing a process by which federal food, agriculture, and health officials would review and report on the possible implications of U.S. agriculture policy for obesity prevention to ensure that this issue will be fully taken into account when policy makers consider the Farm Bill;
- Congress and the U.S. Department of Agriculture (USDA) developing policy options for promoting increased domestic production of foods recommended for a healthy diet that are generally underconsumed, including fruits and vegetables and dairy products, by reviewing incentives and disincentives that exist in current policy;
- as part of its agricultural research agenda, USDA exploring the optimal mix of crops and farming methods for meeting the current Dietary Guidelines for Americans, including an examination of the possible impact of smaller-scale agriculture, of regional agricultural product distribution chains, and of various agricultural models from small to large scale, as well as other efforts to ensure a sustainable, sufficient, and affordable supply of fresh fruits and vegetables; and

- Congress and the Administration ensuring that there is adequate public funding for agricultural research and extension so that the research agenda can include a greater focus on supporting the production of foods Americans need to consume in greater quantities according to the Dietary Guidelines for Americans.

GOAL 3: Transform messages about physical activity and nutrition.

RECOMMENDATION 3

Industry, educators, and governments should act quickly, aggressively, and in a sustained manner on many levels to transform the environment that surrounds Americans with messages about physical activity, food, and nutrition.

Strategy 3-1: Develop and Support a Sustained, Targeted Physical Activity and Nutrition Social Marketing Program

Congress, the Administration, other federal policy makers, and foundations should dedicate substantial funding and support to the development and implementation of a robust and sustained social marketing program on physical activity and nutrition. This program should encompass carefully targeted, culturally appropriate messages aimed at specific audiences (e.g., tweens, new parents, mothers); clear behavior-change goals (e.g., take a daily walk, reduce consumption of sugar-sweetened beverages among adolescents, introduce infants to vegetables, make use of the new front-of-package nutrition labels); and related environmental change goals (e.g., improve physical environments, offer better food choices in public places, increase the availability of healthy food retailing).

For **Congress, the Administration, and other federal policy makers, working with entertainment media,** potential actions include

- providing a sustained source of funding for a major national social marketing program on physical activity and nutrition; and
- designating a lead agency to guide and oversee the federal program and appointing a small advisory group of physical activity, nutrition, and marketing experts to recommend message and audience priorities for the program; ensuring that the program includes a balance of messages on

physical activity and nutrition, and on both individual behavior change and related environmental change goals; and exploring all forms of marketing, including message placement in popular entertainment, viral and social marketing, and multiplatform advertising—including online, outdoor, radio, television, and print.

For **foundations, working with state, local, and national organizations and the news media,** potential actions include

- enhancing the social marketing program by encouraging and supporting the news media's coverage of obesity prevention policies through the development of local and national media programs that engage individuals in the civic debate about local, state, and national-level environmental and policy changes, including such steps as providing resources to enable journalists to cover these issues and enhancing the expertise of local, state, and national organizations in engaging the news media on these issues.

Strategy 3-2: Implement Common Standards for Marketing Foods and Beverages to Children and Adolescents

The food, beverage, restaurant, and media industries should take broad, common, and urgent voluntary action to make substantial improvements in their marketing aimed directly at children and adolescents aged 2-17. All foods and beverages marketed to this age group should support a diet that accords with the Dietary Guidelines for Americans in order to prevent obesity and risk factors associated with chronic disease risk. Children and adolescents should be encouraged to avoid calories from foods that they generally overconsume (e.g., products high in sugar, fat, and sodium) and to replace them with foods they generally underconsume (e.g., fruits, vegetables, and whole grains).

The standards set for foods and beverages marketed to children and adolescents should be widely publicized and easily available to parents and other consumers. They should cover foods and beverages marketed to children and adolescents aged 2-17 and should apply to a broad range of marketing and advertising practices, including digital marketing and the use of licensed characters and toy premiums. If such marketing standards have not been adopted within 2 years by a substantial majority of food, beverage, restaurant, and media companies that market foods and beverages to children and adolescents, policy makers at the local, state, and federal levels should consider setting mandatory nutritional standards for marketing to this age group to ensure that such standards are implemented.

Potential actions include

- all food and beverage companies, including chain and quick-service restaurants, adopting and implementing voluntary nutrition standards for foods and beverages marketed to children and adolescents;
- the Children's Food and Beverage Advertising Initiative and National Restaurant Association Initiative, as major self-regulatory marketing efforts, adopting common marketing standards for all member companies, and actively recruiting additional members to increase the impact of improved food marketing to children and adolescents;
- media companies adopting nutrition standards for all foods they market to young people; and
- the Federal Trade Commission regularly tracking the marketing standards adopted by food and beverage companies, restaurants, and media companies.

Strategy 3-3: Ensure Consistent Nutrition Labeling for the Front of Packages, Retail Store Shelves, and Menus and Menu Boards That Encourages Healthier Food Choices

The Food and Drug Administration (FDA) and the USDA should implement a standard system of nutrition labeling for the front of packages and retail store shelves that is harmonious with the Nutrition Facts panel, and restaurants should provide calorie labeling on all menus and menu boards.

Potential actions include

- The FDA and USDA adopting a single standard nutrition labeling system for all fronts of packages and retail store shelves, the FDA and USDA considering making this system mandatory to enable consumers to compare products on a standard nutrition profile, and the guidelines provided by the Institute of Medicine (2011) being used for implementation; and
- restaurants implementing the FDA regulations that require restaurants with 20 or more locations to provide calorie labeling on their menus and menu boards, and the FDA/USDA monitoring industry for compliance with this policy.

Strategy 3-4: Adopt Consistent Nutrition Education Policies for Federal Programs with Nutrition Education Components

USDA should update the policies for Supplemental Nutrition Assistance Program Education (SNAP-Ed) and the policies for other federal programs with nutrition education components to explicitly encourage the provision of advice about types of foods to reduce in the diet, consistent with the Dietary Guidelines for Americans.

Potential actions include

- removing the restrictions on the types of information that can be included in SNAP-Ed programs and encouraging advice about types of foods to reduce;
- disseminating, immediately and effectively, notification of the revised regulations, along with authoritative guidance on how to align federally funded nutrition education programs with the Dietary Guidelines; and
- ensuring that such full alignment of nutrition education with the Dietary Guidelines applies to all federal programs with a nutrition education component, particularly programs that target primary food shoppers in low-income families (e.g., the Expanded Food and Nutrition Education Program and the Special Supplemental Nutrition Program for Women, Infants, and Children [WIC]).

GOAL 4: Expand the role of health care providers, insurers, and employers in obesity prevention.

RECOMMENDATION 4

Health care and health service providers, employers, and insurers should increase the support structure for achieving better population health and obesity prevention.

Strategy 4-1: Provide Standardized Care and Advocate for Healthy Community Environments

All health care providers should adopt standards of practice (evidence-based or consensus guidelines) for prevention, screening, diagnosis, and treatment of overweight and obesity to help children, adolescents, and adults achieve and maintain a healthy weight, avoid obesity-related complications, and reduce the psychosocial consequences of obesity. Health care providers also should advocate, on behalf of their patients, for improved physical activity and diet opportunities in their patients' communities.

Potential actions include

- health care providers' standards of practice including routine screening of body mass index (BMI), counseling, and behavioral interventions for children, adolescents, and adults to improve physical activity behaviors and dietary choices;
- medical schools, nursing schools, physician assistant schools, and other relevant health professional training programs (including continuing education programs), including instruction in prevention, screening, diagnosis, and treatment of overweight and obesity in children, adolescents, and adults; and
- health care providers serving as role models for their patients and providing leadership for obesity prevention efforts in their communities by advocating for institutional (e.g., child care, school, and worksite), community, and state-level strategies that can improve physical activity and nutrition resources for their patients and their communities.

Strategy 4-2: Ensure Coverage of, Access to, and Incentives for Routine Obesity Prevention, Screening, Diagnosis, and Treatment

Insurers (both public and private) should ensure that health insurance coverage and access provisions address obesity prevention, screening, diagnosis, and treatment.

Potential actions include

- insurers, including self-insured organizations and employers, considering the inclusion of incentives in individual and family health plans for maintaining healthy lifestyles;
- insurers considering (1) benefit designs and programs that promote obesity screening and prevention and (2) innovative approaches to reimbursing for routine screening and obesity prevention services (including preconception

counseling) in clinical practice and for monitoring the performance of these services in relation to obesity prevention; and

- insurers taking full advantage of obesity-related provisions in health care reform legislation.

Strategy 4-3: Encourage Active Living and Healthy Eating at Work

Worksites should create, or expand, healthy environments by establishing, implementing, and monitoring policy initiatives that support wellness.

Potential actions include

- public and private employers promoting healthy eating and active living in the worksite in their own institutional policies and practices by, for example, increasing opportunities for physical activity as part of a wellness/health promotion program, providing access to and promotion of healthful foods and beverages, and offering health benefits that provide employees and their dependents coverage for obesity-related services and programs; and
- health care organizations and providers serving as models for the incorporation of healthy eating and active living into worksite practices and programs.

Strategy 4-4: Encourage Healthy Weight Gain During Pregnancy and Breastfeeding, and Promote Breastfeeding-Friendly Environments

Health service providers and employers should adopt, implement, and monitor policies that support healthy weight gain during pregnancy and the initiation and continuation of breastfeeding. Population disparities in breastfeeding should be specifically addressed at the federal, state, and local levels to remove barriers and promote targeted increases in breastfeeding initiation and continuation.

Potential actions include

- all those who provide health care or related services to women of child-bearing age offering preconception counseling on the importance of conceiving at a healthy BMI;

- medical facilities, prenatal services, and community clinics adopting policies consistent with the Baby-Friendly Hospital Initiative;
- local health departments and community-based organizations, working with other segments of the health sector, providing information on breastfeeding and the availability of related classes to pregnant women and new mothers, connecting pregnant women and new mothers with breastfeeding support programs to help them make informed infant feeding decisions, and developing peer support programs that empower pregnant women and mothers to obtain the help and support they need from other mothers who have breastfed;
- workplaces instituting policies to support breastfeeding mothers, including ensuring both private space and adequate break time; and
- the federal government using Prevention Fund dollars to support implementation of the Baby-Friendly Hospital Initiative nationwide, and providing funding to support community-level collaborative efforts and peer counseling with the aim of increasing the duration of breastfeeding.

GOAL 5: Make schools a national focal point for obesity prevention.

RECOMMENDATION 5

Federal, state, and local government and education authorities, with support from parents, teachers, and the business community and the private sector, should make schools a focal point for obesity prevention.

Strategy 5-1: Require Quality Physical Education and Opportunities for Physical Activity in Schools

Through support from federal and state governments, state and local education agencies and local school districts should ensure that all students in grades K-12 have adequate opportunities to engage in 60 minutes of physical activity per school day. This 60-minute goal includes access to and participation in quality physical education.

For **Congress,** potential actions include

- strengthening the local wellness policy requirement in Section 204 of the *Healthy, Hunger-Free Kids Act of 2010* (Public Law 111-296, 111th Cong., 2d sess. [December 13, 2010], 124, 3183) or the *Elementary and Secondary Education Act* (Public Law 89-19, 89th Cong., 1st sess. [April 11, 1965] 27, 20) by including a requirement for local education agencies to develop and implement a K-12 quality physical education curriculum with proficiency assessments.

For **state legislatures and departments of education,** potential actions include

- enacting policies with appropriate funding to ensure the provision of daily quality physical education at school for all students in grades K-12; and
- developing, requiring, and financially supporting the implementation of K-12 curriculum standards for quality physical education that (1) are aligned with guidance from practice and/or professional associations and appropriate instructional practice guidelines, and (2) ensure that at least 50 percent of class time is spent in vigorous or moderate-intensity physical activity.

For **local education agencies,** potential actions include

- adopting requirements that include opportunities for daily physical activity outside of physical education, such as active transport to school programs, intramural sports and activity programs, active recess, classroom breaks, after-school physical activity programming, and integration of physical activity into curricula lesson plans.

For **local school districts,** potential actions include

- improving and maintaining an environment that is conducive to safe physical education and physical activity.

Strategy 5-2: Ensure Strong Nutritional Standards for All Foods and Beverages Sold or Provided Through Schools

All government agencies (federal, state, local, and school district) providing foods and beverages to children and adolescents have a responsibility to provide those in their care with foods and beverages that promote health and learning. The Dietary Guidelines for Americans provide specific science-based recommendations for optimizing dietary intake to prevent disease and promote health. Implementation of these guidelines would shift children's and adolescents' dietary intake to prevent obesity and risk factors associated with chronic disease risk by increasing the amounts of fruits, vegetables, and high-fiber grains they consume; decreasing their consumption of sugar-sweetened beverages, dietary fat in general, solid fats, and added sugars; and ensuring age-appropriate portion sizes of meals and other foods and beverages. Federal, state, and local decision makers are responsible for ensuring that nutrition standards based on the Dietary Guidelines are adopted by schools; these decision makers, in partnership with regulatory agencies, parents, teachers, and food manufacturers, also are responsible for ensuring that these standards are implemented fully and that adherence is monitored so as to protect the health of the nation's children and adolescents.

For the **USDA,** potential actions include

- adopting nutrition standards for all federal child nutrition programs (i.e., the School Breakfast, National School Lunch, Afterschool Snack, Summer Food Service, and Special Milk programs) that are aligned with guidance on optimal nutrition; and
- adopting nutrition standards for all snacks and beverages sold/served outside of federal child nutrition programs that are aligned with guidance on optimal nutrition.

For **state legislatures and departments of education,** potential actions include

- adopting nutrition standards for foods sold/served outside of federal child nutrition programs that are aligned with guidance on optimal nutrition.

For **school boards and state departments of education,** potential actions include

- developing school district policies (including wellness policies for districts participating in federal child nutrition programs) and related regulations that include nutrition standards for foods sold/served outside of the federal programs that are aligned with guidance on optimal nutrition.

Strategy 5-3: Ensure Food Literacy, Including Skill Development, in Schools

Through leadership and guidance from federal and state governments, state and local education agencies should ensure the implementation and monitoring of sequential food literacy and nutrition science education, spanning grades K-12, based on the food and nutrition recommendations in the Dietary Guidelines for Americans.

For the **federal government,** potential actions include

- USDA developing K-12 food and nutrition curriculum guides that can be used by states and updating information in these guides as appropriate with each periodic revision of the Dietary Guidelines for Americans; and
- as USDA develops regulations to implement Section 204 of the *Healthy, Hunger-Free Kids Act of 2010* (Public Law 111-296, December 13, 2010), including a requirement for local education agencies to adopt and implement a K-12 food and nutrition curriculum based on state and federal guidance.

For **states, state legislatures, and departments of education,** potential actions include

- state legislatures and departments of education adopting, requiring, and financially supporting K-12 standards for food and nutrition curriculum based on USDA guidance;
- state departments of education establishing requirements for training teachers in effectively incorporating nutrition education into their curricula;
- states requiring teacher training programs to include curriculum requirements for the study of nutrition;

- state legislatures and departments of education adopting and requiring proficiency assessments for core elements of their state food and nutrition curriculum standards in accordance with the Common Core State Standards Initiative, and local education agency wellness policies articulating ways in which results of food and nutrition education proficiency assessments can be used to inform program improvement; and
- state and local departments of education, working with local education agency wellness policies, to link changes in the meals provided through child nutrition services with the food literacy and nutrition education curriculum to the extent possible.

REFERENCE

IOM (Institute of Medicine). 2011. *Examination of front-of-package nutrition rating systems and symbols: Promoting healthier choices.* Washington, DC: The National Academies Press.

D

Workshop and Panel Public Sessions

MARKETING APPROACHES PANEL

January 13, 2011
Irvine, CA

Panel Goals:

1. Explore the progress in meeting the goals set forth in the 2006 Institute of Medicine's (IOM's) *Food Marketing to Children and Youth: Threat or Opportunity?*
2. Identify key food and beverage marketing approaches that can accelerate progress in preventing obesity.

OVERVIEW

Ellen Wartella, Northwestern University

RESEARCH

Jerome Williams, Rutgers Business School-Newark and New Brunswick
Kathryn Montgomery and Jeff Chester, American University and Center for Digital Democracy
Kelly Brownell, Rudd Center for Food Policy and Obesity, Yale University

SELF-REGULATION

Elaine Kolish, Children's Food and Beverage Advertising Initiative (CFBAI)
Lisa Gable, Healthy Weight Commitment Foundation (HWCF)
Bill Dietz, Centers for Disease Control and Prevention (CDC)

CASE STUDIES IN IMPLEMENTING COMPREHENSIVE OBESITY PREVENTION PLANS PANEL

March 23, 2011
Irvine, CA

Panel Goals:

1. Hear first-hand accounts from state and local governments and community organizations that have developed and implemented obesity prevention initiatives.
2. Explore the successes, failures, and challenges that groups and individuals have encountered in their efforts.
3. Gain insights that may be useful in selecting recommendations to accelerate progress in obesity prevention.

Susan Combs, Texas Comptroller of Public Accounts
America Bracho, Executive Director, Latino Health Access
Anthony Iton, Senior Vice President, Healthy Communities, The California Endowment
Tom Farley, Commissioner, New York City Department of Health and Mental Hygiene
Karl Dean, Mayor, The Metropolitan Government of Nashville and Davidson County

WORKSHOP ON MEASUREMENT STRATEGIES FOR ACCELERATING PROGRESS IN OBESITY PREVENTION*

March 23-24, 2011
Irvine, CA

Workshop Purpose:

1. Explore and understand the ways that measurement techniques, strategies, and data sources can impede and or promote acceleration of progress toward prevention of obesity.
2. Understand what additional knowledge regarding assessments of environments and policies is needed to measure progress of obesity prevention.

PANEL I: The Physical Activity, Inactivity, and Built Environments: Current and Potential Sources of Measures for Assessing Progress in Obesity Prevention

> *James F. Sallis*, San Diego State University
> *Christine Hoehner*, Washington University

PANEL II: The Food and Nutrition Environments: Current and Potential Sources of Measures for Assessing Progress in Obesity Prevention

> *Karen Glanz*, University of Pennsylvania
> *Susan M. Krebs-Smith*, National Cancer Institute

PANEL III: Cross-Cutting Issues: Current and Potential Sources of Measures for Assessing Progress in Obesity Prevention

> *Robert M. Malina*, University of Texas at Austin and Tarleton State University
> *Robin McKinnon*, National Cancer Institute
> *Roland Sturm*, RAND Corporation

Measuring Progress in Obesity Prevention: Workshop Report can be accessed at http://www.nap.edu.

PANEL IV: Marketing and Industry Measures and Evaluations

>*Victoria Rideout*, VJR Consulting
>*Shu Wen Ng*, University of North Carolina at Chapel Hill
>*Robert C. Hornik*, University of Pennsylvania

PANEL V: State and Community Reach

>*Maya Rockeymoore*, Global Policy Solutions and Leadership for Healthy Communities
>*Laura Kettel Khan*, Centers for Disease Control and Prevention
>*Amy A. Eyler*, Washington University, St. Louis
>*Jamie Chriqui*, University of Illinois at Chicago
>*Brian Cole*, University of California, Los Angeles

PANEL VI: Disparities and Measurement

>*Sarah Samuels*, Samuels & Associates
>*Carlos J. Crespo*, Portland State University
>*Sonya Grier*, American University

CLOSING SESSION: Themes of the Workshop and Next Steps

>*Robin McKinnon*, National Cancer Institute

PANEL ON FARM AND FOOD POLICY: RELATIONSHIP TO OBESITY PREVENTION

May 19, 2011
Washington, DC

Panel Goals:

1. Learn about the current policy and political context surrounding farm and food policies.
2. Explore stakeholder perspectives on the role of agricultural policy and practices and food manufacturer and retailer decision making in obesity prevention.

3. Gain insights that may be useful in determining committee recommendations on accelerating progress in obesity prevention.

INTRODUCTORY SPEAKER: Legislative perspectives on obesity in farm and health policies: What lies ahead in Congress?

Eric Olsen, Feeding America

PANEL I: U.S. Agricultural Policies and Their Influence on Obesity: What Do We Know?

Daryll Ray, University of Tennessee
Helen Jensen, Iowa State University

PANEL II: Food Procurement and Obesity Prevention

Kate Rogers, H-E-B
Andrea B. Thomas, Walmart

PANEL III: Perspectives on Farm and Health Issues

Linda Barnes, Marshalltown Community College
Doug Sombke, South Dakota Farmers Union

CLOSING SPEAKER: Obesity and Farm and Food Policy in the Current Political Context

Jerry Hagstrom, The Hagstrom Report

E

Committee Member Biographical Sketches

Daniel R. Glickman, J.D. (*Chair*) is executive director of congressional programs at the Aspen Institute and senior fellow at The Bipartisan Policy Center in Washington, DC. He previously served as president of Refugees International and chairman and chief executive officer of the Motion Picture Association of America (MPAA). Prior to joining the MPAA in September 2004, Mr. Glickman was director of the Institute of Politics at Harvard University's John F. Kennedy School of Government (August 2002-August 2004). He served as the 26th U.S. secretary of agriculture from March 1995 until January 2001. During his tenure, improving the nation's diet and nutrition and fighting hunger were among the department's priorities. Before his appointment as secretary of agriculture, Mr. Glickman served for 18 years in the U.S. House of Representatives, representing Kansas' 4th Congressional District. During his time in Congress, he was a member of the House Agriculture Committee, including 6 years as chairman of the subcommittee with jurisdiction over federal farm policy issues, nutrition policy, the Food Stamp Program, the School Lunch Program and other child nutrition programs, and the Supplemental Nutrition Program for Women, Infants, and Children (WIC). He also served as chairman of the House Permanent Select Committee on Intelligence. He is co-chair of the Chicago Council on Global Affairs' Global Agricultural Development Initiative and vice chairman of World Food Program USA (formerly the Friends of the World Food Program). Mr. Glickman's service includes membership on the board of directors of the American Film Institute, CME Group, Communities in Schools, the Food Research and Action Center, the National 4-H Council, the William Davidson Institute at the University of Michigan, and the Center for U.S. Global Engagement. He is a member of the Council on Foreign Relations; a member of the Council on American Politics at the Graduate School of Political Management at The George Washington University; and a senior fellow of the Center on Communication, Leadership, and Policy at the Annenberg School for Communication and Journalism at the University of Southern California. In addition, Mr. Glickman is co-chair of AGree, a multifoundation effort to review long-term food and agriculture policy. Mr. Glickman received his B.A. in history from the University of Michigan and his J.D. from The George Washington University. He is a member of the Kansas and District of Columbia Bars.

M. R. C. Greenwood, Ph.D. (*Vice Chair*) is president of the University of Hawaii System, a position she assumed in 2009. Previously, Dr. Greenwood was professor of nutrition and internal medicine, chair of the Graduate Group in Nutritional Biology, and director of the Foods for Health Initiative at the University of California, Davis. She served as chancellor of the University of California, Santa Cruz, from 1996 to 2004, and University of California provost and senior vice president for academic affairs. Prior to her Santa Cruz appointments, Dr. Greenwood was dean of graduate studies, vice provost of academic outreach, and professor of biology and internal medicine at the University of California, Davis. She was chair of the Department of Biology at Vassar College. From 1993 to 1995, she served as associate director for science at the Office of Science and Technology Policy in the Executive Office of the President of the United States. Dr. Greenwood is the author of numerous scientific publications in the areas of nutrition, obesity, and diabetes. She is past president and fellow of the American Association for the Advancement of Science, fellow of the American Academies of Arts and Sciences, and past president of the North American Association for the Study of Obesity. She is past chair of the Institute of Medicine's (IOM's) Food and Nutrition Board, the National Research Council (NRC) Policy and Global Affairs Committee, and the IOM Committee on Dietary Supplement Use by Military Personnel, and is a former member of the National Science Board. Dr. Greenwood received her A.B., summa cum laude, from Vassar College and received her Ph.D. from The Rockefeller University. She is a member of the IOM.

William Purcell, III, J.D. (*Vice Chair*) is an attorney in Nashville, Tennessee, who most recently served as special advisor on Allston and co-chair of the Work Team for Allston in the Office of the President at Harvard University. From 2008 to 2010, he served as director of the Institute of Politics at the Kennedy School of Government at Harvard. He previously was mayor of Nashville, Tennessee, from 1999 to 2007. Mr. Purcell's accomplishments as a civic leader earned him Public Official of the Year honors in 2006 from *Governing Magazine*. In 1986 he was elected to the Tennessee House of Representatives, where he served for five terms, holding the positions of majority leader and chair of the Select Committee on Children and Youth. After retiring from the General Assembly, Mr. Purcell founded and became director of the Child and Family Policy Center at the Vanderbilt Institute of Public Policy Studies. He was a member of the IOM Committee on an Evidence Framework for Obesity Prevention Decision Making. Mr. Purcell graduated from Hamilton College and Vanderbilt University School of Law.

David V. B. Britt, M.P.A., is retired president and chief executive officer of Sesame Workshop. Mr. Britt's professional experience includes executive positions with the U.S. Agency for International Development, the Equal Employment Opportunity Commission, and the Overseas Private Investment Corporation. Since his retirement, Mr. Britt has been engaged in consulting and leadership development for nonprofit organizations. He is currently chair of the board of directors of The Education Trust. Mr. Britt has been a member of the Advisory Board on Social Enterprise at the Harvard Business School, and is a member of the Council on Foreign Relations and the Board of INMED Partnerships for Children. He is a former member of the IOM/NRC Board on Children, Youth, and Families. He served as a member of the IOM Committee on Obesity Prevention Policies for Young Children and of the IOM Committee on Food Marketing and the Diets of Children and Youth. Mr. Britt received a B.A. from Wesleyan University and an M.P.A. from the John F. Kennedy School of Government at Harvard University.

Jamie F. Chriqui, Ph.D., M.H.S., is a senior research scientist and director of policy surveillance and evaluation for the Health Policy Center within the Institute for Health Research and Policy at the University of Illinois at Chicago (UIC) and a research associate professor in political science at UIC. She has more than 21 years' experience conducting public health policy research, evaluation, and analysis, with an emphasis on obesity, substance abuse, tobacco control, and other chronic disease-related policy issues. Her research interests focus on examining the impact of law and policy on community and school environments, as well as individual behaviors and attitudes. Her current research focuses heavily on sugar-sweetened beverage taxation, school district wellness policies, and community policies related to the physical activity and food environments. Dr. Chriqui directs all state, local, and school district policy research activities for the Robert Wood Johnson Foundation–supported Bridging the Gap program and is principal investigator or co-investigator on several National Institutes of Health (NIH)–funded research grants. She serves on numerous obesity-related advisory and expert panels and is widely called upon for her expertise in obesity policy-related issues. Prior to joining UIC, Dr. Chriqui served as technical vice-president of the Center for Health Policy and Legislative Analysis at The MayaTech Corporation and, previously, as a policy analyst at the National Institute on Drug Abuse. She holds a B.A. in political science from Barnard College at Columbia University; an M.H.S. in health policy from the Johns Hopkins University School of Hygiene and Public Health; and a Ph.D. in policy sciences (health policy concentration) from the University of Maryland, Baltimore County.

Patricia Crawford, Dr.P.H., R.D., is director of the Dr. Robert C. and Veronica Atkins Center for Weight and Health, Cooperative Extension nutrition specialist in the Department of Nutritional Science and Toxicology, and adjunct professor in the School of Public Health at the University of California, Berkeley. Dr. Crawford directed the longitudinal National Heart, Lung, and Blood Institute's Growth and Health Study, a study of the development of cardiovascular risk factors in black and white girls, as well as the Five-State FitWIC Initiative to Prevent Childhood Obesity. She has developed numerous obesity prevention materials, including the *Fit Families* novella series for Latino families and Let's Get Moving, an activity program for those who work with young children. Dr. Crawford has served on a number of advisory committees, including the California Legislative Task Force on Diabetes and Obesity. Her current studies include evaluations of large community-based obesity initiatives and school-based policy interventions. Dr. Crawford is currently a member of the IOM Standing Committee on Childhood Obesity Prevention and has served as a member or chair of three IOM obesity-related planning committees. She earned a B.S. from the University of Washington and a doctorate in public health and an R.D. from the University of California, Berkeley.

Christina Economos, Ph.D., M.S., is associate professor of nutrition and New Balance Chair in Childhood Nutrition at the Friedman School of Nutrition Science and Policy at Tufts University. She also serves as director of ChildObesity180. Her research focuses on the interactions among exercise, diet, and body composition. Her translational research includes theory-based obesity prevention interventions with ethnically and socioeconomically diverse children, adolescents, and their families in urban and rural communities across the United States. Dr. Economos was principal investigator for the Shape Up Somerville (SUS) program and currently leads several large obesity prevention intervention trials. The SUS program targeted behavior change in children through community-based, environmental change in a low-income, racially/ethnically diverse population. Dr. Economos has held positions in public health nutrition, including at the Massachusetts Department of Public Health. She serves on numerous state and national advisory boards. She was a consultant on the Youth Subcommittee for the 2008 Physical Activity Guidelines for Americans and is a member of the Public Policy Committee of the American Society for Nutrition. Dr. Economos served as a member of the IOM Committee on an Evidence Framework for Obesity Prevention Decision Making. She earned her M.S. at Columbia University and her Ph.D. at the Friedman School for Nutrition Science and Policy at Tufts University.

Sandra G. Hassink, M.D., launched the Pediatric Weight Management Clinic at Alfred I. duPont Hospital for Children in Wilmington, Delaware, in 1988. The clinic is part of the Division of General Pediatrics, which cares for children from infancy to young adulthood and uses a multidisciplinary, family-based approach to obesity. Dr. Hassink is now director of the Nemours Obesity Initiative and works both in the clinical division treating obese pediatric patients and in Nemours Health and Prevention Services. She has served as clinical consultant for the Primary Care Quality Collaborative on childhood obesity and has helped develop obesity-related policy at the community and state levels. Dr. Hassink has collaborated in basic research efforts to identify pathophysiologic mechanisms of obesity, centering on the role of leptin, and has lectured widely in the field of pediatric obesity. In addition to her other responsibilities, she currently chairs the ethics committee at Alfred I. duPont Hospital for Children. Dr. Hassink is on the board of directors of the American Academy of Pediatrics (AAP), has been a member of the AAP Task Force on Obesity, and is currently chair of the AAP Obesity Leadership Workgroup. She authored *A Parent's Guide to Childhood Obesity; Pediatric Obesity: Prevention, Intervention, and Treatment Strategies for Primary Care*; and *Clinical Guide to Pediatric Weight Management*. Dr. Hassink received her medical degree from Vanderbilt Medical School and a master's degree in pastoral care and counseling from Neumann College.

Anthony B. Iton, M.D., J.D., is senior vice president for healthy communities at The California Endowment in Oakland. In this role, he directs the foundation's 10-year Building Healthy Communities: California Living 2.0 initiative, an effort to create communities where children are healthy, safe, and ready to learn. Prior to assuming this role, Dr. Iton served as both health officer and director of the

Public Health Department for Alameda County (Oakland, California), beginning in 2003. There he oversaw the creation of an innovative public health practice designed to eliminate health disparities by tackling the root causes of poor health commonly found in California's low-income communities. Dr. Iton also served for 3 years as director of health and human services and school medical advisor for the City of Stamford, Connecticut. Concurrently, he served as a physician in internal medicine for Stamford Hospital's HIV clinic. He also has served as a primary care physician for the San Francisco Department of Public Health. Dr. Iton's work has been published in numerous public health and medical journals, and he is a regular public health lecturer and keynote speaker. He earned his B.S. in neurophysiology from McGill University; his M.D. from the Johns Hopkins University School of Medicine; and his J.D. from the University of California, Berkeley.

Steven H. Kelder, Ph.D., M.P.H., is Beth Toby Grossman Distinguished Professor in Spirituality and Healing and co-director of the Michael & Susan Dell Center for Healthy Living at the University of Texas School of Public Health in Austin, Texas. Dr. Kelder has directed NIH- and Centers for Disease Control and Prevention (CDC)–funded research projects to develop and evaluate school-based programs that address risk behaviors among children and adolescents with the aim of reducing chronic disease, including promotion of healthy eating and physical activity and prevention of tobacco use and osteoporosis. He has been principal investigator directing efforts to disseminate the Coordinated Approach To Child Health (CATCH) program, which has been adopted by elementary schools nationwide, including more than 2,500 elementary schools in Texas, potentially reaching more than 1 million children in the state. Dr. Kelder has authored or co-authored numerous scientific papers and book chapters over the past 15 years covering topics related to the design and analysis of epidemiological studies and health promotion interventions. He teaches graduate courses in epidemiology, social and behavioral aspects of behavior change, community nutrition education, epidemiology of child and adolescent health, and obesity and public health. Dr. Kelder received his Ph.D. in behavioral epidemiology and M.P.H. in community health education from the University of Minnesota, and his B.S. in marketing and economics from Northern Illinois University.

Harold W. (Bill) Kohl, III, Ph.D., M.S.P.H., is professor of epidemiology and kinesiology at the University of Texas Health Science Center-Houston and in the Department of Kinesiology and Health Education at the University of Texas at

Austin, College of Education. Dr. Kohl is also faculty at the Michael & Susan Dell Center for the Advancement of Healthy Living in Austin. He is founder and director of the University of Texas Physical Activity Epidemiology Program, where he is responsible for student training, research, and community service related to physical activity and public health. Dr. Kohl's previous service includes directing physical activity epidemiology and surveillance projects in the Division of Nutrition, Physical Activity, and Obesity at CDC. His research focuses on the specific area of epidemiology related to physical inactivity and obesity, in adults but also in children. Dr. Kohl also studies the effect of the built environment on physical activity and is currently researching a planned development that implements "smart growth" techniques designed to support physically active lifestyles. He received an M.S.P.H. from the University of South Carolina School of Public Health in epidemiology and biostatistics and a Ph.D. from the University of Texas Health Science Center-Houston School of Public Health in community health studies.

Shiriki K. Kumanyika, Ph.D., M.S.W., M.P.H., R.D., is professor of epidemiology in the Department of Biostatistics and Epidemiology and Pediatrics (Gastroenterology, Nutrition Section) and associate dean for health promotion and disease prevention at the University of Pennsylvania Perelman School of Medicine. Dr. Kumanyika's interdisciplinary background integrates epidemiology, nutrition, prevention, minority health, and women's health issues across the life course. The main themes in her research have concerned the role of nutritional factors in the primary and secondary prevention of chronic diseases, with a particular focus on obesity, sodium reduction, and related health problems such as hypertension and diabetes. She has a particular interest in the epidemiology and prevention of obesity among blacks. Dr. Kumanyika has served on numerous national and international advisory committees and expert panels related to nutrition and obesity. She is co-chair of the International Obesity Task Force, the policy and advocacy arm of the International Association for the Study of Obesity, and serves as a consultant to the World Health Organization's Department of Nutrition for Health and Development. Dr. Kumanyika has served as a member of the IOM Food and Nutrition Board, chair of the IOM Committee on an Evidence Framework for Obesity Prevention Decision Making, and a member of the IOM Committee on Prevention of Obesity in Children and Youth. She is currently chair of the IOM Standing Committee on Childhood Obesity Prevention. She received a B.A. from Syracuse University, an M.S.W. from Columbia University, a Ph.D. in human nutrition from Cornell University, and an M.P.H. from Johns Hopkins University. She is a member of the IOM.

Philip A. Marineau, M.B.A., is operating partner with LNK Partners, a private equity firm in White Plains, New York. Mr. Marineau is also currently chairman of the board of Shutterfly, an online photo sharing and greeting card company, and holds numerous other board positions, including positions with Kaiser Permanente, the Meredith Corporation, and Georgetown University. At LNK Partners, his experience guides the firm's investments, which are exclusively in the consumer and retail sector. Mr. Marineau has had a 33-year career working in the major name brand consumer retail business. He was president of Quaker Oats, where he worked for 23 years. After his time at Quaker, he served as president of Dean Foods, a dairy company, from 1996 to 1997. He then served as president of Pepsi-Cola North America, from 1997 to 1999. After leaving Pepsi, he served as president and chief executive officer of Levi Strauss, the global apparel company, from 1999 to 2006. Mr. Marineau received his M.B.A. from Northwestern University and his B.A. in history from Georgetown University.

Victoria Rideout, M.A., is president and founder of VJR Consulting, a private consulting firm specializing in media research and social marketing strategy. Until 2010 she served as vice president of the Kaiser Family Foundation and director of the foundation's Program for the Study of Media and Health. Ms. Rideout has directed more than 30 studies on topics concerning media and health, including a 10-year study tracking the evolving nature of media use among children and youth, research quantifying the amount and nature of food advertising to children on television and the Internet, surveys on teenagers' use of the Internet for health information, content analyses of public service advertising on television, and several studies documenting the influence of health-related content in entertainment television. Her research has been published in peer-reviewed journals such as the *Journal of the American Medical Association, Pediatrics*, the *Journal of Public Policy and Marketing, Health Affairs*, and *American Behavioral Scientist*, and has been widely reported on in the news media. Ms. Rideout has also negotiated ground-breaking partnerships with the television networks MTV, BET, and UPN, securing high-profile, multi-million-dollar donations of media time to conduct youth-oriented public education campaigns. The public service ads, original long-form programming, and online content she helped develop through these partnerships received many awards, including a National Emmy Award for best public service campaign. Ms. Rideout received her B.A. from Harvard University and her M.A. from the Maxwell School of Public Affairs at Syracuse University.

Eduardo J. Sanchez, M.D., M.P.H., FAAFP, is vice president and chief medical officer for Blue Cross and Blue Shield of Texas. He served as director of the Institute for Health Policy at the Austin Regional Campus of the School of Public Health in the University of Texas Health Science Center at Houston, and before that as commissioner of the Texas Department of State Health Services. As commissioner and chief health officer for the State of Texas, Dr. Sanchez led a statewide, comprehensive obesity prevention initiative and oversaw the creation of the 2006 Texas Obesity Policy Portfolio and the release of a Texas obesity cost projection comparing 2000 with 2040. He also oversaw Texas' behavioral health programs, disease prevention and bioterrorism preparedness programs, family and community health services programs, and environmental and consumer safety and health-related regulatory programs. Dr. Sanchez practiced clinical medicine in Austin from 1992 to 2001 and served as health authority and chief medical officer for the Austin-Travis County Health and Human Services Department from 1994 to 1998. He served as chair of the IOM Committee on Childhood Obesity Prevention Actions for Local Governments, and as a member of the IOM Committee on Progress in Preventing Childhood Obesity and the IOM Committee on a Comprehensive Review of the HHS Office of Family Planning Title X Program. He is a current member of the IOM Standing Committee on Childhood Obesity Prevention. Dr. Sanchez received his M.D. from the University of Texas Southwestern Medical School in Dallas, an M.P.H. from the University of Texas Health Science Center at Houston School of Public Health, and an M.S. in biomedical engineering from Duke University. He holds a B.S. in biomedical engineering and a B.A. in chemistry from Boston University. Dr. Sanchez is a fellow of the American Academy of Family Physicians and is certified by the American Board of Family Medicine.

Ellen Wartella, Ph.D., is Al-Thani Professor of Communication and professor of psychology and human development and social policy at Northwestern University. She directs the Center on Media and Human Development in the School of Communication at Northwestern. Previously, she was distinguished professor of psychology at the University of California, Riverside (UCR), and served as executive vice chancellor and provost at UCR. Dr. Wartella is co-principal investigator on a 5-year, multisite research project entitled Integrative Research Activities for Developmental Science (IRADS) Collaborative Research: Influence of Digital

Media on Very Young Children, funded by the National Science Foundation. She was co-principal investigator on the National TV Violence Study and co-principal investigator on the Children's Digital Media Center project, funded by the National Science Foundation. Dr. Wartella serves on the National Educational Advisory Board of the Children's Advertising Review Unit of the Council of Better Business Bureaus, the board of directors for the World Summit on Media for Children Foundation, the PBS KIDS Next Generation Media Advisory Board, the board of trustees for Sesame Workshop, and advisory boards for Harvard's Center on Media and Child Health and The Rudd Center for Food Policy and Obesity at Yale University. She is a member of the American Psychological Association and the Society for Research in Child Development and is past president of the International Communication Association. Recent honors include election as fellow of the American Association for the Advancement of Science and the Steven H. Chaffee Career Productivity Award from the International Communication Association. Dr. Wartella has served on the IOM/NRC Board on Children, Youth, and Families and the IOM Committee on Food Marketing and the Diets of Children and Youth. She also served as chair of the IOM Committee on Examination of Front-of-Package Nutrition Rating Systems and Symbols. Dr. Wartella received a B.A. with honors in economics from the University of Pittsburgh and M.A. and Ph.D. degrees in mass communications from the University of Minnesota, and completed her postdoctoral research in developmental psychology at the University of Kansas.